ULTRA-LOW FIELD NUCLEAR MAGNETIC RESONANCE

ULTRA-LOW FIELD NUCLEAR MAGNETIC RESONANCE

A New MRI Regime

Robert H. Kraus Jr., PhD

Chief Scientist, Samitaur Medical Technologies

Honolulu, HI

Michelle A. Espy, PhD

Scientist, Los Alamos National Laboratory

Los Alamos, NM

Per E. Magnelind, PhD

Scientist, Los Alamos National Laboratory

Los Alamos, NM

Petr L. Volegov, PhD

Scientist, Los Alamos National Laboratory

Los Alamos, NM

OXFORD
UNIVERSITY PRESS

OXFORD
UNIVERSITY PRESS

Oxford University Press is a department of the University of Oxford.
It furthers the University's objective of excellence in research, scholarship,
and education by publishing worldwide.

Oxford New York
Auckland Cape Town Dar es Salaam Hong Kong Karachi
Kuala Lumpur Madrid Melbourne Mexico City Nairobi
New Delhi Shanghai Taipei Toronto

With offices in
Argentina Austria Brazil Chile Czech Republic France Greece
Guatemala Hungary Italy Japan Poland Portugal Singapore
South Korea Switzerland Thailand Turkey Ukraine Vietnam

Published in the United States of America by
Oxford University Press
198 Madison Avenue, New York, NY 10016

Library of Congress Cataloging-in-Publication Data
Kraus, Robert H., Jr. (Robert Henry), author.
Ultra-low field nuclear magnetic resonance : a new MRI regime / Robert H. Kraus Jr., Michelle A. Espy, Per E. Magnelind, Petr L. Volegov.
p. ; cm.
Includes bibliographical references and index.
ISBN 978-0-19-979643-4 (alk. paper)
I. Espy, Michelle A. (Michelle Anna), author. II. Magnelind, Per E., author. III. Volegov, Petr L., author. IV. Title.
[DNLM: 1. Magnetic Resonance Imaging. WN 185]
RC78.7.N83
616.07′548—dc23
2013023133

9 8 7 6 5 4 3 2 1
Printed in China
on acid-free paper

To those who, through science, would help others.

CONTENTS

Foreword ix

Preface xiii

Acknowledgments xv

Common Acronyms and Abbreviations xvii

1. Fundamental Principles of NMR and MRI at ULF **1**

1.1. Introduction 1

1.2. Characteristics of the NMR Signal 6

1.3. Introducing Signal-to-Noise and Contrast-to-Noise 20

1.4. NMR and MRI at ULF 25

1.5. MRI Effects 33

1.6. New Regimes of Physics Accessible at ULF 38

1.7. Summary of MRI at ULF 39

1.8. Summary of HF and ULF MRI Comparisons 40

2. Nuts and Bolts of ULF MRI **47**

2.1. Introduction 47

2.2. General Concepts of Pre-Polarization Field Generation 51

2.3. Generation of Measurement Field, Gradients, and Spin-flip 55

2.4. Sensing the ULF MR Signals 58

2.5. Magnetic Shielding 71

2.6. Summary 78

3. Magnetic Resonance Phenomena at ULF **83**

3.1. Interaction Between the Electromagnetic Radiation and the Nuclear Spins at ULF 86

3.2. Quantum Mechanical Description of Interaction between the Electromagnetic Radiation and the Nuclear Spins 111

3.3. NMR Relaxation 120

4. Imaging Techniques at ULF **124**

4.1. Introduction 124

4.2. General Imaging Concepts (How to Do MRI) 128

4.3. ULF MRI 141

4.4. Imaging Techniques: Making the Most of What You've Got 165

4.5. On the Plus Side 180

4.6. Conclusions 197

5. Applications in ULF MRI **202**

5.1. Multimodal Imaging of Human Brain Anatomy and Function: MEG and ULF MRI 202

5.2. New Approaches to Image Human Brain Function Uniquely Enabled by ULF MRI 212

5.3. MagViz and ULF NMR Relaxometers 222

5.4. A Final Word 224

Index *229*

FOREWORD

A decade ago in Berkeley, it was shown that the nuclear magnetic resonance (NMR) line width of protons in a liquid could be very narrow in a magnetic field B_0 of a couple of microtesla, even though it was deliberately made highly inhomogeneous by the standards of conventional NMR. In fact, the narrow line width was to nobody's surprise; the important point being the high signal-to-noise ratio (SNR) obtained at a Larmor frequency f_0 of 75Hz. This was achieved by combining two well-known ideas: pre-polarization of the proton spins by a much larger magnetic field B_p that was turned off before the NMR signal was acquired, and the detection of the NMR signal with an untuned detector based on a superconducting quantum interference device (SQUID). Most SQUIDs operate at 4.2K, the boiling point of liquid helium. Unlike a Faraday detector, the SQUID has a frequency-independent response to magnetic flux. These early experiments also demonstrated the simplicity of obtaining the spectra of two nuclear species in a single acquisition using switched magnetic fields and of directly detecting the scalar coupling (*J*-coupling) splitting in heteronuclear spin systems—a unique benefit of the SQUID sensor.

Subsequently, the Berkeley group made the logical step to ULF magnetic resonance imaging (ULF MRI) by adding switched field gradients. Their system, built with lumber and copper wire coils, operated in a magnetic field of 132μT, corresponding to f_0 = 5,600Hz, four orders of magnitude lower than in conventional high-field (HF) MRI. The first image was of a pepper slice. Shortly after, an in-plane resolution of 1mm was demonstrated. This was followed by the three-dimensional *in vivo* image of an arm with an in-plane resolution of 2mm. Subsequently, the group demonstrated the strong dependence of the longitudinal relaxation time T_1 on the concentration of agarose gel in water at low fields, in contrast to the weak dependence at high fields. This observation resulted in the development of ULF T_1-weighted contrast imaging. The large skin depth of metals at ULF enabled the imaging of a pepper in a metal container. The requirement of only modest field homogeneity at ULF made possible undistorted images in the presence of a metal bar, which could, for example, be an orthopaedic screw.

Today, groups at perhaps 20 institutions worldwide are involved in some aspect of ULF NMR and ULF MRI. For example, a line width of 0.034Hz was observed in benzene in the Earth's field, and of 0.34Hz in a *J*-coupling spectrum. An early demonstration was the simultaneous acquisition of the stimulated magnetic signal from the human brain (magnetoencephalography [MEG]) and the ULF NMR signal from protons in the brain, using a single SQUID. Although these signals were in no way correlated, this was an important demonstration of the potential to combine the two modalities into a single acquisition system. Three-dimensional *in vivo* images of the brain were acquired with multiple SQUIDs. Trials at the Albuquerque airport showed the ability of ULF MRI in a T_1-contrast imaging mode to seek out liquids in carry-on luggage. On the technical front, an MRI phantom was successfully imaged using a SQUID on a cryocooler. Alternative sensors to SQUIDs are being explored—for example, "mixed sensors," which combine a superconducting pickup loop with a giant magnetoresistance sensor, and atomic magnetometers.

What are the long-term prospects for this field? In my view, although other as-yet-unheralded applications will undoubtedly emerge, if there is to be a major application it will be in medical imaging. But it will not be easy! HF clinical MRI is a magnificent tool, with perhaps 30,000 machines worldwide. Its great versatility leads to multiple applications, and it can achieve a spatial resolution of 1mm for most parts of the human body in a relative short time. A particular advantage is that specifically designed detection coils—at room temperature—can be placed over any part of the body to optimize detection sensitivity.

What would it take for ULF MRI to compete? It's mostly a question of SNR. The magnetic moment of a given ensemble of spins scales as B_0, and the signal it induces in a tuned pickup coil—by Faraday's law—scales as f_0. Thus, all things being equal, the signal from a tuned detector scales as B_0^2. Given that realizable pulsed pre-polarizing fields are likely to be an order of magnitude lower than the 1.5T field of a clinical system and that ULF MRI involves an untuned detector, the simple fact is that ULF MRI is unlikely to compete with HF MRI in terms of combined speed and spatial resolution. One may argue, with some justification, that a ULF MRI machine is likely to be substantially less costly than a 1.5T machine, but at least in the developed world the radiologist—not to mention the patient—seeks high resolution without an unduly long imaging time. Thus, in my view, if the goal of ULF MRI is to compete head on with HF MRI on its own terms, it is doomed to failure.

Fortunately, ULF MRI has its own virtues that extend beyond raw speed and resolution. An obvious strength is its greatly enhanced T_1 contrast compared with HF MRI. In HF MRI, T_1-weighted contrast imaging is well established but has its limitations. For example, in the case of breast cancer, there is no intrinsic T_1 contrast between cancerous and healthy tissue. This drawback is overcome by injecting a Gd-salt into the bloodstream, which flows preferentially to the tumor. The paramagnetic Gd ions enhance the T_1 relaxation rate, enabling one to image the tumor. Although this technique yields high resolution of the tumor, the rate of false positives has inhibited its becoming a screening technique for breast cancer. The use of the contrast agent works well for brain tumors but not at all for prostate cancer, which is the second leading cause of cancer deaths among American men.

The intrinsic difference in T_1 at low fields for different tissue types has been long known; it is the development of ULF MRI that has enabled one to take advantage of it. Although ULF T_1-weighted contrast imaging is well established in phantoms, in tissue it is in its infancy. Studies at Berkeley on *ex vivo* prostate tissue surgically removed from cancer patients, however, have established that T_1 in tumors is substantially shorter than in normal tissue. Simulations suggest that this T_1 difference is sufficient to produce *in vivo* images with sufficient contrast-to-noise ratio and spatial resolution to be clinically significant. Clearly, only clinical trials can establish the effectiveness of this technique, which relies on the intrinsic difference of T_1. If it were possible to image prostate cancer with ULF MRI, one could hope to use it, for example, to assess the extent of the disease in newly diagnosed patients, to provide a map to guide biopsy should it be deemed necessary, and to monitor changes in the prostate during active surveillance or therapies such as brachytherapy (implantation of radioactive seeds), thereby obviating the need for repeated biopsies. An obvious question is the applicability to other kinds of cancer. Could ULF MRI be used to screen for breast cancer? Or to detect ovarian cancer—which is notoriously difficult to detect at an early stage? Again, only clinical trials can address these questions.

A second forward-looking application of ULF MRI is its combination with systems for MEG. These systems, containing typically 300 SQUIDs, are used to detect stimulated or spontaneous magnetic fields from neurons in the brain in real time. They are used, for example, for presurgical mapping of brain tumors, the locating and presurgical mapping of sites of focal epilepsy, and the progression of recovery from brain trauma such as brain injury or stroke. To interpret the magnetic source image, an MRI of the brain is essential. The MEGMRI project, funded by the European Union and involving about a dozen institutes led by Aalto University, Helsinki, aims to incorporate ULF MRI into MEG systems. In principle, this simply involves the addition of appropriate sets of coils to existing MEG systems. The NMR signals are detected by the array of SQUIDs, so that averaging over these sensors can substantially reduce their noise. The notion of obtaining magnetic source and MR images with a single system is very appealing, since it overcomes difficulties in co-registering images obtained with two different systems and could result in substantial cost savings. In practice, the combination of MEG and MRI has many challenges, but there is every reason to believe these will be overcome. If so, these combined technologies could have a significant impact both clinically and commercially.

Currently, the holy grail of ULF MRI is its potential for direct neural current imaging (DNI). The essential idea is that currents flowing in neurons during neural activity produce local magnetic fields that can induce a tiny shift in the phase of the NMR signal over a tiny region. Strenuous efforts have been expended to observe this effect in HF MRI, so far without success. Since ULF MRI operates at a magnetic field four orders of magnitude lower, one expects the relative shift of the NMR signal to be enhanced by the same factor. The realization of DNI would be revolutionary, making real-time, spatially localized observation of neural activity a reality.

What are the challenges in bringing ULF MRI to clinical practice? The single biggest issue is, again, SNR, which scales as the ratio of the NMR signal at the sensor to the noise at the sensor, B_N. The imaging time for a given spatial resolution sales inversely as $(\mathrm{SNR})^2$, and hence as B_N^2/B_P^2. This immutable law should be displayed prominently in every ULF MRI laboratory! To obtain a sensible imaging time, one requires a sensor noise approaching 0.1 $\mathrm{fTHz}^{-1/2}$ (roughly the limit set by body noise) and a polarizing field of at least 0.1T. Both are achievable, but not trivially. A noise of 0.1 $\mathrm{fTHz}^{-1/2}$ is at the limit of what one can detect with an appropriate coil size and a SQUID at 4.2K, and assumes that environmental noise can be reduced to this level. Generating a pulsed magnetic field of, say, 0.15T at the prostate or head that can be turned off in some milliseconds is achievable but requires a water-cooled coil and a power supply providing at least 50kW. Screening out external electrical and magnetic interference, almost certainly with a shielded room, presents a major challenge. When the polarizing field is switched off, large eddy currents in the room can severely distort both B_0 and pulsed gradient fields unless one either cancels the field with a second, counter-wound coil or designs a room that rapidly damps out low-frequency current while retaining a high degree of screening at the imaging frequency. Perseverance by the community will undoubtedly achieve these goals.

Another issue concerns cryogenics. I believe the clinical community is unlikely to embrace a system that requires refilling with liquid helium every few days. Fortunately, reliable cryocoolers are readily available at reasonable cost, and ULF MRI has already been demonstrated with a cryocooled SQUID. An alternative approach would be a refrigerator that automatically refills the cryostat at night.

Finally, one should not underestimate the time and cost required for clinical trials. To undertake a meaningful trial will require a company with deep pockets and, one hopes, a steady stream of federal funding.

The group at Los Alamos National Laboratory has been a major driving force in the development of ULF MRI. Their efforts are reflected in this book, which covers all aspects of the subject in depth, ranging from history and the nuts-and-bolts practicalities of building such a system to ULF resonance phenomena and applications of a variety of imaging techniques to pulse sequences and direct neural current imaging. The book is surely destined to become the standard reference in the field.

John Clarke
Berkeley
May 12, 2011

PREFACE

This book endeavors to provide the background for and current status of the emerging field of ultra-low field (ULF) magnetic resonance imaging (MRI). We lay the groundwork by providing a brief history of MRI at extremely low fields and for why ULF NMR and MRI are of both scientific and practical interest. In particular, we examine the benefits realized at applied magnetic fields that are many orders of magnitude below traditional NMR and MRI. We balance the benefits at ULF with the various anticipated and unanticipated challenges our team and others working in the field have experienced, and a variety of approaches used to deal with these challenges. We present the current status in sufficient detail for the reader to effectively pursue ULF MRI investigations in both medical and material science applications. While the primary focus of this book is MRI, we discuss a variety of nuclear magnetic resonance (NMR) phenomena, particularly as they apply at ULF, because ultimately MRI is simply a spatially encoded measurement of specific NMR phenomena.

Traditional MRI involves applied magnetic fields typically in the Tesla regime. Most clinical imaging instrumentation operates at 1.5T, with more 3T imagers being installed every day. The lowest magnetic fields commonly used in clinical instruments are 0.3T (3kG) in applications where an open geometry is required and lower spatial resolution is acceptable or tolerable. Exploring NMR signals at extremely low fields in the milli-Tesla regime was initially reported about two decades ago, where the NMR signal for water was observed at 10mT. However, it has been only in the last decade or so since the observation of exceptionally narrow NMR line widths for various liquid solutions at a few micro-Tesla was reported. The field of ULF NMR and MRI has seen a tremendous growth of publications and research investment around the world since then. This book describes the current state of the art of ULF MRI in our laboratory and others, and while we make an effort to be thorough and relatively complete, the field is evolving rapidly and new ideas are constantly being pursued and reported. We will share practical insights into ideas being pursued and conclude the book with a number of promising concepts for ULF applications that have yet to be investigated and are, as yet, unproven.

Our book focuses on the practical aspects of ULF MRI that will enable the reader to practice in the field. Only a few of the most relevant derivations of first principles of ULF NMR and MRI are provided, with a focus on those specifically relevant to the regime of ULF (e.g., concomitant gradients) and those we thought were lacking elsewhere. Others are provided in the bibliography. We attempt to present a thorough discussion of concomitant gradients because of the large effect they can have on MRI at ULF. While they have been mentioned in high field MRI texts, concomitant gradients have been either treated with simple approximations or entirely ignored.

We present a detailed discussion of current state-of-the-art instrumentation that is unique to ULF MRI. The most common sensor to acquire the NMR signal for ULF MRI is the superconducting quantum interference device (SQUID). SQUIDs are the most sensitive magnetic field sensors in wide use today but require cooling with liquid cryogens (liquid nitrogen or liquid helium). Furthermore, SQUIDs require extraordinary expertise and measures to operate in a typical ULF MRI environment. While we thoroughly cover the techniques needed to employ SQUID sensors in ULF MRI, we also discuss the ongoing search for robust, noncryogenic sensors with the required sensitivity to the desired signal. We present the tradeoffs for currently available sensors. Our discussion of the instrumentation also includes all other aspects of the hardware used in ULF MRI systems, together with experimental techniques and practical insights into how it all works.

We have interspersed relatively general material throughout the book to provide a complete and self-consistent picture for the reader, but we also rely heavily on many excellent references and readily available sources as needed to provide a comprehensive picture of the field. We have made an effort to carefully define nomenclature and thoroughly describe methods to avoid the confusion that can occur between the many sources of NMR information, particularly as one switches between high-field and ULF MRI. A comprehensive table of acronyms and abbreviations is also provided.

Working at the forefront of a new field is exhilarating, educational, and competitive. Many novel features and capabilities of ULF MRI have been discovered, yet we are certain that only the proverbial surface of the field has been scratched. There is far more yet to be discovered and learned, and we wish you, the reader, the very best of luck and insight.

Robert H. Kraus Jr.
Michelle A. Espy
Per E. Magnelind
Petr L. Volegov

ACKNOWLEDGMENTS

We wish to acknowledge the Los Alamos National Laboratory (Los Alamos National Security, LLC) for the research support through the Laboratory Directed Research and Development program, the National Institutes of Health, and the U.S. Department of Homeland Security. In addition, one of us (RHK) wishes to thank Samitaur Medical Technologies and to acknowledge the support and interest of the principals of SMT in advancing medical technology for all humanity. We would also like to thank the many people with whom we have had stimulating and insightful discussions regarding this book. While there are far too many people to individually name here, we would like to specifically acknowledge Prof. John Clarke, Prof. Martin Burghoff, Prof. Risto Ilmoniemi, Ms. Miranda Intrator, Prof. Stefan Posse, Dr. John George, Dr. John Mosher, Dr. Leon Heller, Dr. Don Tucker, Dr. Sergei Turovets, Dr. Jaakko Nieminen, Dr. Rainer Körber, and Mr. Shaun Newman for their many valuable insights, critiques, suggestions, and contributions during the preparation of this book.

We must also acknowledge the many members of our research team (fondly known as the "SQUID Team"), past and present, who have contributed so much to the field of ULF MRI and biomagnetism.

We also wish to make a special acknowledgement and express our sincere appreciation to our colleague Dr. Andrei Matlashov for his critical role in all aspects of the Los Alamos experimental capability in ULF NMR and MRI. Without him, we certainly wouldn't have had much to write about!

Finally, there can be no acknowledgement or "thank you" sufficient to express the gratitude and appreciation we feel for those most important to us: our families, who have sacrificed countless hours for the sake of this book.

COMMON ACRONYMS AND ABBREVIATIONS

We include a list of common acronyms, abbreviations, and symbols used in this book. We ask the reader to be aware that sections of the book where detailed mathematical derivations are presented may use symbols and letters in formulae that are not consistent with this table. We have, however, attempted to clearly define every symbol and character at the first instance of use in the context of the derivation.

2D	Two-dimensional
3D	Three-dimensional
A	Context dependent: Amp or Nuclear mass number (number of protons and neutrons in a given nucleus)
Å	Ångström, 10^{-10}m
AC	Alternating current (time-varying current)
ADC	Analog-to-Digital converter
AM	Atomic Magnetometer (or Atomic Magnetometry)
ASL	Arterial spin labeling, a MRI technique used to measure blood flow that can be used to deduce brain function
B_0	MRI magnetic field, typically both the polarization and measurement field used in high-field MRI
B_m	Measurement magnetic field
BOLD	Blood Oxygen Level Dependent, a MRI technique used to deduce brain activity
B_p	Polarization magnetic field used in MRI.
BW	Bandwidth
CNR	Contrast-to-noise ratio
CSF	Cereberal spinal fluid
DC	Direct current (constant current)
DNI	Direct neural imaging, a method to directly measure the neural activity (presumably in the brain). Our team coined the acronym to refer to the direct imaging of neural currents using ULF MR

e	Elementary charge
EEG	Electroencephalography
EIT	Electrical impedance tomography
EPI	Echo-planar imaging
f	Frequency, when used as a variable or quantity, typically in Hz.
FAIR	Flow-sensitive alternating inversion recovery, a MRI technique to used to measure blood flow that may be associated with function
FC	Field cycling, typically refers to techniques for varying the NMR or MR field
FFT	Fourier Transform (or Fast Fourier Transform)
FID	Free Induction Decay
FLAIR	Fluid attenuated inversion recovery
FLASH	Fast low-angle shot
fMRI	Functional magnetic resonance imaging
FOV	Field-of-view, often (thought not always) synonymous with volume of interest
G	(non-italicized) Gauss, unit of magnetic field equal to 10^{-4} T
G	Magnetic field gradient (usually includes a direction: G_x, G_y, G_z).
GMR	Giant magneto-resistive or giant magnetoresistance
h	Planck's constant (6.626×10^{-34} J-sec)
H	Magnetic field strength
$\hbar$	$h/2\pi$ or the reduced Planck's constant (1.055×10^{-34} J-sec)
HF	High Field, typically referring to >0.3 T imaging field in HF MRI
HTC	High (critical temperature) superconductor, typically designates materials with superconducting critical temperature well above ~4 K. also high-T_c
Hz	Hertz, cycles per second
I	Context dependent: Current or spin quantum number
J	Current density
J	(non-italicized) Joule
k	The mathematical space convient for imaging, "k-space"
K	Kelvin
k_B	Boltzmann's constant (1.381×10^{-23} J/K)
L	Inductance (also used as image size in Ch. 4 derivations)
LANL	Los Alamos National Laboratory
LF	Low (magnetic) Field, commonly referring to MRI fields below 0.3T. We define LF MRI as the regime between ULF MRI and HF MRI.
LHe	Liquid helium
LN	Liquid Nitrogen
LSB	Least Significant Bit, the lowest significant bit in a digital acquisition system
LTC	Low (critical temperature) superconductor, typically ~4 K and below. Also low-T_c

M	Magnetization, may be a vector (**M**) quantity, scalar (M) or a vector component (e.g. M_x)
MAGVIZ	The name given to the ULF MR relaxometry technique used to differentiate materials based on relaxation profile
MEG	Magnetoencephalography
MR	Magnetic Resonance
MREIT	Magnetic Resonance electrical impedance tomography
MRI	Magnetic Resonance Imaging
MSR	Magnetically Shielded Room
N	Number in a given population (such as number of spins)
nc-MRI	Neural current MRI—designates methodologies used in MRI to detect signatures directly associated with neural activity (such as rapid dephasing).
NEMA	National Electrical Manufacturers Association, See also www.nema.org
NMR	Nuclear Magnetic Resonance
NQR	Nuclear quadrupole resonance
PET	Positron emission tomography (medical imaging modality using radioisotopes)
PSD	Power Spectral Density
R	Resistance
Rad	Radian
RF	Radio frequency, often referred to as "rf" elsewhere
RFI	Radio frequency interference
ROI	Region of Interest (see VOI/volume of interest)
S	Context dependent: Shielding factor (various subscripts designate specific type), or the NMR signal measured from a specific region or volume.
SD	Standard deviation
SENSE	Sensitivity Encoding - a method for using multiple sensor to improve imaging speed or signal-to-noise
SMASH	Simultaneous acquisition of spatial harmonics—a method for using multiple sensor to improve imaging speed
SNR	Signal-to-noise ratio
SOC	Streams of commerce, refers to commonly available packaging of commodities
Spin	Quantum mechanical spin, typically referring to nuclear spin in this book
SQUID	Superconducting Quantum Interference Device
T	(non-italicized), Tesla, unit of magnetic field equal to 10,000 G
T	Context dependent: Temperature or time when used as a variable
t	Typically refers to a time, often denoted by a subscript (e.g. t_g - time gradient field is applied, t_a - acquisition time, etc.)
T_1	Longitudinal (or spin-lattice) relaxation time
T_2	Transverse (or spin-spin) relaxation time

T_c	Critical temperature, typically referring to the temperature at which a material becomes superconducting
ULF	Ultra-low magnetic field (erroneously "ultra-low frequency")
V	(Context dependent) Voltage or Volume
VOI	Volume of interest, typically the imaging region of interest in MRI
Voxel	Volume element, typically referring to a specific size element from which a signal is derived
Z	(non-italicized) refers to the nuclear atomic number
Z	Impedance
μ_0	Free space permeability
γ	Gyromagnetic ratio (depends on isotope/nucleus)
μ	Relative permeability
μ-metal	Mu-metal, generally refers to any high magnetic permeability material
δ	Skin depth—the thickness of a material needed to reduce a signal by $1/e$
σ	Electrical conductivity
χ	Magnetic susceptibility
Ω	Ohm, measure of resistance
ω	Frequency (general)
ω_L	Larmor Frequency

ULTRA-LOW FIELD NUCLEAR MAGNETIC RESONANCE

CHAPTER 1

FUNDAMENTAL PRINCIPLES OF NMR AND MRI AT ULF

1.1 INTRODUCTION

Magnetic resonance imaging (MRI, originally called nuclear magnetic resonance [NMR] imaging) has for nearly four decades been a tool synonymous with high-tech and high-resolution imaging [1]. While MRI applications are most widely known in the medical field [2], applications are also many and varied outside the medical community. A few examples include anthropology [3], paleontology [4], evolution [5,6], material analysis [7,8], and analyzing food quality and safety [9–11]. Widely known for its medical diagnostic capability, MRI is also a powerful research tool because of a wide variety of unique capabilities that include high resolution, localized spectroscopy, isotopic specificity, etc. The popularity of MRI in general, and in comparison to x-ray–based imaging methods in particular, has also been bolstered by the fact that it employs no ionizing radiation and that MRI can often differentiate materials with virtually identical density and chemical composition (called "contrast"). For example, soft tissue contrast that can differentiate white and gray matter in the brain is commonplace for MRI while virtually beyond the capability of x-ray. While the number and breadth of MRI techniques and applications have exploded in the four short decades since Lauterbur and Mansfield demonstrated the method in the 1970s, the field has driven to ever-higher magnetic fields in the quest for more signal, better signal-to-noise ratios (SNRs), and ever-greater spatial resolution. This book provides the rationale and the techniques for applications in which bigger may not always be better.

At the heart of all MRI is the NMR signal. In the simplest form, an MRI is constructed as a spin density (typically for protons in most MRI applications) image. This is referred to as a "proton density-weighted" (or "spin density-weighted") image. For example, because the proton spin density in tissue is far greater than bone, a large spin density signal is generated by tissue and a correspondingly small signal from bone. Figure 1.1 illustrates a single-slice MRI for a human hand derived primarily from the proton spin density where the brightness (lighter regions of the image) indicates the density of protons in a given volume of the image. The area around the hand (i.e., air) has little or no proton spin density whereas the tissue (flesh) has a significant proton population. The dark gaps in the fingers occur at the joints and are the result of the short relaxation time of the cartilage. This difference is known as T_2 contrast, a concept we will discuss later.

Anatomical images are typically generated by exploiting the differences, often quite small, in NMR signal between various tissue types (e.g., white vs. gray matter) and

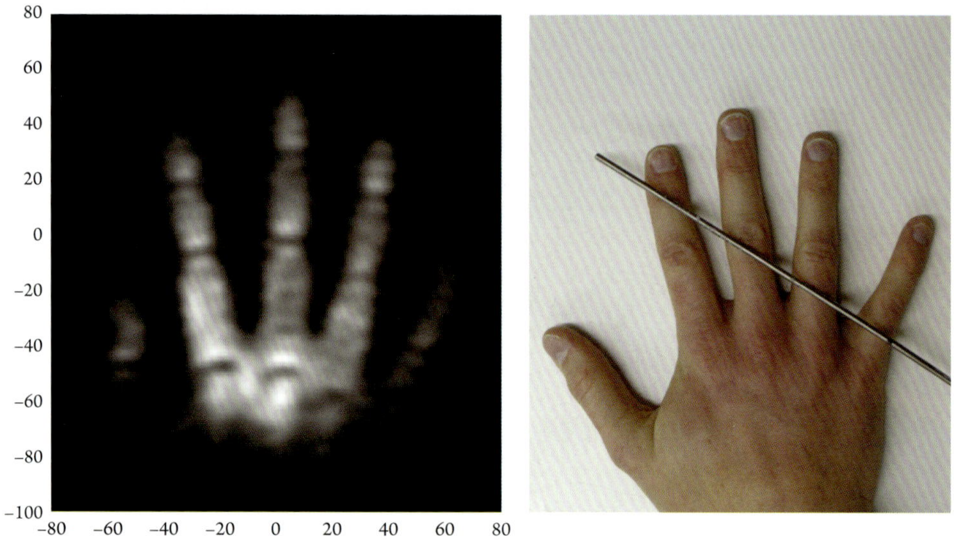

FIGURE 1.1 (Left) MRI of hand at ULF with Ti rod. The image is primarily a proton density-weighted image where brightness is roughly a measure of proton density. The proton spin density weighted MR image was acquired at 94μT after pre-polarization at 30mT with a spatial resolution of approximately 2mm. While the left panel is a simple MRI acquired at ULF, it is extraordinary because it could not have been acquired in a typical MRI scanner due to the presence of the Ti rod. (Right) Photograph of the hand for which the MRI was acquired, showing a 4mm-diameter titanium rod that was placed on top of the hand during acquisition of the ULF MRI. The presence of such metal in typical MRI scanner would have made the acquisition of the MRI in the left panel virtually impossible, as we shall describe later in the book.

fluids (e.g., blood, cerebrospinal fluid [CSF], etc.). Imaging human tissue most commonly exploits the difference between tissue parameters of spin density (e.g., Fig. 1.1), spin-lattice relaxation, spin-spin relaxation, flow, and diffusion. MRI in other applications relies on the same basic techniques where differences in a specific NMR phenomenon are imaged and associated with specific material type. For example, imaging fat content in meat relies on the fact that the spin density and relaxation times in fat are significantly different than other tissue types. These differences in NMR phenomena result in a contrast or difference between materials and tissue types that can be exploited with the appropriate techniques to generate the desired image.

Contrast can (and often is) a very dynamic phenomenon, changing with time as a consequence of the inherent NMR phenomena themselves or as a result of physiological processes. In recent years, MRI has been applied to observe the temporal evolution of NMR signals/signatures combined with the spatial information. One of the most common and powerful examples of this method is functional MRI (fMRI), in which the time evolution of blood oxygenation, blood flow, and blood volume as a function of location have been used to deduce function in the human brain [12]. While fMRI has become an exceptionally powerful tool, it is still limited by temporal resolution and an indirect association with the underlying neural activity. Nevertheless fMRI has provided an unprecedented map of the functional architecture of the cortical areas that are the substrate of higher brain function.

The differences in the NMR signal for the various tissue types and fluids are spatially encoded through the application of magnetic field gradients. The final MRI image is developed from the analysis of the resulting signal (described later in the book and in references [13,14]) acquired by a variety of possible sensors. The specific NMR phenomenon (e.g., relaxation time, spin diffusion, etc.) imaged is elicited by the specific pulse sequence applied. These are discussed in detail later in the book.

Improving spatial resolution, reducing imaging time, and increasing the sensitivity to differences between materials (e.g., tissue types, fluids, etc.) are the key drivers in the scientific and technological advancement of MRI. A common need in each of these key drivers is ever-greater signal from a given volume of the sample (or voxel) and the SNR to differentiate one voxel from its neighboring voxels. We will briefly examine here the primary contributing factors to the NMR signal that underpins the MRI and the relationships to variables, particularly those that can be controlled by the imaging system. Noise is a more complex topic and will be covered in later chapters. Suffice it to say that the quest for ever-greater signal has driven most of the advances in MRI over the last few decades.

The phenomenon that underlies NMR is the rotation of nuclear magnetic (dipole) moments about a magnetic field. While it is not feasible to detect the rotation of a single nucleus, the NMR signal observed in spectroscopic NMR and MRI arises from a population of nuclei, similarly aligned and rotating in phase about a magnetic field that is roughly uniform across the sample. Because the nuclear magnetic moment, μ, is proportional to the nuclear spin, S, every nucleus with non-zero spin can produce a NMR signal. While virtually every known element has an isotope (isotopes for a given element have the same "Z" or number of protons in the nucleus but differing number of neutrons and consequently atomic mass number "A") that has a non-zero spin, only a handful are commonly used in NMR and even fewer in MRI. The vast majority of MRI is based on the NMR signal of the proton (^1H, the most abundant form of hydrogen) because the magnitude of the NMR signal per nucleus (the NMR "sensitivity," see Table 1.1) is larger for ^1H than any other known isotope. Furthermore, hydrogen is the most abundant element in the human body (measured as number of nuclei). Water makes up approximately 75% of the human body and every water molecule includes two hydrogen nuclei, not to mention the hydrogen contained in fats and proteins. Consequently, there are more hydrogen nuclei in the human body with which to generate the observed NMR signal.

Traditional MRI involves applied magnetic fields typically in the Tesla (T) regime. Most modern clinical imaging instrumentation operate at 1.5T to 3T. The lower extreme of magnetic fields commonly used in clinical instruments, the so-called "low-field" regime, is 0.2T to 0.3T (3kG). These instruments are commonly used in applications where an open geometry is required and lower spatial resolution is acceptable or tolerable. In general, the MRI technology is moving toward ever-larger magnetic fields, with more 3T clinical imagers being installed every day. The primary driver for this trend toward increasing magnetic fields is the increased signal realized as a function of the applied "polarizing" field, which results in faster imaging and higher resolution, along with other benefits that result with more signal. However, these larger fields come at a cost, monetary and otherwise. Larger fields require physically larger and heavier magnets that place ever-increasing demands on the facility to house these instruments. Increasing MRI fields also result in numerous safety challenges that become more severe with increasing fields. We compare various aspects of high- and low-field MRI in more detail later.

The development of "low-field" (LF) MRI systems in the 1980s thorough the early 21st century were initially driven by the desire to reduce patient anxiety by enabling open-magnet designs, as opposed to the physically constraining cylindrical design of most high-field

(HF) MRI systems. Such systems could also be used in operating rooms: the open design allowed access to the patient and had reduced effects on surgical instruments and electronics. The LF systems were also far less noisy during surgery. Clinics were further enticed by the reduced capital and operational costs of LF systems. Such systems typically operated in the range of 0.2T to 0.5T using normal (non-superconducting) magnetic field coils. A recent review by Hayashi et al. pointed to not only the reduced cost and patient anxiety factors but also the greater safety of operation as the primary drivers for developing LF medical scanners [15]. Hayashi noted that reducing capital and operational costs was an important driver, but patient anxiety and safety issues were the most significant drivers to develop LF MRI. Blanco et al. reviewed low-field applications of interventional and intraoperative MRI and reported significant benefits of LF MRI and virtually no impediments [16]. Blanco et al. found that the cylindrical design of the HF MRI presented significant limitations to patient access. Additionally, the high magnetic field and RF heating presented serious safety concerns. In contrast, LF (around 0.2T) MRI significantly reduced the limitations, most significantly by providing ample imaging resolution and speed and easy patient access because of the open-magnet designs. In a related study, de Salles et al. reported the importance of 0.2T open geometry interventional MRI to visualize the brain during stereotactic surgical procedures [17].

The detailed data and trends for installed MRI systems are somewhat sparse, but using data from 1983 through 2001 based on European Forum on Magnetic Resonance Research & Applications estimates, we can see general trends. Two distinct trends are evident for installed MRI systems in the United States and Europe: the highest field of installed MRI systems is increasing since the first systems were installed in the 1980s, and the fraction of installed systems operating at fields at or above 1.5T is growing. The highest field of commercial systems has increased from 1.5T in 1995 to 3T in 2002 and is currently 7T in 2011. The number of installed HF MRI systems has grown steadily since the early 1990s as shown in Figure 1.2. Current projections show the HF market share will grow to exceed 80% of the whole-body MRI systems in 2020. In contrast, the number of low- and medium-field MRI installations has not grown as quickly. The primary HF driver of larger signal and better spatial resolution appears to outweigh the medium- and low-field drivers of patient comfort and access and cost in the majority of cases. It will be interesting to watch how worldwide shortages in liquid helium, new MRI systems designed with rare-earth magnet materials, and MRI methods described in this book affect this trend.

At the same time, it has become practical in the last decade to perform MR at fields far smaller even than the so-called "low field," systems, indeed in the range of mT to μT: the *ultra-low field (ULF)* regime. For the purpose of this book, and because there is some variation in the literature regarding the definition of ULF, we will explicitly define it here: ULF is the magnetic field at which one acquires the NMR/MRI signal in the regime of applied magnetic fields below 10mT (100G). We explicitly use *field* as the defining parameter for ULF MRI and not frequency (ULF in some cases refers to ultra-low frequency, but not here). This is also a good point to define another convention that differentiates ULF MRI from traditional HF MRI. HF MRI (and even the vast majority of LF MRI systems) use a single static magnetic field (1) to polarize the sample and (2) acquire the NMR signal. This is a matter of both practicality and safety: practicality because superconducting magnets (and the occasional permanent magnet system) cannot readily be turned on and off, and safety because the huge dB/dt that would result, if you could turn such systems on and off, would induce hazardous physiological currents in patients and subjects. Consequently, most HF and LF MRI applications refer to only one magnetic field: B_0. In contrast, the

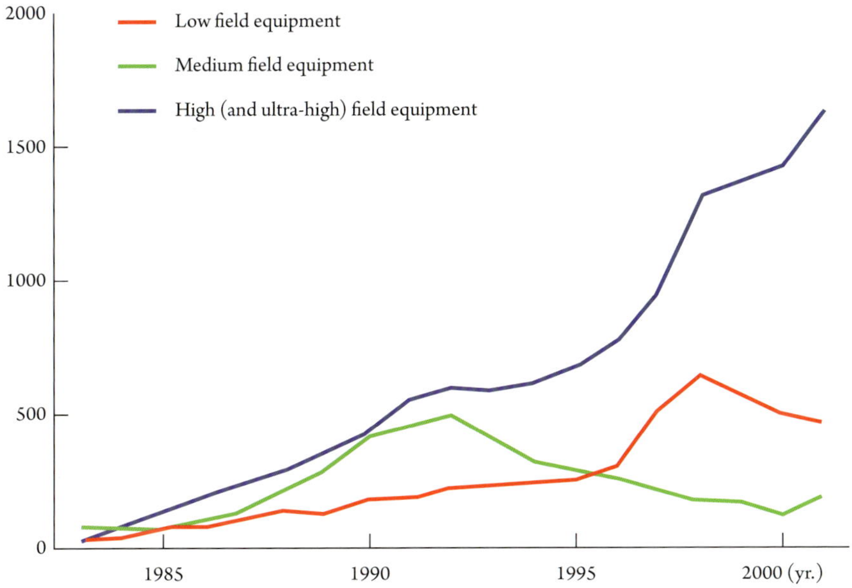

FIGURE 1.2 Trends in installed MRI systems in the United States. Field regimes are defined as: low (<0.5T), medium (0.5–1.2T), or high (>1.2T). From Rinck P., *Magnetic Resonance in Medicine. The Basic Textbook of the European Magnetic Resonance Forum*, 6th ed. 2012. Electronic version 6.1. www.magnetic-resonance.org. © 2012 by TRTF/EMRF, used with permission.

ULF magnetic field regime readily allows manipulation of the fields used to both polarize the sample and to measure the NMR signal. This flexibility in magnetic field manipulation, including when a patient or subject is in the ULF MRI instrument, results in one of the key strengths of the technique. This necessitates that we define two different (and rarely static) magnetic fields commonly used in ULF MRI: B_p (the "polarization field" used to initially polarize the sample) and B_m (the "measurement field" at which the NMR signal is acquired).

In the following sections, we shall see that the greatest challenge for ULF MRI is to acquire sufficient signal to enable reconstruction of a usable image. Figure 1.1 demonstrates that techniques to tease out sufficient signal to acquire useful ULF MRI have been clearly developed, but it is unlikely that ULF MRI will ever demonstrate spatial resolution that *generally* competes with that attainable at traditional HF MRI. Nonetheless, there may be benefits to acquiring MRIs at low fields that are driving the development of ULF MRI and that must be weighed against the simplistic scaling of signal with applied field. These benefits include open and accessible system geometries, lower system cost, virtually nonexistent susceptibility artifacts, and dramatically lower field homogeneity requirements [18–22]. There may be special cases in which ULF MRI can demonstrate better material discrimination and spatial resolution relative to HF MRI due to the field dependence of certain contrast mechanisms (contrast is discussed in a later section). There are indications that the contrast between some materials and tissue types may be significantly greater at ULF than at HF [23–25]. Improved contrast may enable discriminating different materials or tissue types at ULF that is not possible at HF or provide higher imaging resolution at ULF. Finally, ULF MRI may be the only way to image brain function and anatomy at the same time with the same instrument [26,27].

1.2 CHARACTERISTICS OF THE NMR SIGNAL

1.2.1 Scaling of the NMR Signal

It is handy to have an understanding of what NMR frequency regime ULF works in. To translate the ULF magnetic field regime into NMR signal frequencies, we will briefly describe the relationship between the magnetic field and the NMR signal. The NMR signal originates from a population of nuclear spins rotating about a magnetic field. The rotational frequency for a population of spins about the magnetic field is described by the simple relationship:

(Eqn. 1.1) $$\omega_{\mathrm{L}} = 2\pi f_{\mathrm{L}} = \gamma B_{\mathrm{m}}$$

where ω_{L} is the Larmor frequency (ω_{L} is Rad/sec, f_{L} is Hz) at which the spins rotate about the magnetic field at which the signal is measured, B_{m}. And γ is the gyromagnetic ratio,[1] a measure of the polarizability for a nucleus, and varies for every nuclear isotope. It is important to keep in mind that this formalism applies to every population of non-zero spin nuclei in a given sample, regardless of which particular isotope one may be measuring at any given time. Indeed, all non-zero spin nuclei will be responding to the applied magnetic fields according to their specific physical parameters. Most traditional MRI systems use tuned coils that are optimized to detect the high-frequency RF signal for a specific nuclear species at a set magnetic field. While the spin populations for any MRI system are all rotating about the applied magnetic field according to Eqn. 1.1, the design inherent in the high-field MRI sensors is rarely able to measure the NMR signal from more than a single isotopic population. Sensors for high-field MRI scanners are most commonly tuned to detect the NMR signal from protons because of the abundance of protons in the body.

The gyromagnetic ratios, γ, for a few of the most important isotopes used in NMR and MRI are listed in Table 1.1, along with their commonly quoted sensitivity values, which describe the NMR signal amplitude relative to protons (^{1}H) for typical Faraday induction sensors. The sensitivity for a given isotope scales as:

(Eqn. 1.2) $$\gamma^{3}_{\mathrm{isotope}} / \gamma^{3}_{\mathrm{proton}}$$

The cubic dependence results from the linear dependence of the magnetic moment on γ, the population difference between spin states depending linearly on γ, and finally the signal voltage generated by a Faraday induction pickup being proportional to the Larmor frequency ω_{L}, consequently also to γ. It is crucial to point out that the last factor of γ is dropped when the NMR signal is measured by non-inductive magnetometers such as superconducting quantum interference devices (SQUIDs) or atomic magnetometers. Some NMR data tables list the "receptivity" for isotopes, which is the sensitivity (in Table 1.1) multiplied by the natural abundance.

While there are a vast number of nuclei accessible to NMR and MRI, virtually every MRI instrument used for tissue imaging measures the NMR signature of protons because of the high sensitivity and large abundance of protons in tissue. Table 1.1 also lists the natural and biological abundance of a few of the isotopes most commonly used in NMR and MRI. Some of the isotopes included in Table 1.1 have little or no biological abundance,

[1] This quantity is also known as a magnetogyric ratio, reflecting the fact that it is a ratio of the magnetic moment of a nucleus to its angular momentum.

but some isotopes (e.g., ^{3}He and ^{129}Xe) can be readily and safely introduced into biological organisms to enhance imaging in certain applications. For example, hyperpolarized ^{3}He is used for lung MRI. Motivated by the poor image quality of lung MRI, hyperpolarized noble gasses were demonstrated to hold great promise in assessing human lung structure and function [28,29]. The isotope ^{129}Xe can also be hyperpolarized and is used in a broad range of biological applications [30]. Nonetheless, because of its abundance and high sensitivity, ^{1}H remain the mainstay for all MRI, from ULF to HF. The gyromagnetic ratio for protons (the most abundant form of hydrogen) is approximately 42.6MHz/T. Thus, the NMR frequency range for ^{1}H in the ULF regime (defined above as magnetic fields below 10mT) is less than 426kHz or roughly below 500kHz. However, because we have defined the ULF regime in terms of field, the NMR *frequency* regime at ULF will vary widely for different isotopes. For example, the ULF frequency regime for ^{19}F is less than 401kHz (quite similar to ^{1}H), while for ^{14}N the ULF frequency regime is less than 31kHz. Finally, we note simply in passing that the sign of γ indicates the order of energy levels that are split in a magnetic field. For positive γ, the energy level with the largest z-quantum number is the lowest energy state.

Returning now to the challenges presented by performing MRI at ULF, it is well known that the inherent NMR signal is dramatically reduced relative to traditional HF MRI. This is an extension of the trend that impedes resolution and slows imaging time at LF, consequently it is potentially even more serious at ULF. The reduced SNR associated with LF

TABLE 1.1 NMR Properties for Selected Isotopes

NUCLEUS	SPIN (I)	NATURAL ABUNDANCE (%)	BIOLOGICAL ABUNDANCE (% OF MASS)	γ (10^6 RAD/T-SEC)	$\gamma/2\pi$ (MHz/T)	SENSITIVITY (REL. ^{1}H)
^{1}H	½	99.985	10.	267.513	42.576	1
^{2}H	1	0.015	0.0015	41.065	6.536	9.65×10^{-3}
^{3}He	½	0.000138	-	-203.78	-32.434	0.44
^{7}Li	3/2	92.5	3×10^{-6}	103.96	16.546	0.29
^{13}C	½	1.10	0.198	67.263	10.705	1.59×10^{-2}
^{14}N	1	99.634	3.0	19.331	3.077	1.01×10^{-3}
^{15}N	½	0.366	0.011	-27.116	-4.316	1.04×10^{-3}
^{17}O	5/2	0.048	0.025	-36.264	-5.772	2.91×10^{-2}
^{19}F	½	100.0	0.004	251.66	40.053	0.834
^{23}Na	3/2	100.0	0.15	70.761	11.262	9.25×10^{-2}
^{31}P	½	100.0	1.0	108.29	17.235	6.63×10^{-2}
^{39}K	3/2	93.26	0.23	12.483	1.987	5.08×10^{-4}
^{43}Ca	7/2	0.135	0.002	-18.001	2.865	6.40×10^{-3}
^{129}Xe	½	26.4	-	-74.00	-11.78	2.12×10^{-2}

The spin, I, is given in units of $\hbar$, ($\hbar = h/2\pi$, where h is Planck's constant). The natural abundance, γ, and sensitivity are taken from reference 115 (a particularly valuable reference for NMR and MRI). The biological abundance is typical abundance in the human body (values are elemental abundance from reference 116 multiplied by isotopic abundance).

measurements can be at least partially compensated for by using stronger pre-polarizing fields and SQUID sensor technology in place of the traditional Faraday pickup. While any application of ULF MRI will need to examine a broad range of tradeoffs, working in the ULF regime has some advantages that may be important compared to traditional MRI, both in medicine and a variety of other emerging applications, as we shall explore in later chapters. Before delving into the details of the various tradeoffs between ULF and HF MRI, we will briefly examine how the basic physics behind MRI depends on the magnetic fields used.

Every MRI is derived from the measured NMR signal and how that signal can be used to differentiate materials such as tissue types. Most MRI technology endeavors to improve image quality by increasing signal; however, larger signal, greater SNRs, and better "contrast" all contribute directly to improved image quality. We shall briefly examine the underlying physics needed to appreciate these contributions to image quality.

We will now briefly examine the factors contributing to the NMR signal to understand how the signal scales with the applied magnetic field (a far more thorough treatment can be found in the book by Abragam [31]). The primary and universal contributor to the NMR signal is the magnitude of the magnetization of the sample that rotates about the ambient magnetic field vector. The bulk magnetization is a result of the polarization of spins by the externally applied magnetic field. Consider the quantum model for a population of spins, each with associated magnetic moment, μ, and nuclear spin, I, in an ambient magnetic field B_p (the subscript "p" designates the magnetic field applied for the purpose of polarizing the spin population). The magnetic dipole moment, μ, for an individual spin in this model is given by:

(Eqn. 1.3)
$$\mu = -g_N \beta_N I = \hbar \gamma_N I$$

where γ_N is the nuclear gyromagnetic ratio, γ_N is the nuclear "γ" factor, and β_N is the nuclear magneton. In the quantum model, an external magnetic field interacts with the spin (the Zeeman interaction) and splits the field-free energy level into states described by:

(Eqn. 1.4)
$$E_m = m\hbar \gamma_N B_p$$

where the energy states are described by the magnetic quantum number, m, which can have values from $-I, -I+1, \ldots +I-1, +I$. Consequently, the number of energy levels available for a given nucleus depends on the nuclear spin. For protons, there are two energy levels with $m = -\frac{1}{2}$ and $+\frac{1}{2}$, with an energy spacing between the two levels of $\delta E = \hbar \gamma_N B_p$. The transition energy between the two states of the proton is associated with a photon that has an angular frequency of:

(Eqn. 1.5)
$$\omega = \gamma B_p$$

which we note as being the same relationship as the classical Larmor frequency, ω_L, presented in Eqn. 1.1. We again remind the reader that it will be important to differentiate the magnetic field at which an NMR signal is measured (designated by the subscript "m") and the magnetic field used to polarize the spin population (designated by the subscript "p") in later discussions. The spin angular frequency depends on the applied field, regardless of the designation.

We now consider the large population of spins (e.g., nuclei) that provide the signal measured in NMR and MRI applications. Let us take some population of spins and place them in a uniform external magnetic field, B_p. The spins will be divided between available states according to the Boltzmann distribution: the number of spins in a given state is proportional to $\exp(-E_m/k_B T)$. It can be shown that for any given transition with an energy difference δE, the excess fraction of spins in the lower energy level is roughly

(Eqn. 1.6)
$$\frac{\Delta N}{N_0} = \frac{1 - e^{\frac{-\delta E}{k_B T}}}{1 + e^{\frac{-\delta E}{k_B T}}} \approx \frac{\delta E}{2k_B T} = \frac{\hbar \gamma B_p}{2k_B T}$$

This population difference between different spin energy levels results in a net sample polarization that, when properly manipulated, can result in a measurable time-varying magnetic field. A practical example using Eqn. 1.6 with typical values for the parameters will illustrate the key challenge for measuring NMR signals. Let us consider 1cm^3 of water that contains approximately $N_0 = 6.69 \times 10^{22}$ protons (spins). It is obvious that in the absence of a magnetic field, the energy levels are not split, and hence there is no population difference and consequently no signal. In the presence of a polarizing magnetic field, the energy levels are split and a population difference develops that depends upon both the magnetic field and the temperature. Consider what happens when we subject our 1cm^3 of water to a substantial 1T (10,000G) polarizing magnetic field at room temperature (293K). This will result in a population difference of the protons in the water sample between the two states of

(Eqn. 1.7)
$$\frac{\Delta N}{N_0} \approx \frac{\hbar \gamma B_p}{2k_B T} = 3.49 \times 10^{-6}$$

where k_B=1.381 × 10^{-23} J/K and $\hbar = h/2\pi = 1.055 \times 10^{-3}$ J-sec, and γ is in the Rad/T-sec form (267.513 for protons). This extremely small population difference (even at 1T) results in two important effects that are used in NMR and MRI. First and foremost, the population difference results in a net polarization of the sample that produces the observable NMR signal. In addition, the excess population in the lower energy state provides the quantum-level structure and population that is excited by an external source ("RF field" at traditional HF), allowing manipulation of the polarization. This manipulation of the spin population is the basis for most of the pulse sequences used in both NMR spectroscopy and MR imaging, discussed in later chapters. The polarization at equilibrium can be calculated by summing the magnetic dipole moments over the volume of interest. The volume of interest in MRI is typically the volume element or voxel that ultimately describes the imaging resolution. If we use Curie's law in the limit where the magnetic energy is far less than the thermal energy (true for any normal range of temperatures and magnetic fields used in medical imaging), the magnetic moment vector at equilibrium, $\mathbf{M}_0$, is aligned with the external field, $\mathbf{B}_p$:

(Eqn. 1.8)
$$\mathbf{M}_0 = \frac{N\hbar^2 \gamma^2 I(I+1)\mathbf{B}_p}{3k_B T}$$

where the volume of interest contains N spins of spin I. Using the standard form of the constants and expressing γ in Rad/T-sec, we compute $\mathbf{M}_0$ in units of J/T = A·m^2 (the typical current-area form of a magnetic dipole). For example, if we place 1cm^3 of pure water at 293K into a B_p = 1T field and wait for the spin population to reach equilibrium, we can calculate

$\mathbf{M}_0$ for this sample based on 6.69×10^{22} protons, each with spin ½ and $\gamma = 267.513 \times 10^6$ Rad/T-sec, to be $\mathbf{M}_0(1\text{cm}^3\ H_2O\ @293K) = 3.29 \times 10^{-9}$ J/T.

The measured NMR signal is not of the moment itself but rather the time-varying magnetic field produced by the moment at some distance from the voxel source that is detected and measured by the sensor of choice. The total flux density (field) produced by some polarized voxel at the pickup coil (and using the geometrically simplifying assumptions that the source is far smaller than the pickup, and the size of the pickup is much less than the distance from the source) can be simply expressed as:

(Eqn. 1.9)

$$B_{\text{Sens}} = \frac{\Gamma_{\text{PU}}\mu_0\mathbf{M}_0}{d^3}$$

where Γ_{PU} is a geometry factor and d is the distance between the polarized voxel and a point on the sensor. The NMR signal produced by this field depends on the detailed characteristics of the sensor and is discussed in Section 1.4.3 and more extensively in Chapter 2. Eqn. 1.9 illustrates the field at the sensor scales with (1) a geometric factor, Γ_{PU}, that depends on the geometry of the pickup coil and the orientation of the magnetic moment vector relative to the pickup and (2) the inverse cube of the distance between the signal source and sensor.

Equation 9 illustrates a key relationship in NMR and MRI: the polarization of a sample from which the NMR signal is derived scales linearly with $\mathbf{B}_p$. Additionally, the total magnetic moment scales with the number of spins (N), and in an imaging sense, translates to the spin density or the number of spins in a given voxel. A voxel is the computational volume elements into which a region of interest is divided to both acquire and analyze the MRI signal. Finally, we note that while the polarization (and consequently the magnetic moment) also scales inversely with temperature, lowering the temperature is practically restricted to some material applications and is not particularly useful when imaging living biological systems. While temperature is not likely to be an important variable for controlling net polarization in living biological systems, temperature induces other effects that are important in MRI and will be discussed later. The challenge in all NMR is to maximize the spin state population difference and the total number of spins to maximize the polarization in each voxel and, hence, the measurable signal. However, the desire for any imaging technique such as MRI is to improve spatial resolution. As the spatial resolution increases, the volume of a voxel decreases and the total number of spins contributing to the signal from that voxel decreases proportionately. These factors become the overwhelming driver for increasing $\mathbf{B}_p$.

This is an appropriate point at which to point out that the number of spins, N, contributing to the sample magnetic moment is the mole fraction of the *isotope* of interest, which may be significantly smaller than the mole fraction of the element. For example, while the vast majority of hydrogen is made up of NMR active protons (>99.9%), only 1.1% of the carbon in the body is NMR-active ^{13}C—because $I(^{12}C) = 0$. Furthermore, less than 0.05% of the oxygen in the body is NMR-active ^{17}O—because $I(^{16}O) = 0$. In addition to the number of spins (nuclei) that contribute to the NMR signal for a given isotope, the magnitude of the NMR signal also depends on the sensitivity that describes the polarizability of a given isotope relative to protons. Many tables of isotopic NMR properties that are aimed at biological applications list the "receptivity" rather than the sensitivity. The receptivity is the product of the sensitivity and the typical biological abundance of the given isotope. Table 1.1 lists the sensitivity that exclusively relates to the nucleus and includes no factor or correction for isotopic abundance.

1.2.2 Manipulating and Measuring the Polarization

Underlying all of the many factors that contribute to image quality is the ability to measure the NMR signal from the spin population. In the vast majority of MRI applications, the NMR signal is measured by a magnetic sensor that couples to the sample net (or bulk) magnetic moment as it rotates about an applied measurement field, B_m, in accordance with Eqn. 1.1. In traditional MRI at HF, the field at which the NMR signal is measured, B_m, is the same as the large fixed polarizing field, B_p; as a result, $B_p = B_m$, commonly referred to as simply B_0 at HF. The same field is used for both polarization and measurement because the orientation of the field cannot be readily changed, nor is it practical or safe to switch the field on and off. The magnetic field orientation for HF magnets is dictated by a magnet design that consists of fixed coils and, in some cases, pole pieces. The stored energy in HF magnets is extremely large (typically tens of megaJoules, or about 10 sticks of dynamite), which presents technological challenges to quickly dump the energy and adds significant expense in terms of wasted energy (or significant capital cost for systems to recover and reuse that energy). In almost all HF systems, the need to dump these massive quantities of energy occurs only in the relatively rare occasions of a superconducting magnet "quench." These events are most commonly caused by some small portion of the superconducting coil becoming resistive, which causes energy to be locally deposited that warms more of the coil, which causes more energy to be deposited, and so on. This sequence of events (though exceedingly rare) occur in milliseconds finally resulting in large and rapid changes in magnetic field that induce significant physiological currents that can cause discomfort and pain that may even result in neurological and tissue damage.

A measurable NMR signal is produced by the precession of $\mathbf{M}_0$ about $\mathbf{B}_m$ that is detected by an appropriately oriented sensor through which the magnetic flux changes with the precession of $\mathbf{M}_0$. A variety of different techniques are used to orient the sample magnetic moment, $\mathbf{M}_0$, orthogonal to the measurement field, $\mathbf{B}_m$. ULF MRI affords tremendous flexibility in manipulating all of the fields used, one of the many benefits to ULF. This flexibility provides a number of approaches to manipulate both $\mathbf{M}_0$ and $\mathbf{B}_m$ to set up the appropriate relative orientation, discussed in Chapter 4. The options for systems with a fixed $\mathbf{B}_p = \mathbf{B}_m$ are far more limited and require the reorientation of the $\mathbf{M}_0$ vector away from the fixed system field to allow it to produce a measurable signal. To use a consistent nomenclature for single fixed-field systems and ULF MRI systems, we designate the fixed field as $\mathbf{B}_p$ during the polarization phase (Fig. 1.3, panel a). This field is relabeled $\mathbf{B}_m$ immediately after the spins are reoriented to induce the bulk magnetic moment to precess about the field in such a way as to provide a measurable signal. Differentiating $\mathbf{B}_p$ and $\mathbf{B}_m$ will facilitate later discussions of various "evolution fields" that are used to induce desired contrast mechanisms. This allows the following discussion to apply equally to traditional HF MRI in which there is a single fixed field and to ULF MRI, where $\mathbf{B}_p$ and $\mathbf{B}_m$ are variable in both magnitude and orientation. By far the most common approach to reorient the spin population, first reported by Hahn [32–34], is to apply a relatively short AC or rotating magnetic field, $\mathbf{B}_{RF}$, (called "RF" owing to the commonly high-frequency nature of the applied field) to the spin population at an orientation orthogonal to the fixed system field ($\mathbf{B}_{RF} \perp \mathbf{B}_p$). The frequency of the applied $\mathbf{B}_{RF}$ is matched to the Larmor precession frequency, $\omega_L = \gamma B_p$, of the spin population. $\mathbf{B}_{RF}$ rotates the sample polarization away from the z-axis at an angular velocity that is proportional to the magnitude $|\mathbf{B}_{RF}|$, so that after a time t_{RF}, $\mathbf{M}_0$ is rotated by an angle:

(Eqn. 1.10)
$$\Theta = \gamma B_{RF} t_{RF}.$$

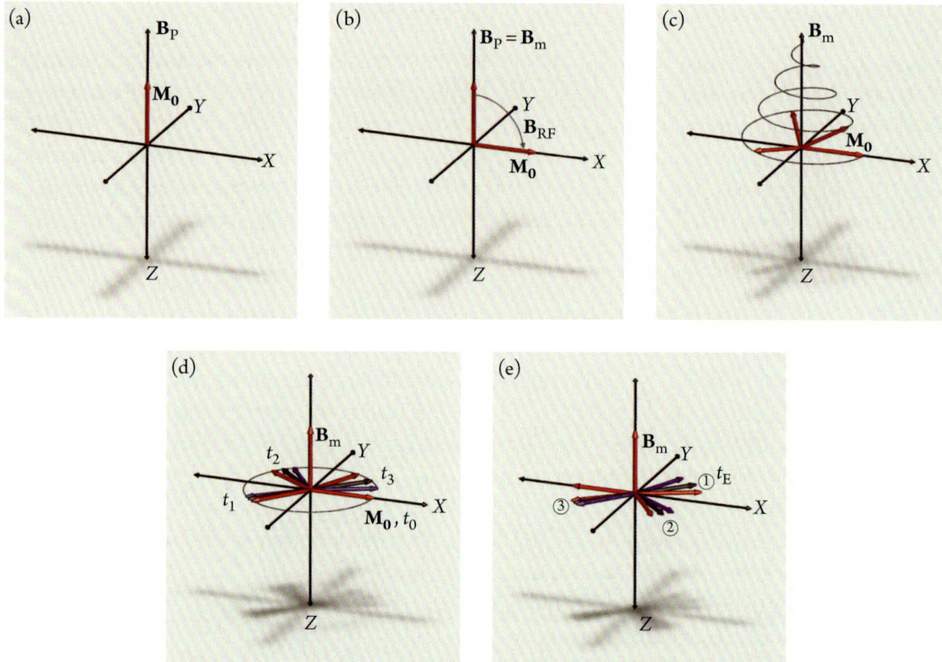

FIGURE 1.3 Spin-echo sequence. Panel a: $\mathbf{M}_0$ along $\mathbf{B}_p$ at t = 0. Panel b: $\mathbf{M}_0$ rotated by 90 degrees away from $\mathbf{B}_m = \mathbf{B}_p$ at $t = t_1$, by applied RF pulse. Panel c: Ensemble of spins rotating about applied field $\mathbf{B}_m$ (= $\mathbf{B}_p$) at $t = t_2$ where the ensemble is relaxing toward the applied field. Panel d: While relaxing, the ensemble of spins also spreads out (dephases) with time, as illustrated by the projection of $\mathbf{M}_0$ on the *X-Y* plane at three times. Panel e: After application of a spin-flip pulse, the ensemble partially rephases after time $t = t_3$.

The magnetic moment $\mathbf{M}_0$ is reoriented normal to $\mathbf{B}_p$ as illustrated in Figure 1.3, panel b. After removal of $\mathbf{B}_{RF}$, the component of $\mathbf{M}_0$ normal to $\mathbf{B}_p$ rotates about the fixed field, producing the measurable NMR signal (assuming an appropriately oriented sensor, discussed in Section 1.2.5).

1.2.3 Introducing Relaxation

The process of applying $\mathbf{B}_{RF}$ for a sufficient time to rotate $\mathbf{M}_0$ until it is normal to $\mathbf{B}_p$ is commonly referred to as applying a $\pi/2$ (pi-over-two) pulse having the effect of "tipping" the spins by 90 degrees. After the $\mathbf{B}_{RF}$ is turned off, the measurable signal is produced by the projection of the bulk magnetic moment on the *X-Y* plane (defined as the plane normal to $\mathbf{B}_m$) precessing about $\mathbf{B}_m$. The signal decreases with time in what is called the free induction decay (FID), shown in Figure 1.4. The frequency of the decaying sinusoid is the Larmor frequency at the measurement field: $\omega_L = \gamma_N B_p$. The decay of the measured NMR signal (FID) is attributed to three effects: (1) the "relaxation" of the magnetic moment, $\mathbf{M}_0$ (that was tipped away from $\mathbf{B}_m$), back toward the equilibrium orientation along $\mathbf{B}_m$ (as illustrated in Fig. 1.3, panel c; (2) the spin population dephases as it rotates about $\mathbf{B}_m$ because of small variations in the local

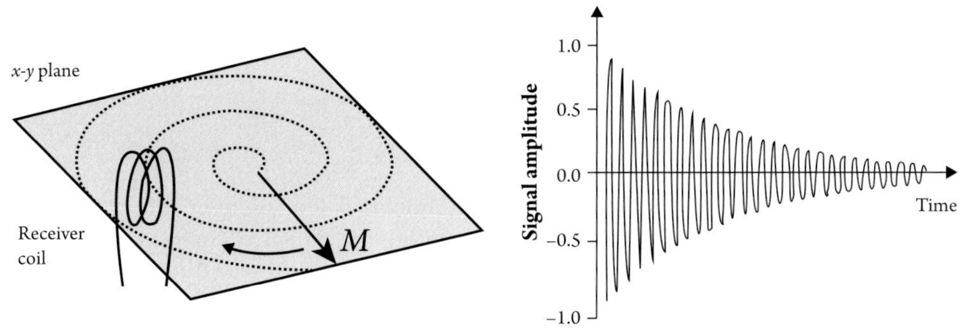

FIGURE 1.4 NMR signal immediately after π/2 pulse. The decay of the signal is caused by both longitudinal and transverse relaxation mechanisms and is called the free induction decay (FID).

magnetic field experienced by each spin; and (3) dephasing due to inhomogeneities in the applied field. The combined dephasing effects are illustrated in Figure 1.3, panel d, at three times: t_1, t_2, and t_3.

The first effect is commonly referred to as spin-lattice relaxation because it involves transition between energy levels of the spin system requiring an energy reservoir—typically named the "lattice" or "bath"—into which energy transferring out of the spin system is deposited. This energy transfer is facilitated by fluctuating magnetic fields orthogonal to the measurement field. The transitions between energy states associated with this process randomize orientation of the spins in the *X-Y* plane, having the effect of reducing $\mathbf{M}_{XY}$, the projection of $\mathbf{M}_0$ on the *X-Y* plane, with time (Fig. 1.3, panel c).

The second effect, commonly referred to as spin-spin relaxation, is characterized by microscopic magnetic field variations parallel to the measurement field; hence the spins have different precession rates, resulting in randomization of their relative angles with time. A simple example of this microscopic magnetic field variation is the fields associated with dipole-dipole interaction of the spins. The decay of the NMR signal associated with these two processes is called transverse relaxation. The rate of this relaxation is defined by properties of the sample material and generally speaking is not affected by the quality of the applied measurement field.

The third effect is associated with an inhomogeneous measurement field, again resulting in different precession rates for different spins and associated with this spread of the relative angles. Reduction of the NMR signal associated with this effect is not a property of the material under study and generally speaking is avoidable by proper design of the experimental apparatus or/and measurement sequence. Both spin dephasing mechanisms, effects 2 and 3, have the effect of spreading out the spins as they rotate about $\mathbf{B}_m$, causing the total superposed spins that contribute to the magnetic moment, $\mathbf{M}_0$, to be reduced over time (see Fig. 1.3, panel d).

Let us consider the longitudinal and transverse relaxation mechanisms separately. We know that applying $\mathbf{B}_p$ causes the spin population to be divided between available quantum states according to the Boltzmann distribution that quantitatively describes the division of the spin population between the available states. When $\mathbf{B}_p$ is removed, the populations return to the zero-field equilibrium distribution at an exponential rate described by the spin-lattice or longitudinal relaxation time constant, T_1. Physically, this is the time required for the energy tied up in the excess spin populations to be redistributed to the lattice—hence the name "spin-lattice" relaxation. We use here the typical convention in which the *z*-axis is defined along $\mathbf{B}_{\mathrm{p}}$ and the time evolution of the magnetic moment caused by spin-lattice relaxation is described by

(Eqn. 1.11)
$$\mathbf{M}_Z(t) = \mathbf{M}_{Z,t=0}\left(1 - e^{-t/T_1}\right)$$

where we use $\mathbf{M}_{Z,t=0}$ to designate the projection of the magnetic moment along z at $t = 0$. This is the same mechanism responsible for the relaxation of $\mathbf{M}_0$ (that was tipped away from $\mathbf{B}_{\mathrm{m}}$, as described above) back toward the equilibrium orientation along $\mathbf{B}_{\mathrm{m}}$.

The second major contributor to the decay of the NMR signal is the spin-spin relaxation, which is caused by the dephasing of the spins due to different magnetic fields experienced by each spin. Spins that experience a slightly larger local magnetic field will rotate slightly faster (Eqn. 1.1), and those in a slightly smaller local field will rotate slightly slower (Fig. 1.3, panel d; the red vector represents the spin rotating slower and the blue one faster). These differences in the precession frequency cause a "destructive interference" over the ensemble that reduces the net polarization and consequently the NMR signal over time. Dephasing of the spin population reduces the total $\mathbf{M}_0$. This dephasing effect is the result of interactions at the microscopic and macroscopic scales. The microscopic scale is dominated by interactions between the neighboring spins in the sample that induce spin-spin relaxation (or decay) of the net magnetic moment with time. These interactions occur in the form of neighboring nuclei in a single molecule or those nuclei that are brought into proximity of one another by molecular motion. The spin-spin interactions reduce the transverse magnetization of a sample and are characterized by the time constant T_2. Inhomogeneities in the applied magnetic field (whether due to the applied field itself or spurious fields from other sources) are primarily responsible for the macroscopic-scale interactions that result in transverse relaxation. Taken together, the sources of transverse dephasing result in a transverse relaxation time constant T_2^*. The rate at which the transverse NMR signal decreases is described by

(Eqn. 1.12)
$$\mathbf{M}_{XY}(t) = \mathbf{M}_{XY,t=0}\cos(\omega_L t)e^{-t/T_2^*}$$

where $\mathbf{M}_{XY,t=0}$ designates the magnitude of the initial magnetic moment transverse to the measurement field, $\mathbf{B}_{\mathrm{m}}$. The *cos* term describes the rotation of the magnetic moment at ω_{L}, the Larmor precession frequency of the spins in the measurement field. Finally, we employ the common assumption that the total transverse relaxation time constant, T_2^*, can be separated into a purely molecular component, T_2, and a macroscopic inhomogeneity component, T_{IH}:

(Eqn. 1.13)
$$\frac{1}{T_2^*} = \frac{1}{T_2} + \frac{1}{T_{\mathrm{IH}}} + \frac{1}{T_\chi} + \frac{1}{T_{\mathrm{other}}}.$$

There are a variety of contributors to the observed (total) T_2^* shown in Eqn. 1.13 including relaxation due to variations of magnetic susceptibility through the sample (T_χ) and other effects (T_{other}) that we discuss later.

The observed FID for any NMR signal is the time evolution of the projection of the bulk magnetic moment on the *X-Y* plane. Hence, the measured signal is proportional to the product of both transverse and longitudinal relaxation mechanisms. Therefore, we can describe the time evolution of the measurable magnetic moment as

(Eqn. 1.14) $$\mathbf{M}_{XY}(t) = \mathbf{M}_{0,t=0}\cos(\omega_L t)e^{-t/T_2^*}(1-e^{-t/T_1}).$$

It should be noted that T_1 is always longer than T_2, and at HF the total relaxation is usually dominated by T_2 effects, while in the ULF regime T_1 is typically similar to T_2.

1.2.4 Introducing Pulse Sequences (the Spin Echo)

In addition to the $\pi/2$ pulse, Hahn first reported applying an RF pulse at resonance with ω_L of the spin population that causes the spins to "flip" in the plane of rotation such that their relative order in the population is reversed, as in a mirror image. The motivation for flipping the spin population was that the ensemble would tend to "rephase" as it evolved in a static (though imperfect) magnetic environment. The effect of this so-called "π pulse" is illustrated in panel 3 of Figure 1.3. We described the evolution of the spin population that is initially polarized by $\mathbf{B}_p$ (panel a), after which a $\pi/2$ pulse tips the polarization away from the fixed $\mathbf{B}_p$ (panel b, where we also use the designation $\mathbf{B}_p = \mathbf{B}_m$). The spin population rotates about the fixed field and evolves in time as described in Eqn. 1.14 (panel c representing the T_1 effect and panel d illustrating a T_2 effect). In panel d, we see that the spin population has a distribution of phase velocities, with the red and blue vectors representing the slowest and fastest, respectively. After some evolution time, t_E, a π pulse is applied to the spin population, causing the spins to flip in the plane of rotation, resulting in the slowest spins (red) being at the front of the ensemble and the fastest (blue) at the rear. After the π pulse inverts the spin population, the ensemble continues to evolve as before; however, because the spins that are rotating faster (blue) are at the rear of the ensemble and those rotating slower (red) are at the fore, the ensemble "rephases" over time. The practical result is the magnetic moment and associated signal increase (for a while) as the ensemble rephases and the destructive interference is reduced. Once the spins with the fastest phase velocity catch up to those with the slowest velocity, the ensemble again dephases and the signal diminishes. This RF "π pulse" was originally described by Hahn and is widely practiced in modern MRI. The signal lost to spin-spin relaxation and recovered by application of a π pulse is called the "spin echo" and is illustrated in Figure 1.5. This style of echo is also known as a "pancake" echo because it is like

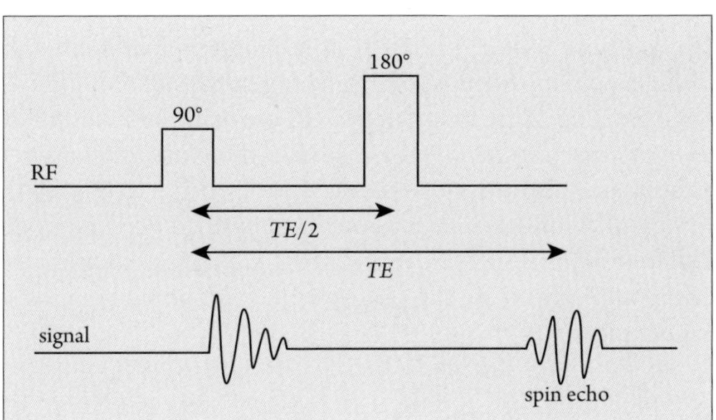

FIGURE 1.5 Illustration of the spin-echo pulse sequence and the resulting NMR signal.

flipping a pancake and the relative positions of the spins are inverted (i.e., lagging spins end up as leading spins).

The degree to which the magnetic moment increases and the signal is recovered after application of the π pulse is limited by the T_1 relaxation and other factors such as diffusion and flow. The spin-lattice relaxation is not affected, and no signal lost to this relaxation mechanism is recovered in the spin echo. Furthermore, only the portion of the transverse relaxation that is lost to the microscopic, purely spin-spin interactions is fully recovered by application of the π pulse. For example, dephasing caused by inhomogeneities in the applied field is not likely to be recovered by the ensemble because molecular and/or ensemble motion will cause the spins to sample different fields during the period of time before and after the π pulse, resulting in imperfect rephasing. By separating out the portion of the signal that can be fully recovered in the spin echo, one has a much better approximation of the T_2 (purely spin-spin) relaxation time.

Developing different pulse sequences to manipulate the spin ensemble in specific ways is a vast area of active research in HF MRI and an important tool in the developing field of ULF MRI. Pulse sequences are developed for a vast array of purposes, such as enhancing specific tissue or fluid contrast, imaging blood flow, or maximizing sensitivity to slight differences in paramagnetism, which serves as the basis of fMRI. While most of the pulse sequences developed for HF MRI involve the application of high-frequency RF pulses, the flexibility in manipulating the magnitude and direction of $\mathbf{B}_\mathrm{p}$ and $\mathbf{B}_\mathrm{m}$ provides additional "knobs" with which to design pulse sequences at ULF.

1.2.5 Sensing the NMR Signal

The most common sensor used to measure the rotating magnetic moment (time-varying field) that is the NMR signal in traditional HF NMR and MRI is the Faraday coil. The name of the pickup is derived from Faraday's law, which describes the fundamental relationship between voltage (*emf*) and a changing magnetic field. This is most simply described as

(Eqn. 1.15)
$$emf = \frac{d\Phi}{dt} = -N_{\mathrm{PU}} A \frac{dB_\perp}{dt}$$

where $d\Phi/dt$ is the time-varying total flux in a pickup coil, often described in terms of the simplistic case of a sensor consisting of N_{PU} turns of average area A in a time-varying magnetic field (flux density). We use $dB_\perp/dt$ to designate the magnetic field that threads through the pickup coil; hence, it is the normal component of the field, averaged over the coil area.

For illustrative purposes, we calculate $\mathbf{B}$ at a simple planar sensor produced by the polarized voxel with dipole moment $\mathbf{M}_0$ located some distance from the sensor. Recalling that only the component of $\mathbf{M}$ that produces field normal to the sensor couples flux into the pickup coil, we assume for this simple case that the planar pickup is tangential to $\mathbf{B}_0$ and that a $\pi/2$ pulse has just been applied to tilt $\mathbf{M}_0$ orthogonal to $\mathbf{B}_0$ (Fig. 1.3, panel b) and the pickup coil. We also assume the spin population has had no time to relax. Because we wish to simply illustrate general spatial dependences, we further simplify the calculation by assuming the voxel is directly below the pickup coil. For this simple case we can calculate the flux density at the pickup as

(Eqn. 1.16)
$$\mathbf{B}_{\mathrm{pu}} = \frac{\mu_0}{2\pi(a^2+d^2)^{3/2}}\mathbf{M}_0 = \frac{\mu_0}{2\pi(a^2+d^2)^{3/2}} \frac{N_V \hbar^2 \gamma^2 I(I+1)\mathbf{B}_\mathrm{p}}{3k_B T}$$

where $\boldsymbol{B}_{\mathrm{pu}}$ is the magnetic field at the pickup coil. The voxel is roughly centered a distance d from the circular pickup coil of radius a, consisting of one turn $(N_{\mathrm{PU}} = 1)$. We see that both the size of the pickup and the distance between the voxel and the pickup are significant factors in determining the flux coupled into the pickup. They play important roles in analyzing tradeoffs for various MRI applications where single large pickups may be compared to an array of smaller pickups. We can now estimate the peak-to-peak amplitude of the voltage in our Faraday pickup as

(Eqn. 1.17)

$$V_{\mathrm{PP}} \propto M_0 \omega_{\mathrm{L}} \propto \gamma^3 B_{\mathrm{p}} B_{\mathrm{m}}$$

where B_{p} is the polarization field responsible for aligning the spins and generating the sample magnetic moment and B_{m} is the field at which the signal is acquired. While not typical for HF MRI, we distinguished the polarization field from the measurement field to again provide consistency with later discussions of ULF MRI. In traditional NMR and MRI applications using Faraday sensors where $B_{\mathrm{p}} = B_{\mathrm{m}} = B_0$, the signal amplitude (voltage) is said to depend on B_0^2. This has been yet another driver for higher magnetic fields in traditional MRI and, similarly, a detriment to lower fields.

The most common sensors used at ULF are SQUIDs. The SQUID was first demonstrated in 1964 as a DC-coupled device consisting of two Josephson junctions by Jaklevic et al. [35]. In 1970 Zimmerman, Thiene, and Harding [36] demonstrated a single-Josephson-junction RF-coupled SQUID. The SQUID is the most sensitive magnetic flux detector known, approaching the quantum limit in sensitivity, and has been tailored for a vast array of applications [37]. An important distinction between SQUIDs and Faraday sensors used in MRI applications is that the signal amplitude (S) from the latter depends on frequency ($S_{\mathrm{Faraday}} \propto dB/dt$), while the SQUID is used as a direct magnetic flux-to-voltage converter that is independent of frequency ($S_{\mathrm{SQUID}} \propto B$). Furthermore, we note that while $B_{\mathrm{p}} = B_{\mathrm{m}} = B_0$ is assumed for virtually all HF MRI applications, many implementations of ULF MRI utilize B_{p} that is orders of magnitude larger than B_{m}. The sensitivity of the SQUID sensor, together with a polarization field that can be far larger than the measurement field, enables sufficient signal to provide unique opportunities for ULF MRI that may otherwise seem beyond the realm of possibilities. Myers et al. published a study (see reference [54]) comparing the SNR performance of SQUID sensors and Faraday pickups for measuring NMR signals as a function of frequency in which the tradeoffs were found to depend strongly on geometry, specific application, and frequency. They reported that in general the frequency tradeoff point between SQUID and Faraday coil sensors would be around 50 to 100kHz. Our own work indicates the equivalence point may be at significantly lower frequencies for some applications (see, for example, Chapter 2), showing that the tradeoff analysis is complex.

Independent of whether the application is HF or LF MRI, the orientation, size, number, and spatial sensitivity of the magnetic sensors are important system design considerations. The orientation and size of sensors dictate the coupling to both the signal of interest (the rotating bulk magnetic moment of the sample) and various noise sources that affect the all-important SNR for HF and ULF applications alike. The number of sensors and sensor size play a crucial role in tradeoff studies that include spatial sensitivity, imaging time, and SNR [38,39]. Finally, the spatial sensitivity of the sensor is particularly relevant to ULF applications where the SQUID sensor can be coupled to pickup coils with a variety of spatial sensitivities that most commonly include magnetometers, first-order gradiometers, and second-order gradiometers. Each of these issues and related trade-offs will be discussed in various contexts in later chapters.

A casual observer may conclude that ULF MRI is going off in a direction that is contrary to the primary drivers in MRI. We will examine in detail the drivers for ULF MRI and why one would pursue a technology that appears to contradict the popular wisdom for MRI. In addition, we will examine the impediments for ULF MRI and present the approaches that mitigate them. The two primary mitigating approaches to compensate for the reduction of NMR signal at ULF are: (1) using the pre-polarization methods originally proposed by Packard will significantly increase sample polarization and, consequently, the signal; and (2) using SQUIDs to measure the NMR signal both applies the most sensitive magnetic field sensor known and does not suffer a frequency penalty at low fields. We note that while SQUIDs are a boon to ULF MRI, they cannot be used at HF (or even in the >0.3T LF regime) because they would be destroyed by these high magnetic fields.

1.2.6 MRI: Spatially Encoding the NMR

We have shown that MRI in the ULF regime provides a large degree of variability in the magnetic fields used to polarize the sample, manipulate the spin population, and read out the NMR signals compared to the HF regime, where B_0 is fixed and consequently limits B_{RF}. The approach to applying magnetic field gradients that encode position in the measured NMR signal has, thus far, been quite similar between ULF and HF. Directional gradients are superposed with B_m in such a way that a gradient along one axis alters the NMR frequency as a function of position along that axis and a gradient applied orthogonally alters the phase of the NMR signal relative to position along the orthogonal axis.

Figure 1.6 illustrates how a gradient that increases in strength along the x-axis (G_x) is superposed with the spatially uniform magnetic field at which the NMR signal is measured ($B_m = B_0$). The spins in the sample experience a slightly different local magnetic field that varies with position along the x-axis ($B(x) = B_m + \Delta x \cdot G_x$). This means that the Larmor frequency for the spins will vary depending on position:

(Eqn. 1.18) $$\omega_L(x) = \gamma B(x) = \gamma(B_m + \Delta x \cdot G_x)$$

The spatial encoding of information along the second (y) axis is illustrated in Figure 1.6, where a gradient along the y-axis (G_y) is superposed with both B_m and G_x. In most applications, G_y is introduced as a time-varying gradient.

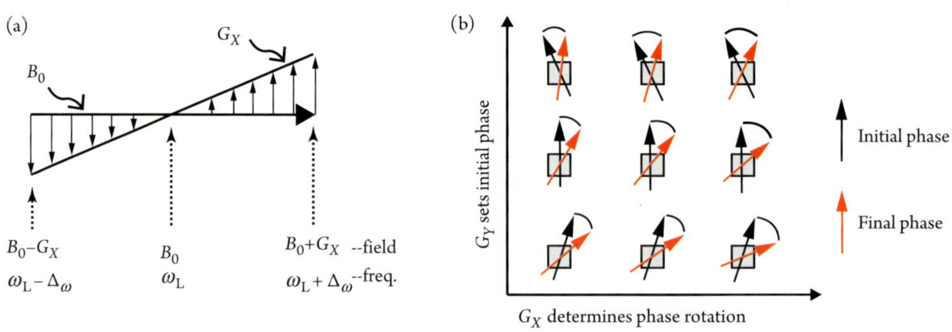

FIGURE 1.6 (a) Illustration of the spatially uniform B_0 superposed with a linear gradient (G_x). ω_L of the spins varies with position according to: $\Delta\omega = \Delta x\, G_x$; where the $\Delta\omega$ gives position. (b) Illustration of how the addition of a time-varying gradient along the y-axis will encode different phases.

The accuracy with which the MRI signal can be spatially encoded using magnetic field gradients depends directly on the inherent peak width (often defined in terms of the full width at half maximum [FWHM]) of the NMR signal in the absence of a gradient. The FWHM determines the accuracy with which a frequency can be measured, and that, in turn, determines the accuracy with which we can calculate the position based on the applied gradient. The spatial accuracy, Δx (m), with which a measured NMR signal can be localized (in the x-dimension) is expressed as

(Eqn. 1.19)
$$\Delta x = \frac{2\pi\Delta f}{\gamma G_x}$$

where Δf is the FWHM line width of the NMR peak in the absence of a gradient (in Hz) and G_x is the strength of the applied magnetic field gradient (T/m).

The inherent line width is the NMR line width measured for a given system in the absence of applied gradients. This inherent line width is proportional to the inverse of the measured relaxation time, $1/T_2^*$, which is largely the result of the "natural" line width, proportional to $1/T_2$, and field inhomogeneity effects that contribute to the measured relaxation time. In most NMR and MRI experiments, the line broadening resulting from various instrumental causes is negligible.

This relationship highlights one of the distinct benefits of ULF MRI: the line broadening caused by inhomogeneities in the magnetic field reduces spectral resolution, reducing information in the spectrum. This is immediately evident from Eqn. 1.1, where we see that the variation in local Larmor frequency arises from local field inhomogeneities:

(Eqn. 1.20)
$$(\omega_L + \Delta\omega_L) = \gamma(B_m + \Delta B)$$

where $\Delta\omega_L$ is the variation in the Larmor frequency that is attributed to inhomogeneities ΔB relative to the applied measurement field, B_m. We note that the line width scales with *absolute* inhomogeneity, consequently the relative homogeneity (or fractional inhomogeneities), become ever smaller and harder to attain as the total field increases. For example, at $B_m = 100\mu T$ with 0.1% field homogeneity (relatively simple with simple, uncorrected and unshimmed coils), the frequency variation, and inhomogeneity-induced peak broadening, across the sample would be about 4Hz. Attaining this same level of frequency variation for a 1.5T system would require better than 0.1ppm field homogeneity. While this level of homogeneity is feasible in HF systems across a voxel, it is extraordinarily difficult across any sizable field of view (let alone an entire sample volume). To reiterate, as the field at which the NMR is measured decreases, while the absolute homogeneity remains constant, the relative homogeneity constraints are relaxed. The fact that extraordinarily narrow line widths could be experimentally observed and used for spectroscopic measurements was first reported by McDermott et al. at 1.8μT [see reference 84] and extended to 40nT measurement fields by Burghoff et al. [see reference 94].

As the field at which the NMR signal is measured decreases, ω_L decreases and the voltage generated in a Faraday coil declines linearly with field in accordance with Eqn. 1.17. This scaling of sensor output with ω_L is not true for SQUIDs; in fact, the amplitude of the SQUID output signal depends only on the total magnetic flux coupled into the pickup and is entirely *independent* of the frequency. We reiterate and emphasize this point largely because of the vast number of HF systems in use and the assumption in virtually every NMR and MRI text that the pickup coil is a Faraday-type induction pickup.

There are a variety of approaches to acquire the data for a full 3D image. One is to directly sample all three dimensions of "*k*-space" and another is to build up the third dimension with a series of multiple "slices" of 2D images. Slice selection is simply a specialized case of applying the $\pi/2$ pulse while a gradient is superposed with the uniform field. As shown in Figure 1.6, panel a, the Larmor frequency varies across the sample, and when the $\pi/2$ pulse is applied, only the spins in a small "slice" of the sample match the frequency of the $B_{RF}(\omega)$. All other spins rotating at different local ω_L are unaffected by the $B_{RF}(\omega)$. Hence, signal for successive application of gradients will originate only from this slice of the sample. We will describe a variety of imaging approaches used for ULF MRI in far more detail in Chapter 4.

Gradients provide the key to almost all approaches for MR image reconstruction that assume linear magnetic field gradients across the sample [40]. The basic assumption is that signal within a specific frequency window can be associated with a planar region of the sample, commonly referred to as a slice. A significant problem encountered at ULF is potentially large distortions caused by concomitant gradients—that is, gradients in the directions transverse to the desired (longitudinal) gradient. Maxwell's equations predict that any coil system generating desired gradients will also generate undesired gradients of transverse components. For HF MRI applications, ($B_0 \geq 1$T), typical values of the transverse gradients relative to the applied magnetic field are extremely small and the frequency variation is reasonably assumed to be proportional only to the longitudinal gradients.

For ULF MRI, if we assume operating parameters of $B_m \approx 10^{-4}$T, $dB/dz \approx 10^{-4}$T/m, and a relatively small sample volume of $D \approx 0.2$m, the shift of the Larmor frequencies caused by the concomitant (transverse) gradients can be shown to be 10% of total frequency shift due to the primary gradient, even for a small ROI [41–43]. Concomitant gradients in ULF MRI will clearly result in significant distortions of the frequency and phase encoding relative to the simple planar model of gradients that will result in correspondingly large displacement and distortion artifacts that must be accounted for in any ULF MRI approach. Understanding and accurately correcting the distortion artifacts that result from concomitant gradients is a key aspect of ULF MRI and is fully discussed in Chapter 4.

Finally, large arrays of smaller pickup coils have been used to spatially encode the NMR signal using a variety of techniques, some borrowed from magnetoencephalography (MEG) and electroencephalography (EEG) [44]. One of the first applications of multiple pickup coils demonstrated in HF MRI was to reconstruct images for the full field-of-view (FOV) from undersampled or incomplete *k*-space data from each pickup. The SMASH (simultaneous acquisition of spatial harmonics) [45] and SENSE (sensitivity encoding) [46] methods are two such approaches. The application of the SENSE parallel imaging technique to ULF MRI was first published by our group in 2008 [47] and demonstrated accelerated image acquisition of the living human brain. Parallel MRI techniques are used to increase the imaging speed, which leads to reduced patient scan times and, for some applications, improved temporal resolution at both HF and ULF. Alternatively, these techniques can improve spatial resolution, assuming the same imaging time as single pickup methods.

1.3 INTRODUCING SIGNAL-TO-NOISE AND CONTRAST-TO-NOISE

The preceding discussion has focused entirely on the dependence of the NMR signal amplitude on factors such as the applied magnetic field and the number of spins in a given region of interest. While signal amplitude is fundamental to all MRI, the ability to reconstruct a usable image also depends on high SNR and contrast-to-noise ratio (CNR). This is particularly true of medical MRI, as we shall discuss in depth. The SNR is a quantitative measure of how large the NMR signal for a given voxel is relative to the various sources of noise for a given instrument and acquisition protocol. As the SNR decreases, it becomes increasingly difficult or even impossible to reconstruct a usable image from the information available in the acquired signal. Perhaps second only to signal amplitude and SNR, the quality of an image depends on the "contrast" and CNR, which measure the signal difference between materials we wish to differentiate in the image. Accurate determination, either experimentally or theoretically, of both SNR and CNR involves a detailed analysis of the acquisition system, protocol, and material being imaged that is far beyond the scope of this book. We will, however, introduce the important aspects of these topics here and delve into some of the details particularly relevant to ULF MRI in later chapters. It is particularly important to understand the variables that contribute to SNR and CNR in order to optimize system design and acquisition protocol for the best possible image quality.

SNR and CNR are crucial metrics of ultimate image quality that can significantly impact the complexity of system design and acquisition protocol. These metrics are important tools for measuring system improvement as we compare acquisition protocols, different sensors, and various noise-reduction methodologies. We would, however, urge caution against any simplistic approach to using these metrics (particularly CNR) to compare systems that operate in different field and frequency regimes without careful examination and understanding of the variables. We will only scratch the surface of this complex topic (worthy of a book in and of itself) here and in later chapters to provide the reader with a qualitative sense of how SNR and CNR vary between ULF and HF. These metrics are perhaps most useful and important in optimizing image quality for a given system by providing an understanding of the relationship between system and imaging protocol parameters and image quality.

As we showed in the preceding section, the signal obtained with traditional Faraday-type pickups scales with ω_L (and ω_L depends linearly on the applied field). Noise, however, also increases with the frequency and field. Nonetheless, the MRI SNR is reported to have a net increase that scales approximately with $\omega_L^{3/2}$ [31,48,49], or in a more recent report, linearly with frequency under specific imaging conditions [50]. Two primary sources contribute to the measurement noise in NMR and MRI: the sensor noise and the subject (sample) noise. The noise that arises from the sample itself cannot be readily controlled, especially in the case of living subjects, where significant cooling of the subject is not a viable alternative. The noise resulting from the pickup can be controlled with a number of approaches, including simply cooling the pickup [51] or using superconducting pickups (see, for example, reference [54] for a comparison of noise in SQUID pickups with Faraday induction pickups), or noise can be controlled and SNR gains realized with an optimization of parallel sensor arrays [52]. Thus, the noise originating from the subject represents the lower noise limit toward which the design point for sensor noise should focus. There will be little gain in SNR realized for sensors that produce significantly less noise than the subject.

We will start with an admittedly simplistic and cursory word about comparing system performance, especially among disparate systems, by simply comparing published values of measured SNR. The most common practice to experimentally determine the SNR for a given system and imaging sequence is to divide the amplitude of the signal from a voxel within the volume of interest by the signal from a voxel of equivalent volume outside the region of interest. While this practice is common, it presents many challenges, and the literature (HF MRI in particular) rarely reports measurements with sufficient detail to reproduce them or understand exactly what they represent. A common practice in reporting experimental SNR for MRI is to determine the "signal" from a voxel in the sample region acquired very early in the sequence and the "noise" from a voxel outside the sample region. There are several difficulties with this practice: first, the locations of the signal and noise voxels are rarely accurately specified. While the results in an individual report may be consistent, such an approach is difficult to apply consistently across techniques and methods. Furthermore, the acquisition is often early in the sampling sequence and will not be representative of the SNR through the imaging sequence used to form the image. Finally, the noise voxel is commonly acquired at the extreme margin of the imaging FOV, which may be separated from the sample region by a significant margin, resulting in a deceptively low estimate of the noise.

1.3.1 Signal-to-Noise

Calculating the SNR in MRI is extremely complex, with numerous noise sources and additional variables that depend on the details of the acquisition methodology (e.g., pulse sequence, acquisition times, etc.) for which an analytic expression is extremely difficult to derive [53]. We will examine only the simpler aspects of estimating SNR here, focusing on the most important scaling factors, and leave more detailed discussion to later chapters and other sources. The primary sources of noise in measuring NMR signals from physiological samples are (1) the electrical resistance of the signal pickup and associated amplifier and (2) the electrical resistance of the volume being imaged (e.g., tissue). Numerous other noise sources include the presence and variability of physiological magnetic materials (e.g., hemoglobin), physiological electrical sources (currents generated in muscles and neurons), magnetic and conducting materials in or near the volume of interest, and ambient noise near the imaging frequency. Beyond these key noise sources, there are innumerable other possible sources that may need to be considered. Further complicating the noise picture is that each of these noise sources has its own thermal and frequency spectrum. The primary purpose of this section is to briefly examine the complexities of SNR and dispel the belief that SNR scales in any simple fashion with ω_L. While the noise sources other than sensor or physiological noise can be significant, we will ignore them because they are neither universal nor always predictable.

A key consideration in evaluating SNR is whether the noise for a given imaging system and protocol is dominated by sensor noise or sample noise. Furthermore, it is important to evaluate whether the sample noise is dominated by inherent or induced sample noise. Regardless of the application, the goal for optimal sensor design should be to reduce the contribution of the sensor noise below the nominal subject noise.

Any discussion of the SNR must explicitly include the specific type of sensor being used [54], in addition to the pickup geometry. Until recently, it was generally assumed that the MRI pickup would be a Faraday-type induction sensor. As we shall see in the next section, the application of SQUID sensors to MRI, particularly at ULF, has been steadily increasing since the 1990s. Two significant differences between Faraday-type and SQUID-based sensors relevant to this discussion are the sensitivities to the NMR signal and the inherent sensor noise. The signal from the Faraday pickup scales as $S_{\text{Faraday}} \propto \omega_L M_0$, whereas the SQUID signal is independent of frequency: $S_{\text{SQUID}} \propto M_0$. This relationship clearly favors the Faraday sensor at higher frequencies (fields), while SQUIDs do not pay a penalty at lower frequencies. In terms of sensor noise, the primary source of noise for the Faraday coil is the Johnson noise inherent in all resistive pickups, whereas the SQUID is a superconducting device with effectively no resistive noise.

Sensor noise for normal resistive conductors is largely due to Johnson noise that scales with resistivity and temperature. Johnson noise originates with thermal electronic motion that induces voltage fluctuations in the conductor. The RMS Johnson voltage noise, V_J, is given by

(Eqn. 1.21)
$$V_J \propto \left(4k_B T \Delta f R\right)^{1/2}$$

where R is the resistance of the circuit, T is the absolute temperature, and Δf is the noise measurement frequency bandwidth (in Hz). Additionally, at frequencies for which the skin depth is less than the conductor size, the effective resistance of the circuit increases as $\omega^{1/2}$, further contributing to the noise at high frequencies. Cooling the sensor will reduce the noise by reducing the thermal and, for most materials, the resistivity contributions to the noise. For example, cooling a copper pickup from typical room-temperature (298K) operation to liquid nitrogen temperature (77K) reduces the thermal contribution to the voltage noise by a factor of approximately two and the resistivity factor by about 2.8 (the resistivity of copper decreases a factor of 8 between 298K and 77K). The Johnson noise in superconducting sensors is effectively zero, but there are other noise sources that are discussed later. While these represent a few simple tradeoffs, the total picture is quite complex. Two recent studies that attempted to address these questions, at least in part, were published by Darrasse and Ginefri [51], in which a wide variety of normal-conducting to superconducting pickups for Faraday induction sensors were studied, and Myers et al. [54], where SQUID-based pickups were compared to Faraday sensors over the range of ULF to LF NMR of protons. These studies demonstrate that while sensor type (Faraday vs. SQUID) and pickup conductivity are important considerations, numerous other factors, including sensor geometry and configuration, both in absolute terms and relative to the sample, are important. Furthermore, pickups coupled to SQUID sensors, particularly when designed for low-frequency applications, are typically gradiometric in design. Gradiometer pickups are exceptionally important for reducing sensitivity to ambient noise (which increases at lower frequencies) coupled into the SQUID. The drawback for gradiometers is that they lose sensitivity as a function of distance to a volume of interest far more rapidly than magnetometers. The spatial sensitivity of gradiometers adds yet another complicating factor to simple and direct comparisons of different types of sensors.

The primary sources of noise in measuring NMR signals from physiological samples are (1) the electrical resistance of the signal pickup and (2) electrical resistance in the sample (tissue). Other noise sources include the presence and variability of physiological magnetic materials (e.g., hemoglobin), physiological electrical sources (currents generated in muscles and neurons), magnetic and conducting materials in or near the volume of interest, and many more that must be considered. One simple definition of the SNR of the acquired NMR signal is

(Eqn. 1.22)
$$\mathrm{SNR} \propto \frac{S_{\mathrm{NMR}}}{\sigma}(t_{\mathrm{Seq}})^{1/2}$$

where S_{NMR} is the NMR signal amplitude for the ROI at the time of signal acquisition. σ is the root-mean-square (RMS) standard deviation of the reference background signal. t_{Seq} weights the instantaneous signal amplitude by the acquisition time. t_{Seq} is a unitless time factor that depends on specific details of the imaging pulse sequence used [55,56]. For example, if the acquisition time is on the order of the relaxation time or longer, the expression for t_{Seq} becomes rather complex. In practice, this is acquired for some voxel in close proximity to the region being imaged but containing no sample. The typical assumption is that the region containing sample is relatively large; consequently, even though the voxel is outside the sample area, the pickup will still be sensitive to the sample noise and other sources of noise.

1.3.2 Contast-to-Noise

Contrast and the associated CNR are second only to signal and SNR in importance for determining ultimate image quality. Contrast generally describes the signal difference between materials one wishes to differentiate in the image. For example, contrast in x-ray–based imaging is primarily due to density and the atomic number (Z) of material constituents because x-ray absorption scales with density and Z. Bones are denser than soft tissue and consist of large quantities of calcium that results in a higher average Z for bone in comparison with soft tissue. This is why the x-ray contrast between bones and soft tissue is large whereas the contrast between different tissue types (e.g., white matter and gray matter in the brain) is extremely small. In comparison, white matter, gray matter, cerebrospinal fluid (CSF), and blood are the key materials one typically wishes to differentiate in an MRI of the brain. Contrast between different tissues in the brain (and elsewhere in the body) results from a variety of factors, chief among which are the differences in the NMR relaxation times, T_1 and T_2, and the proton density $\rho(^1\text{H})$ for each tissue type. However, the contrast between two different tissue types will differ with time because the signal from each tissue type decays exponentially with the relaxation time characteristic for that tissue. Consequently, the timing of the imaging sequence is a key parameter for determining and optimizing the CNR for a given image. The take-home message here is that CNR is not a readily calculable parameter, nor can it be trivially optimized.

Unlike x-ray–based imaging modalities such as CT, where the signal is normalized to Hounsfield standard in which the value for water is set to zero, no such reference exists for MRI. Consequently, the CNR is used to provide a measure of how much the measurement signal varies between different tissue types in comparison to the typical variations due to imaging noise. These differences will ultimately result in the computed image intensity that determines the image resolution between different tissue types. For the purpose of our discussion here, we chose a simple definition for the CNR that is described by [57]

(Eqn. 1.23)

$$\text{CNR} \propto \frac{S_A - S_B}{\sigma}(t_{\text{Seq}})^{1/2}$$

where S_A and S_B are the signal amplitudes for tissue types "A" and "B." σ is the RMS standard deviation of the reference background signal while acquiring a single plane (slice) at each phase-encoding step. t_{Seq} is a time factor, similar to that in Eqn. 1.22 in that it depends on the specific timing of the imaging pulse sequence used [58,59]. The physiological noise from each tissue type in this simple definition of CNR is assumed to be the same, which is clearly not accurate; however, the variability of S_i between typical tissue types is far larger. We must remember that the signal amplitudes, S_i, in Eqn. 1.23 include complex dependencies on B_p, B_m, $\rho(^1\text{H})$, T_1, T_2^*, t, and other variables. In particular, while the CNR dependence on magnetic field at high fields is typically ignored, these effects may become dominant for certain tissue types in the ULF regime. In fact, ULF MRI affords the unique ability to vary either or both B_p and B_m during the imaging sequence, which may increase contrast and CNR for certain tissue types.

The CNR is one approach to quantifying the acquired signal quality and analyzed images that depends on the signal variability between tissue types. It directly relates to how easily different tissue types can be distinguished and what is the smallest feature of a given tissue type that may be distinguished from a neighboring volume element of a different tissue type. The distinction between SNR and CNR is that while the *signal* from two different tissue types may be far larger than inherent system noise (large SNR), the difference between the signals from two different tissue types may be extremely small (small CNR). Further complicating the question of differentiating tissue types of some given size is the fact that it depends on the human observer (radiologist) as much as any quantitative measure of CNR. A more detailed discussion of CNR and the dependence of CNR on magnetic field is presented in Chapter 4.

Now that we have outlined the foundational principles of NMR, let us examine the history of MRI at ULF.

1.4 NMR AND MRI AT ULF

1.4.1. A Brief History of NMR at ULF

The observation of proton NMR at or near the Earth's field (~50μT) was first suggested in the 1953 winter meeting of the American Physical Society by Packard and Varian [60] and by Bloom and Mansir [61]. While this work was published only as abstracts, Packard and Varian reported measuring the free induction decay of protons in a 0.5l sample of water at the Earth's field (~0.05mT) at a Larmor frequency of 2185Hz after pre-polarizing the spins in a 10mT field. Bloom and Mansir reported having measured both spin-lattice and spin-spin relaxation times for water at ~0.2mT using a pre-polarization field at 10mT. While no additional material appears to have ever been published for these abstracts, Bloom [62] reported in 1956 both spin-lattice and spin-spin relaxation measurements for solutions of $MnCl_2$ at applied fields from the Earth's field (50μT) up to ~0.7T. They reported that while T_2 remained largely unchanged over this range of applied fields, the T_1 varied by a factor of five between 20kHz and 200kHz (0.5mT–5mT). The variation of both T_1 and T_2 relaxation times as a function of magnetic field is a unique approach to differentiating a wide variety of materials (contrast) at ULF in comparison with traditional high fields.

One very interesting application of these early ULF NMR experiments was to use the proton Larmor frequency to deduce the magnitude of the Earth's magnetic field at a specific location. In a brief letter to the editor of *Nature,* Waters reported using Packard's prepolarizing technique to measure the proton Larmor frequency of 1.997kHz, from which he deduced the Earth's field (at the location of the measurement) to be 46.9μT [63]. The technique in all of these early papers of Earth's field proton NMR, while not detailed in all cases, applies a pre-polarizing field, B_p (typically referred to as B_0 in the original papers), to the sample for at least a few spin-lattice relaxation times to maximize the sample polarization. $\mathbf{B}_p$ is oriented transverse to the Earth's field in most cases so that when it is removed non-adiabatically the resulting proton magnetic moment precesses about the Earth's magnetic field vector (effectively $\mathbf{B}_m$ in these studies). An excellent review of many of the early investigations of liquid NMR at measurement fields at or near the Earth's magnetic field was published by G. Bene [64] in 1980, quite a long time before the application of SQUID sensors to NMR and MRI.

Bene motivated these early investigations of NMR in the ULF regime primarily with the arguments that these systems were transportable and required far less power. One particularly fascinating experiment reported by Bene that has relevance to physiological functional applications was attributed to Benoit, in which the NMR signal for water was measured in a flow-based system. The fluid was pumped through a tube that initially passed through a 2T polarizing magnet and subsequently through a 100μT measurement field in which the precession was measured.

1.4.2 A Brief History of MRI at ULF

Lauterbur [65] reported the first MRI (then called a zeugmatograph) in 1973 using a back-projection technique to resolve small water-filled phantoms. The image was produced by superposing a magnetic field gradient on a 1.4T primary field (60MHz proton Larmor frequency). Spatial localization of a two-chambered water-filled phantom was demonstrated by both spin-population density and spin-lattice relaxation differences. Lauterbur suggested, largely based on the differences in tissue NMR previously reported by Damadian [66], that this imaging technique could be used to differentiate biological tissue types by the differences in spin density and relaxation time. MRI research, development, and application since this first report has proceeded at a meteoric pace. The first two decades of MRI research and development almost exclusively used fields in the Tesla regime and continually strove for the largest practical fields to reduce imaging time and increase spatial resolution. In 1977, Peter Mansfield greatly enhanced the application of gradients in the magnetic field and developed the mathematical methods to analyze the data that enabled a practical (echo-planar) imaging technique [67].

For nearly two decades after Lauterbur demonstrated the first MRI, virtually the entire publication record of MRI technological development showed an unswerving trend toward larger magnetic fields. In 1990, Stepišnik et al. proposed an approach that bucked this traditional trend toward ever-increasing fields for MRI of samples at room temperature [68]. Stepišnik et al. motivated their work by pointing out that the exceptional field uniformity requirements and cost of HF MRI magnets were limiting the widespread availability of these instruments for medical applications. As an alternative, they suggested that extremely low-field MR imaging was plausible. They successfully acquired an NMR signal with a 2,500-turn solenoidal coil (recall from Eqn. 1.15 that the signal scales with N_{PU}) in the Earth's magnetic field (~50μT) using a non-adiabatic pre-polarization technique similar to that reported by Packard and Varian [60]. While the authors reported that the SNR of their system was too low to acquire an anatomical image, an image of a four-cell ($1cm^3$/cell) water phantom was generated. The phantom image was a proton density image and consequently was easier to acquire than an image based on relaxation contrast, which is required for most anatomical images. This is likely the root cause of the inability to acquire anatomical images since the proton density difference between different soft tissues is typically small. It is particularly interesting to note that Stepišnik et al. reported the necessity of shielding the pickup coil from RF noise with a 10mm-thick aluminum box, an interesting point we shall return to shortly.

Macovski and Conolly [69] reported an analysis of a variety of LF MRI approaches. While the paper provided no experimental data, they report that a pulsed pre-polarizing field with an oscillating bias field is the most promising approach for ULF MRI. A significant impediment to efficient ULF MRI explored through the mid-1990s was the noise inherent in room-temperature (or normal conductor) sensors used to measure the NMR signal. These Faraday-type sensors were most commonly large, bulky coils, necessitated by the fact that many turns were needed to produce a measurable signal. The voltage in such coils, as shown in Eqn. 1.15, is induced by the time-varying magnetic field as the bulk magnetic moment precesses about the ambient field vector present in the sample. While the number of turns in a pickup coil (N_{PU} in Eqn. 1.15) helps to compensate for the small signal amplitude and loss of voltage induced in the coil by the low precession frequency, the noise inherent in the coil increases with the number of turns because it is proportional to the amount of conductor present, ultimately reducing the SNR.

1.4.3 ULF NMR with SQUID Sensors

Until the 1990s ULF NMR (and the speculation of ULF MRI), the only pickups used for NMR in any field regime were Faraday-type pickups. As we noted, Macovski and Conolly only considered Faraday pickups with a large number of turns to provide sufficient sensitivity and did not consider SQUIDs as possible candidates for MRI sensors. SQUIDs, as their name implies, are superconducting devices that are typically operated in a liquid helium bath (4.2K at sea level) and, in virtually all low-noise applications, are coupled to superconducting pickups. The only noise sources in a typical DC-SQUID are the shunt resistors that produce a device design-dependent thermal noise. A simple expression for the noise energy was given by Clarke [70], but suffice it to say that modern SQUIDs can demonstrate noise performance of a few $\hbar$, approaching the quantum limit. Hence, not only are SQUIDs supremely sensitive to magnetic field variations, but the inherent noise in SQUID sensors is virtually nonexistent in comparison to resistive Faraday pickups. SQUIDs are currently the most common sensor for acquiring ULF MRI signals; however, other sensors such as atomic magnetometers are being investigated and will be discussed in Chapter 2.

An excellent review by Greenberg points to the advent of SQUIDs as being a significant driver of the revitalization of interest in LF NMR [71]. There are numerous reports of having used SQUIDs, either as amplifiers or as direct flux-to-voltage converters, to measure NMR signals prior to 1990 (see, for example, the Greenberg review). However, these early reports were entirely for samples at or below ~4K and, in most cases, using ^{3}He. The low temperature of the sample allowed placing it in close proximity to the pickup or SQUID sensor. While these early experiments were of limited value in terms of practical NMR, especially for biological samples (due to sample temperature and the use of rare isotopes), they pointed to an important new technology with exquisite sensitivity to measure the rotating magnetic field associated with NMR. The experiments using a SQUID to directly measure the time-dependent NMR signature were particularly important because they demonstrated not only the extraordinary sensitivity of the SQUIDs but also the fact that the direct flux-to-voltage conversion was independent of ω_L. This removes a γB_m from Eqn. 1.17, resulting in a signal amplitude (V_{PP}) that depends only linearly on magnetic field, and that field is the polarization field, B_p, that we have already noted may be orders of magnitude larger than B_m. Another powerful benefit of using SQUIDs as the magnetic field sensor is that they are broadband devices with uniform sensitivity across the entire frequency range at which they operate. This broadband behavior is, however, not retained when the SQUID is operated as an amplifier coupled to a frequency-tuned pickup coil.

The first application of a DC SQUID to measure the FID NMR signal from a room-temperature sample consisting of a water-$CuSO_4$ solution was reported by Seton et al. in 1992 [72]. They motivated their work with the aim of developing low-field MRI that reduces patient RF absorption and improved tissue discrimination due to greater differences in spin-lattice relaxation times (T_1) for different tissue types that resulted in larger contrast at low fields. Finally, they pointed out that induced currents in tissue that is mildly conducting are dramatically reduced at LF, resulting in lower patient noise contribution to SNR. Seton's apparatus used a static magnetic field $B_p = B_m = 10$mT, following the technique of traditional HF MRI. The proton Larmor frequency at this field is $\omega_L = 425$kHz. An alternating field with resonance frequency matched to ω_L was used to align the spin vector orthogonally to the static field ($\pi/2$ pulse) to measure the proton NMR signal. The spin preparation protocol for this early ULF NMR experiment was an LF equivalent of established HF techniques.

Seton et al. employed SQUID sensors to measure these weak NMR precession signals with extraordinary sensitivity. The SQUID sensor is inductively coupled to a pickup loop (also typically superconducting) that couples the magnetic field to the SQUID. The pickup loop built by Seton was roughly based on the published work of Hilbert [73] and Freeman [74] that included a magnetic sensing loop in series with a capacitor that was used to tune the circuit to the Larmor frequency with high $Q = 4{,}500$. While the SQUID sensor is itself inherently broadband (from DC to GHz) with uniform sensitivity, coupling the SQUID to a tuned circuit introduces a nonlinear frequency dependence to the circuit. An important benefit of tuned circuits is the high sensitivity to a specific frequency range of interest provided by the circuit. This benefit is realized only at frequencies above a few kHz, and the heightened sensitivity falls off as the signal frequency deviates significantly from the design frequency [75]. Modern SQUID sensors are approximately two orders of magnitude more sensitive than those used by Seton; consequently, more recent published work and our team have used untuned sensors with uniform sensitivity across the entire frequency operating range of the sensor (DC to many MHz).

One consequence of the extraordinary sensitivity of SQUID sensors to magnetic fields is that when they are exposed to large magnetic fields or large changes in magnetic field, the sensors suffer a temporary dead time (period of time during which no meaningful signal can be acquired). In some cases, permanent damage to the devices may even result. Hilbert and other early investigators incorporated *Q* spoilers (a form of switch) in their pickup coils to minimize dead time and avoid permanent sensor damage. The *Q* spoilers allowed the user to largely decouple the SQUID sensor from the magnetic field during the application of different magnetic fields during the preparation of the spins prior to the NMR measurement. This helped prevent damage by large static magnetic fields and large changes in magnetic field. Chapter 2 discusses modern implementations of "switches" to isolate the SQUID from various magnetic fields used in ULF MRI systems. In his 1992 report, Seton chose not to add this complexity to his pickup. To minimize coupling between the sensor and the primary field, he carefully aligned the plane of his pickup parallel to the applied magnetic field. In addition, Seton adapted a technique commonly used for noise rejection in SQUID applications in which a gradiometer pickup is coupled to a SQUID [76]. Gradiometer pickups tend to be sensitive to non-uniform fields while largely insensitive to uniform fields across the gradiometer. In practice, gradiometers will be sensitive to nearby sources that tend to produce non-uniform field distributions across the gradiometer, while the geometry of the sensor is relatively insensitive to distant sources or sources that produce uniform magnetic fields across the gradiometer. The sensor used by Seton consisted of a multi-turn first-order gradiometer with 1cm diameter pickups separated by 2.5cm (baseline). Such a sensor is sensitive to sources in close proximity to the gradiometer (a few cm) but becomes relatively less sensitive to distant sources or magnetic field coils designed to produce uniform fields. Finally, the SQUID sensor itself was enclosed in a superconducting shield that prevented it from being directly affected by the external fields. These and other sensor tradeoffs are discussed in detail in Chapter 2.

There are aspects of Seton's early apparatus that are worth examining in terms of what may or may not make sense for modern implementations of ULF MRI systems. Seton noted the choice to remove the aluminized Mylar superinsulation from the tail of the cryostat because he determined it absorbed too much of the 425kHz NMR signal. While little quantitative explanation is given for this decision, it is interesting given that the skin depth at this frequency in aluminum is about 125μm. The thickness of the aluminum layer on cryogenic superinsulation is typically less than 1μm, so the absorption of 425kHz electromagnetic signals by even 30 to 40 layers of superinsulation (typical for liquid helium cryostats) is less than 25% due to a total Al thickness of less than 30μm. This choice is interesting to contrast with Stepišnik's decision to use 10mm-thick aluminum shielding around his pickup to reduce RF noise [68]. While Stepišnik reported measuring the NMR signature in the Earth's magnetic field ($\omega_L \approx 2$kHz), the shielding represented ~5 skin thicknesses at 2kHz that would induce a ~99% signal loss (see discussion in Section 1.5.1, below). The practical lessons here are that cryogenic superinsulation with evaporated metal films will provide thermal insulation and a measure of RF isolation. It will, however, also reduce the NMR signal (see Section 1.5.1), but this is not likely to be a significant effect until ω_L reaches 1MHz or more. Another consideration in SQUID applications, discussed in Chapter 2, is the Johnson noise associated with the conducting layers of superinsulation. This may have been a contributing factor (though not mentioned in his papers) to Seton's decision to remove the superinsulation.

Relaxation times (T_1, T_2, and T_2^*) are another important factor to consider when designing ULF MRI experiments. For example, Seton reported using a water-$CuSO_4$ solution as the NMR sample, where the $CuSO_4$ is added to decrease the solution T_1 relaxation time. This had the effect of appreciable signal loss due to the shortened relaxation time during the SQUID ring-down period. The longer relaxation time provided by pure water would have seemed advantageous in this instance. Finally, the tuned pickup used by Seton adds the complexity of a frequency-dependent response function of the sensor and limits the effective bandwidth. Modern SQUID sensors are sufficiently sensitive and low-noise that they are most commonly coupled to untuned pickups that retain the inherent frequency independence and extraordinarily wide bandwidth (DC to many MHz) of the SQUID sensor.

Ultimately, the pioneering work reported by Seton in 1992 was very encouraging and informative. Even with the separation between the room-temperature sample and the superconducting pickup imposed by the cryostat, a SNR of at least 10 was reported. This encouraging SNR was observed after a significant period of signal loss due to the ring-down of the SQUID sensor.

Between 1995 and 1996 Kumar et al. reported measuring NMR signals for a wide variety of room-temperature samples with an untuned pickup coupled to a DC-SQUID sensors [77,78]. The goal of this work was to demonstrate the broadband sensitivity of DC-SQUIDs, which has significant spectroscopic implications and applications. While the paper did not address MR imaging, the broadband sensitivity of untuned SQUID sensors has major implications. The broadband sensitivity of a DC-SQUID can *simultaneously* detect NMR signatures from numerous nuclei while also allowing for NMR signal acquisition at a wide variety of magnetic fields. Kumar et al. reported measuring the NMR signature from ^{1}H, ^{19}F, ^{23}Na, and ^{31}P at fields from 7mT to 26mT with broadband DC-SQUID coupled pickups (untuned). One of the most important measurements, in our opinion, reported by Kumar was the *simultaneous* acquisition of ^{1}H and ^{19}F NMR signals from a mixture of water and hexafluorobenzene at ~7mT. While the Larmor frequencies of ^{1}H and ^{19}F differ by only ~6% ($\omega_L(^{1}H)$ = 301kHz and $\omega_L(^{19}F)$ = 283kHz), simultaneous acquisition with the same sensor is not possible with tuned pickups. These papers clearly demonstrated that the broadband performance of SQUID sensors coupled to untuned pickups provides many opportunities in spectroscopy. In addition, we note the additional implication that while application of strong gradient fields for imaging could shift ω_L outside the sensitivity band of tuned pickups, the entire frequency range induced by the gradient field from $(\omega_L - \Delta\omega)$ to $(\omega_L + \Delta\omega)$ is readily measured by DC-SQUIDs coupled to untuned pickups.

Kumar et al. appear to also have been the first group to measure the NMR signature from room-temperature samples of animal tissue with a SQUID sensor [77]. While it was an interesting first demonstration that implies the ability to ultimately perform MRI, it was accomplished by placing a small excised tissue sample into a narrow cryostat bore tube. We also note the work reported by Schlenga in which the NMR signal from a sample of mineral oil at room temperature was measured by a high-T_C (YBCO at 77K) SQUID magnetometer-based system in a field of about 2mT [79]. While the results of this work are an important indicator of the applicability of high-T_C devices to ULF NMR and MRI, our group has found current low-T_C technology is far more robust and more sensitive than the high-T_C counterparts. Consequently our research has utilized low-T_C devices almost exclusively.

1.4.4 ULF MRI with SQUID Sensors

In 1995, Seton reported using a SQUID preamplifier coupled to a tuned pickup coil to measure LF NMR signals and reconstruct an image [80]. The work was motivated by the fact that the SNR can be dominated by thermal noise from the sensor that is coupled into a low-noise amplifier. By placing both the pickup and preamplifier into liquid helium (at ~4.2K), the thermal noise can be reduced by nearly an order of magnitude. This implementation is simply a Faraday pickup coil in a tuned circuit that produces an output in accordance with Eqn. 1.17. At low fields and frequencies, it suffers from the loss of signal due to the reduced ω_L, as discussed previously. This approach is inherently different than sensing the signal with a pickup that is directly coupled to a SQUID for which the output signal amplitude does not depend on ω_L. The real importance of this work was the demonstration of the first 2D reconstruction of an MR image of a water phantom acquired with a SQUID-based sensor system at 10mT field ($\omega_L = 425$kHz).

Two years after Seton et al.'s initial low-field MRI work, they reported the first MR images of living human anatomy acquired with a low-temperature Faraday pickup coupled to a SQUID preamplifier [81,82]. The anatomical image was also acquired at 10mT field ($\omega_L = 425$kHz). A key purpose of these papers was to compare the effect of sensor noise on image quality. They compared images analyzed for NMR data acquired by both room-temperature and cryogenic pickup coils. It is immediately evident that the noise from the room-temperature pickup severely degraded the quality of the analyzed MR image in comparison to that acquired by the cryogenic pickup. Both the FOV and the spatial resolution were far worse in the image acquired with the room temperature pickup. This difference was clearly evident in the phantom images, and was even more pronounced in the anatomical images. A foundational contribution of these papers is to critically examine and compare the sensor and sample noise sources and their temperature dependence.

The image of the water phantom acquired by the cryogenic pickup in which 8mm-diameter tubes separated by 2mm were clearly resolved, indicates that the spatial resolution was on the order of 2mm (though not quantitatively analyzed by the authors). The water phantom images are almost certainly based only on proton density contrast, with no reason to believe relaxation contrast had any role. Seton et al. also presented the first anatomical image of a human wrist in which the radius and ulna bones are evident and there is some indication of the tendons as well. Based on the simple pulse sequence used and the extremely short T_2 for highly oriented tissue such as tendon [83], the anatomical images are likely the result of some combination of proton density contrast (differentiating the bone from forearm tissue) and T_2 contrast that will differentiate the tendons from the rest of the forearm tissue.

Again, we note a few practical aspects of Seton's work that are relevant to current design considerations. An important system design consideration is the orientation of all applied magnetic fields to the sensors. In these later papers, the system was designed such that the coils responsible for applying $\mathbf{B}_{RF}$ were oriented both normal to $\mathbf{B}_0$ *and* tangential to the pickup coil, thereby minimizing the coupling of $\mathbf{B}_{RF}$ to the SQUID. Given that the design of the magnet producing $\mathbf{B}_0$ was an electromagnet with 25cm pole pieces separated by 8cm to allow cryostat tail to be situated between the poles and close to the sample, it is surprising that the Barkhausen noise (a result of magnetic domain transitions in the iron), even at constant fields, is not a significant noise component in the sensors. Seton et al. also motivated the use of $CuSO_4$ solutions as a means to reduce imaging times by decreasing the repolarization (T_1) times but failed to analyze the commensurate reduced SNR with time during the imaging sequence.

The SQUID-based MRI performed through most of the 1990s operated almost exclusively in the 10mT regime and also used the approach developed for HF MRI in which a static polarization and measurement field is used and the sample polarization is tipped away from $\mathbf{B}_0$ by an applied $\mathbf{B}_{RF}$. The first important report of NMR signals measured by SQUID sensors at B_m in the ULF regime was presented by McDermott et al. [84]. This work was motivated by the importance of NMR spectroscopy, and while the chemical shift is dramatically reduced at ULF (chemical shift scales with applied field), scalar coupling ("*J*-coupling") is independent of field. Furthermore, because of the extremely narrow line widths (~1Hz, even for inhomogeneous fields) attainable at ULF, more spectroscopic information relating to the covalent bonds may be attainable at ULF than at HF. While this publication was spectroscopically focused, it became the seminal paper that initiated a resurgence of interest and publications in MRI (and NMR) at ULF, in opposition to the broad trend toward higher fields.

Dozens of papers reporting on investigations of LF and ULF NMR and MRI, typically measured with SQUID-based instrumentation (both low-T_C and high-T_C), appeared in 2004 alone, and the annual paper count has continued to grow. The investigations in 2004 were motivated by a wide variety of drivers. The tremendous cost, numerous safety issues, potential benefits inherent in ULF MRI, and basic scientific interest have driven the exploration and development of this new technology. Our own work was initially motivated by the need to combine anatomical MRI with our longstanding MEG measurements of human brain function. Because MEG [85] is purely a measure of neural activity in the brain, providing no anatomical information, it is necessary to superpose the spatial distribution of functional activity onto an anatomical map of the brain to correlate function with anatomy. The standard approach to accomplish the anatomical/functional superposition is to acquire the MEG with one instrument and the anatomical brain map with a standard clinical MRI. Common physical fiducials are mapped and located with both MEG and MRI systems and are used to co-register the two datasets. This approach, however, has substantial inherent error. While our team developed novel MEG systems with superb localization accuracy [86,87], it still required and was limited by superposing the functional image with anatomical images. This became one of the main drivers for our effort to develop ULF MRI so that the same SQUID sensor array could be used to acquire both the MEG signal and the anatomy via ULF MRI. Our team initially demonstrated acquisition of proton NMR and reconstruction of 1D and 2D MR images for phantoms and living animals at 2 to 25μT using a system that had also been used to acquire MEG in separate experiments [88]. Our first published demonstration that MEG and ULF NMR can be simultaneously acquired for reconstruction of functional and anatomical images using a common sensor array appeared in 2004 [89,90]. Our group also demonstrated that simultaneous acquisition of magnetocardiography (MCG) and magnetomyography (MMG) with NMR is also possible [91]. Our team also investigated the compelling application of using ULF MRI to *directly* measure MR consequences of neuronal signals (see also Section 1.6.1). An attempt to observe a relaxation effect in the simultaneous MMG/NMR and MCG/NMR acquisition that could be correlated with the biomagnetic fields was ultimately inconclusive in this early work.

All of our early ULF NMR and MRI work used a similar magnetic field protocol distinct from that used in earlier work. Samples were initially pre-polarized in $\mathbf{B}_p$ for a time greater than T_1 while the SQUID electronics were effectively turned off. The measurement field, $\mathbf{B}_m$, was continuously present and orthogonal to $\mathbf{B}_p$. Because $\mathbf{B}_m$ is orders of magnitude smaller than $\mathbf{B}_p$, the total field vector during application of $\mathbf{B}_p$ was effectively unaffected by $\mathbf{B}_m$. At time $t = 0$, $\mathbf{B}_p$ was non-adiabatically switched off in a very short time (~1ms). This prevented the polarization from following the total field as it transitions from $\mathbf{B}_p$ to $\mathbf{B}_m$ (as it would do if the field were ramped down adiabatically). After $\mathbf{B}_p$ was removed, the SQUID electronics were activated and the precession of $\mathbf{M}_0$ about $\mathbf{B}_m$ was measured. The SQUID sensor requires a period of time to recover ("dead time"), both as a result of the electronics turn-on transient and the decay of the cryostat magnetization. This dead time was typically less than 2ms, much smaller than T_1 or T_2 of all materials measured. Note that no $\mathbf{B}_{RF}$ is required to tip the spin population because the experimental apparatus applies $\mathbf{B}_p$ orthogonal to $\mathbf{B}_m$, and the non-adiabatic removal $\mathbf{B}_p$ retains the orientation of $\mathbf{M}_0$ along $\mathbf{B}_p$ so that $\mathbf{M}_0$ is naturally aligned orthogonal to and precesses about $\mathbf{B}_m$. In all of our early work, $\mathbf{B}_p$ was typically from a few to tens of mT and $\mathbf{B}_m$ was in the range of 1 to 100μT (equivalent to proton ω_L from 40Hz to 4kHz).

Following up on their seminal paper in *Science*, Clarke's group (McDermott et al. [92]) published an extensive study of ULF NMR and MRI over a broad range of B_m from ~1μT to ~2mT. The work demonstrated a number of powerful drivers for NMR and MRI at ULF, including (1) simultaneous multi-nuclear detection (^{31}P and ^{1}H in which $\omega_L\{^1H\} \approx 2\times\omega_L\{^{31}P\}$) enabled by the broadband nature of SQUID sensors; (2) dramatic narrowing of NMR line width (~3 orders of magnitude) and commensurate increase in SNR between 1.8mT and 1.8μT; and (3) both spin density and T_1-weighted ULF MRI. The MRI resolution claimed for this study was 1mm where the resolution along some dimension $\mathbf{r}$ is defined as in Eqn. 1.19, where $r = x$ and $\Delta\omega = 2\pi\Delta f$.

This definition of resolution does not take into consideration the SNR or the similar CNR, both of which have a significant impact on the realizable resolution, as noted previously. An additional practical note about the cryostat used by McDermott in this latest study is the exotic design of the thermal shield in the cryostat. A combination of alumina rods and aluminized polyester cloth was used to provide the thermal shield while dramatically reducing Johnson noise at the SQUID pickups [93]. In addition to the lower fields at which the NMR signal was measured (132μT for the MRI), the pulse sequence used by McDermott applied separate polarization and measurement fields. The spin population was polarized in B_p = 300mT for a time (typically $>T_1$), which was then adiabatically removed. The spin population reoriented with the much weaker B_m = 132μT during the adiabatic ramp-down of B_p, then required a $\pi/2$ pulse to provide the measurable precession signal. A 2D image was reconstructed by 48 1D projections in a gradient of 100 to 200μT/m for both a mineral oil phantom and a slice of a bell pepper. The contrast in these images results from regions of the phantom or pepper that contain a large proton (spin) density relative to those regions that have little or no proton density. Lastly, McDermott et al also demonstrated a T_1-contrast image in which geometrically spaced boluses of water with different T_1 (tuned by the addition of Gd-DOTA) were imaged and the NMR signal was shown to differentiate with time, as the signal from the boluses with short T_1 decayed more rapidly than those with longer T_1. Demonstrating the potential to develop relaxation-based contrast images at ULF is a critical component for virtually all biological MRI because neighboring tissues have very small proton density differences. Therefore, an MR image in which different tissue types can be distinguished must rely on other sources of contrast such as relaxation. The paper concluded with a brief mention that concomitant gradients at very small measurement fields can produce significant image distortions. The experimental parameters of measurement field and FOV were chosen to ensure that the distortions were smaller than the desired imaging resolution. In Chapter 3 we present methods for correcting some of the distortions that result from concomitant gradients that have been derived by our group and others.

We conclude our overview of the recent history of ULF MRI with a study by Burghoff et al. [95] where they pushed the frontiers of "ultra" in ULF NMR. They measured proton NMR from a water sample in an experiment that applied B_p = 250μT that was then non-adiabatically removed. The spin population immediately began to precess about B_m = 40nT–4μT. The experiments were conducted in one of the world's best (if not *the* best) magnetically shielded rooms (MSRs) in Berlin, Germany, that reduced the residual field to less than 10nT. The SQUID sensor was reported to have a dead time of approximately 0.3 ms, but the first 200 ms of data were discarded due to the magnetization decay from various sources after $\mathbf{B}_p$ was removed. The importance of this study was to demonstrate that ULF NMR could observe the natural line width for proton NMR of H_2O and was reported to be 0.17Hz for $\omega_L \approx$ 2Hz. This was possible only because the contribution of field inhomogeneities to the line width at these exceptionally low fields was deduced to be a few mHz at most. The impact of this work is to suggest that high-precision NMR spectroscopy and molecular structure determination can be performed at ULF by virtue of the J-coupling between dissimilar nuclei. Burghoff et al. demonstrated a complex ULF NMR spectrum for the heteronuclear molecule trifluoroethanol (CF_3-CH_2-OH) acquired at ~1μT. A homonuclear molecule would exhibit a single ^{1}H peak because chemical shift is virtually impossible to observe at such low fields since it scales with B_m. We will examine other recent studies and the evolution of techniques for ULF MRI in successive chapters of this book.

1.5 MRI EFFECTS

Both HF and ULF MRI utilize time-varying magnetic fields in the form of either AC fields (fields that vary at a regular frequency, typically according to a sinusoid) or pulsed fields (fields that are turned on or off along a prescribed time ramp). In HF MRI, these most prevalent time-varying fields are the so-called "RF fields" used to manipulate the spin population. Efficient coupling between the applied RF field and the spin population is only realized when the frequency of these RF fields is matched to the Larmor frequency of the spin population, which is commonly tens or even hundreds of MHz (hence, the "RF"). HF MRI also uses various pulsed fields; for example, the gradient fields are switched on and off according to the prescribed pulse sequence. In fact, the field switching in HF MRI systems is the source of the deafening noise that requires most subjects to use some form of hearing protection. The most prevalent time-varying field at ULF is the pulsed pre-polarization field (B_p), which is turned on and off according to a prescribed time ramp. ULF MRI may also use AC fields to manipulate the spin population, much as in HF MRI; however, the frequencies used are typically in or below the kHz regime. Unlike HF MRI, where RF fields are essential to tip the spin population away from the main polarization field, ULF MRI employs a multitude of pulse sequences, some of which require no AC to manipulate the spin population. The magnitude of the fields used at ULF are such that most field switching produces no audible sound in ULF MRI and only the non-adiabatic removal of B_p may be barely audible.

The interactions of time-varying (AC or pulsed) magnetic fields with matter depend on the strength, the rate (frequency) of the field variation, duration, and the electromagnetic properties of the material. The scaling of these interactions with field strength and frequency and whether AC fields are even used at all are at the heart of many differences between HF and ULF MRI. In this section we will briefly explore some of the differences caused by the interaction of dynamic magnetic fields with conducting materials that result in eddy currents, electric potentials, and heating. We discuss only the most basic relationships here to illustrate how these various effects differ between the HF and ULF field regimes. A far more thorough treatment can be found in the textbook by Smythe [95].

1.5.1 Induced Currents and Fields

Currents are induced in conducting materials in the presence of any time-varying magnetic field, dB/dt, that can be caused by transient magnetic fields or AC magnetic fields. Simply changing the position of a conducting material in a non-uniform field is essentially equivalent to inducing a transient magnetic field in the material. The induced currents depend on the magnitude of dB/dt, and material properties, including conductivity and magnetic permeability (properties for a few materials are shown in Table 1.2). The duration for which the material is exposed to a changing magnetic field will, for some characteristics, have a cumulative effect.

Smythe describes how the currents induced in a material themselves produce magnetic fields that oppose the local dB/dt (from the external source). The induced magnetic field has two consequences important to MRI: (1) it locally distorts the applied magnetic field distribution and (2) the induced magnetic fields serve to reduce the field that penetrates into the conductor. The induced magnetic field superposes with the applied field, causing significant distortions. These distortions are a key reason why HF MRI is typically never conducted in the presence of conducting materials. This limitation is far less severe for ULF MRI because AC fields are not always used and the low frequency dramatically reduces the effect. As we demonstrated in Figure 1.1, ULF MRI can readily be performed in the presence of conducting materials.

The second consequence of the magnetic fields induced in conductors is that they cancel, in part, the external field and the total magnetic field decreases with depth into the material. In a perfect conductor, the induced field produces a perfect mirror image of the applied field such that the two fields cancel at the surface of the perfect conductor and effectively no magnetic field penetrates the material. For materials with a finite conductivity,

TABLE 1.2 Various Material Conductivities

$B_0(^1H)$	2.35μT	0.24mT	24mT	2.4T
CONDUCTIVITY	0.1kHz	10kHz	1MHz	100MHz
Copper		5.80×10^{7}		
Aluminum		3.66×10^{7}		
Titanium		1.80×10^{6}		
Stainless (SS 316)		1.35×10^{6}		
CSF	2.00	2.00	2.00	2.114
Blood	0.70	0.70	0.822	1.233
Soft tissue		0.173		
Muscle		0.11		
Gray matter	8.90×10^{-2}	0.115	0.163	0.559
White matter	5.81×10^{-2}	6.95×10^{-2}	0.102	0.324
Fat		$4. \times 10^{-2}$		
Bone		5.4×10^{-3}		

For highly conductive materials, the frequency dependence is minimal and only one conductivity is given.

the magnetic field penetrates into the conductor. The penetration skin depth is a quantity that describes how far the field penetrates, or conversely how effectively conductors absorb electromagnetic signals. The penetration depth is approximately

(Eqn. 1.24)
$$\delta = 1/\sqrt{\pi\sigma\mu f}$$

where δ is the penetration or skin depth (m), f is the frequency of the electromagnetic signal (Hz), σ is the electrical conductivity of the absorber (S/m), and μ is the magnetic permeability of the absorber (H/m). Magnetic permeability is commonly expressed as "relative permeability" in which case $\mu = \mu_r \times \mu_0$, where μ_0 is the vacuum permeability equal to $4\pi \times 10^{-7}$H/m. For absorbers with low conductivity (high resistivity) like blood, CSF, and tissue, a somewhat more accurate expression for the skin depth is [96]

(Eqn. 1.25)
$$\delta = 1/\sqrt{\pi\sigma\mu f}\left[\left[1+\left(\frac{2\pi f\varepsilon}{\sigma}\right)^2\right]^{1/2} + \frac{2\pi f\varepsilon}{\sigma}\right]^{1/2}$$

where ε is the electrical permittivity (F/m). Electrical permittivity is commonly expressed as "relative permittivity" in which case $\varepsilon = \varepsilon_r \times \varepsilon_0$, where $\varepsilon_0 = 8.854 \times 10^{-12}$F/m. The fraction of the signal (or applied RF field) that penetrates a conductor with a given skin depth is calculated by

(Eqn. 1.26)
$$\frac{S}{S_0} = e^{-d/\delta}$$

where S/S_0 is the fraction of the initial signal penetrating a conductor of thickness d (m). Using this simple formalism, the penetration skin depth of a NMR signal with a spin precession frequency of 42.6MHz (proton Larmor frequency at 1T) is only about 10μm in aluminum [97]. Consequently, no measurable signal would penetrate even 1mm of aluminum shielding. However, at f = 4kHz, the proton Larmor frequency in the Earth's magnetic field has a skin depth of about 1.3mm. This is just one of the potential benefits of ULF MRI that will be discussed later.

We have calculated the skin depths for the materials listed in Table 1.2 using Eqn. 1.25 and listed them in Table 1.3 for a range of frequencies (0.1kHz, 10kHz, 1MHz, and 100MHz). This table is particularly useful to develop intuitive estimates of signal penetration and screening. For example, a human brain (~15cm of CSF, white matter, and gray matter) has virtually no effect on signals below 1MHz. At or about 100MHz (proton NMR at fields above ~2.5T), the white and gray matter does not significantly attenuate the NMR signal, but the CSF, which is typically a 2mm- to 4mm-thick layer surrounding the brain [98] (for which the 100MHz skin thickness is 3.9cm), will attenuate a 100MHz NMR signal originating in the brain by 40% to 64%. While this is not an intolerable attenuation, it is nonetheless significant and, of course, increases with field strength as the NMR frequency increases.

Let us examine the results reported by Stepišnik [68] to examine a practical implication of the skin depth in NMR and MRI. Recall that a 1cm-thick conducting (aluminum) box was used to reduce the RF noise at the pickup. We can calculate the skin depth using the conductivity ($\sigma = 3.77 \times 10^7$S/m) and magnetic permeability ($\mu = 1.26 \times 10^{-6}$H/m) for

TABLE 1.3 Skin Depth Values (δ, in m) for a Few Selected Materials as a Function of Frequency

$B_0(^1\text{H})$	2.35μT	0.24mT	24mT	2.4T
SKIN DEPTH (m)	0.1kHz	10kHz	1MHz	100MHz
Copper	6.61×10^{-3}	6.61×10^{-4}	6.600×10^{-5}	6.60×10^{-6}
Aluminum	8.32×10^{-3}	8.32×10^{-4}	8.300×10^{-5}	8.30×10^{-6}
Titanium	3.75×10^{-2}	3.75×10^{-3}	3.750×10^{-4}	3.70×10^{-5}
Stainless (SS 316)	4.30×10^{-2}	4.30×10^{-3}	4.300×10^{-4}	4.30×10^{-5}
CSF	3.56×10^{1}	3.55	3.560×10^{-1}	3.89×10^{-2}
Blood	6.01×10^{1}	6.03	6.150×10^{-1}	5.37×10^{-1}
Soft tissue		1.21×10^{1}		
Muscle		1.52×10^{1}		
Gray matter	1.90×10^{2}	1.57×10^{1}	1.440	9.7×10^{-2}
White matter	2.26×10^{2}	2.01×10^{1}	1.790	1.36×10^{-1}
Fat		2.52×10^{1}		
Bone		6.85×10^{1}		

typical aluminum to be about 1.8mm. The source was described to be water in the Earth's magnetic field with a proton Larmor frequency of about 2kHz. A 1cm-thick box would presumably present just over 5 skin thicknesses of conductor between the source and the sensor, reducing the signal, according to Eqn. 1.26, by about 99%. An RF signal from sources such as a low-frequency AM radio (88kHz) would have a skin thickness of about 0.27mm and would be reduced to an undetectable level ($S/S_0 \approx 10^{-16}$). Had the NMR signal resulted for protons in the Tesla regime, no signal would have been measured, as we noted above. Indeed, the fact that Stepišnik measured any signal at all is remarkable.

1.5.2 Induced Heating

Another effect of the currents induced by the time-varying magnetic fields is Ohmic or resistive heating (sometimes also called Joule heating) of the conductor. Any material with finite conductivity through which a current passes will experience heating. While a detailed derivation of the power deposited in a material is beyond the scope of this book, it is educational to examine the important scaling variables. An expression that captures the important scaling variables for P, the power deposited in a conductor as a result of eddy currents induced by a time-varying magnetic field [96], is

(Eqn. 1.27)
$$P \propto \sigma B_{\mathrm{RF}}^2 d^2 \omega^2 \Gamma_{\mathrm{abs}}$$

where B_{RF} is the peak RF (or AC) field, d is the absorber thickness ($d \ll \delta$ is assumed for this simple example), ω is the frequency of the AC field, σ is the conductivity, and Γ_{abs} is the absorber geometry factor. This simple relationship requires that $d \ll \delta$ because it assumes the flux density in the material is constant. If the thickness of the material were similar to or greater than the skin thickness, the flux density would decrease with depth and a more complex numeric integration would be required. The total energy deposited would be the integral of the power over the time the AC field is applied to the sample (or subject).

It should be evident that the power deposited for highly conducting materials is larger than for poorly conducting materials. Consequently, highly conducting materials (metals) in HF MRI systems not only distort the images but also present potential safety hazards because they will experience significant heating as a result of the RF fields. Weakly conducting materials such as biological tissue can also experience appreciable heating at the high fields and high frequencies of modern HF MRI instruments. While the temperature increase of any given tissue will depend on the electrical properties of the tissue, the geometry, and the properties of the RF field, it is also very sensitive to the perfusion of the tissue. The temperature increase for local tissue that is thoroughly perfused (e.g., kidneys, muscle tissue) will be significantly less than tissue that lacks significant blood flow, such as eyeballs [99], leading to concerns about hot spots and safety.

Using the simple scaling shown in Eqn. 1.27, it is easy to conclude that concerns about heating become virtually nonexistent at ULF. First, in many ULF MRI applications, no AC fields are used and the largest energy deposited in the subjects and material is from the switching of the B_p. Even though the instantaneous power may be relatively large (because both B and effective ω can be significant), the total energy deposited results from the power being integrated over milliseconds or less during which fields are being switched. In cases where AC fields are used to manipulate the spin population in ULF MRI, the frequencies are three to five orders of magnitude less than HF MRI; consequently, the power dissipated in the subject or conducting materials is more than six orders of magnitude (a million times) smaller than HF MRI.

1.5.3 Induced Neurostimulation

Finally, the currents induced in a weak conductor such as tissue will also produce time-varying localized voltages. These voltages can stimulate neurons and other cells to produce well-known sensations such as retinal flashes, muscle twitches, and sensory responses (from tingling to painful burning). In fact, human retinal response to time-varying magnetic fields has been known for over 100 years [100] and was commonly experienced by workers moving around large magnets such as those at particle accelerator facilities since the 1960s. The physiological effects of time- and spatially varying magnetic fields, particularly as they relate to MRI, have been extensively reviewed [101–104]. While a significant body of work exists in modeling neural stimulation resulting from time- and spatially varying magnetic fields, primarily as a therapeutic technique (e.g., transcranial magnetic stimulation), the effects in MRI are typically undesired. The degree and extent of the neural stimulation depends on a complex combination of factors including the field strength (B), the rate of change of the field (dB/dt or ω), the shape and direction of the field, and the electrical properties of the affected tissue. Another poorly understood variable is the individual-to-individual variation in cellular and perceptive sensitivity to the fields. The U.S. Food and Drug Administration (FDA) has determined that time-varying magnetic fields (dB/dt) sufficient to cause discomfort or pain pose a significant risk and has proposed standards for exposure to such fields [105]. Current practice, however, relies on manufacturers to suggest standards based on empirically determined thresholds on large subject populations.

Unlike heating, neural stimulation is a fast (non-integral) effect that is largely determined by dB/dt. Both HR MRI and ULF MRI have the potential to induce sufficient dB/dt in subjects to produce a perceptible neural stimulation. In HF MRI the most common mechanism that leads to perceptible neural stimulation is moving the subject too quickly in and out of the fringe field of the magnet, where the movement of the subject through a strong inhomogeneous field produces a large dB/dt in tissue [106]. Fast cycling of other fields used in HF MRI imaging sequences may also result in perceptible neural stimulation [107]. Some applications of ULF MRI use large polarization fields that may be rapidly (non-adiabatically) turned off or ramped down. This rapid ramp of B_p may produce sufficiently large dB/dt to induce perceptible neural stimulation. Procedures must be employed in both HF MRI and ULF MRI to avoid exposing subjects to discomfort brought on by excessively large dB/dt [108,109].

1.6 NEW REGIMES OF PHYSICS ACCESSIBLE AT ULF

Performing NMR and MRI at extremely low fields opens new regimes of physics at low frequencies to be explored. These include electrical impedance tomography using AC fields that can be selectively interrogated by ULF MRI by tuning the spin Larmor frequency to be in resonance with the applied AC electrical field. Additionally, there are regimes in which the frequencies of physical phenomena can overlap the resonant frequency of the spin population at ULF such as DNI, T_1 dispersion at very low frequencies, and narrow line widths (J-coupling). We have selected just a few of the wide array of such possible phenomena and applications to discuss here and in more detail in Chapters 4 and 5; the number of current areas of exploration for ULF MRI, not to mention potential opportunities, far exceeds the scope of this book.

1.6.1 Direct Imaging of Neural Activity at ULF

One of the most exciting prospects is the possibility of *directly* measuring neural activity with a tomographic imaging technique. Arguably, the most common modalities to measure human brain function are fMRI, EEG, and MEG. While EEG and MEG provide extraordinarily high temporal resolution measurements of the direct consequences of neural activity in the brain, they are widely considered to provide poor spatial resolution because the ill-posed inverse problem of electromagnetism does not yield a unique solution to the source of the neural activity [110]. Conversely, while fMRI at high fields can provide exquisite (sub-millimeter) spatial resolution, it is based on hemodynamic changes that are *indirect* measures of the neural activity (e.g., changes in blood oxygenation, blood flow, or blood volume) that provide relatively poor temporal resolution (on the order of a second). ULF MRI provides the prospect of a multimodal imaging approach based on the same sensor array that can (1) measure the anatomy (ULF MRI), (2) directly *image* neural activity through direct neural imaging (DNI) at ULF, and (3) provide the temporal interpolation of the neural activity with MEG from the same SQUID sensors used to measure the ULF MRI and ULF DNI.

The prospect of directly measuring neural activity with ULF MRI is based on the concept that electromagnetic phenomena with significant power in the spectral range of the ω_L may induce significant changes in the spin population. We hypothesized that neural activity in the human brain could provide sufficient electromagnetic energy in a given frequency band to produce a measurable effect on an appropriately prepared spin population [111]. Furthermore, this effect could be localized to regions of the brain where the greatest activity existed using standard ULF MRI methodologies.

Typical B_m for our ULF NMR and MRI work is in the range of 1 to 100μT, with corresponding proton $\omega_L = 40 \sim 4{,}000$Hz. We can readily choose the proton ω_L at which we wish to measure the NMR spectra by adjusting the B_m and because SQUID sensors are broadband sensors with equal sensitivity across the entire operating range (DC to ~MHz). We also note that the power spectra for neural activity extends from a few Hz to a few kHz range [112]. For example, multiple-unit activity, representing spiking of large pyramidal cells and some inhibitory activity, occurs in the frequency range of 400 to 3,000Hz. Local field potentials, which reflect mostly cooperative activity in neural populations, are generally thought to extend from 10 to 90Hz [113]. The exact shape of any given neural activity spectrum will depend strongly on the stimulus causing the cortical activation. Recognizing the overlap between proton Larmor frequency at ULF and the neural activity spectrum leads us to hypothesize that interactions between the spin population and neural activity in cortex can be dominated by resonant mechanisms that are unique to ULF. Demonstrating this mechanism would provide the foundation for an exciting new functional neuroimaging modality: ULF DNI. Moreover, it may be possible, by scanning the Larmor frequency, to target different kinds of neural activity based on frequency. This concept and recent experimental results are discussed in greater detail in Chapter 5.

In addition to providing a unique noninvasive method of directly imaging neural activity, ULF DNI can open the door to understanding the heretofore poorly understood correlation between cellular-level neural activity and noninvasive measures of brain function such as MEG and EEG. The magnetic fields responsible for our resonant DNI approach result from axonal and dendritic currents in proximity to the proton spins. MEG, on the other hand, primarily measures the fields produced by relatively large populations of dendritic currents with a high degree of temporal synchrony. The correlation between the local cellular level fields and those measured centimeters outside the head could be studied by simultaneously measuring ULF DNI and MEG.

1.7 SUMMARY OF MRI AT ULF

The greatest challenge of MRI at ULF is obtaining sufficient signal at high SNR and CNR to produce a useful image. Choosing to perform MRI at ULF as opposed to HF will always require careful consideration of the tradeoffs. Once it has been determined that sufficient signal and CNR can be obtained for ULF MRI to be efficacious in a given application, there are many unique benefits and variables that can be used at ULF. This section will briefly present a sampling of these benefits and later chapters will discuss methods to realize these benefits in various applications. There are certainly many situations in which the signal is insufficient and any enhanced contrast at ULF cannot make up for the lost signal.

The magnetic fields used in ULF applications, even the relatively large polarization field, are orders of magnitude smaller than HF MRI. Consequently, all of the fields and gradients used at ULF are readily manipulated in time and space. HF fields are produced by massive coils and, in the case of most HF B_0 fields, are produced by persistent current superconducting coils that cannot be easily turned off (recall the stored energy of several sticks of dynamite that must be deposited somewhere). Some MRI systems in the 0.1 to 1.0T regime use permanent magnets that simply cannot be turned off at all. Our group and others have built and operated magnetic field coils for ULF MRI that not only can be turned on and off (as in the case of pulsed pre-polarization coils) but also can be dynamically varied in time (to allow spin population evolution at one field and measurement at another) and can also readily change the orientation of the applied field by applying currents to coils in a desired ratio that can literally rotate or even spin the field.

Another unique benefit of ULF MRI is the ability to measure MRI signals in the presence of and even through metal. There are two relevant effects: first, the large skin depth at ULF allows the NMR signal to penetrate large quantities of conductor. The corollary to this is the fact that because the low-frequency signals penetrate significant conductor thickness, very little signal is absorbed per unit thickness of conductor. This fact, combined with the low frequency, results in very small energy deposition in conducting materials and minimal if any heating by the applied fields. ULF NMR allows spin manipulation without the application of any AC fields, and even when AC fields are used, they are of low amplitude and low frequency that induce very little heating. Finally, the currents induced in conductors by applied fields in HF MRI are large and result in induced magnetic fields that severely distort the image and affect the spin population in the vicinity of the metal. At ULF, any applied AC fields are extremely small, the low-frequency nature of the fields further reduces the induced currents, and the resulting induced magnetic fields cause only minor image distortions that can be corrected in post processing.

Chemical shift is a powerful tool in HF NMR spectroscopic MRI for determining or selecting specific chemical structures. It has been widely concluded that chemical shift cannot be observed at ULF. For the protons of hydrogenous liquids, for instance, the chemical displacements are distributed over a frequency band that is at most about 15ppm and more typically 10ppm or less. In the Earth's field (50μT) this represents about 5×10^{-10}T, which, in fact, corresponds to the finest lines observed to date. Consequently, we conclude that while measuring chemical shift at ULF is not impossible, it would be extraordinarily difficult.

1.8 SUMMARY OF HF AND ULF MRI COMPARISONS

We have enumerated many of the benefits of ULF MRI in comparison to traditional HF approaches:

- The very low homogeneity requirements for B_p (image quality does not depend on B_p) greatly simplify coil design and shimming.
- The absolute homogeneity requirement for B_m of ~0.1% simplifies the design of measurement field coils.
- The tremendous flexibility in temporal and spatial application of B_p and B_m is afforded by simple coil designs.
- The reduced peak width reduces required gradients to obtain similar spatial resolution, increases SNR, and can provide molecular structure information (*J*-coupling or even possibly chemical shift).
- Smaller fields are safer, can be turned off, can be used for intraoperative MRI, use less power, and are less expensive.
- Switching of fields and gradients at HF result in deafening noise while most field switching produces no audible sound in ULF MRI with the possible exception of the non-adiabatic removal of B_p which may be audible.
- Readily manipulated fields open the door for pulse sequences that can elicit field-dependent contrast [114], the equivalent of sample spinning (relative to the field), directional fields and gradients, etc.
- SQUID sensors do not lose sensitivity with decreasing field and frequency.
- SQUID sensor arrays can be used for array acquisition of MRI to increase speed and/or resolution.
- SQUID sensors can be used to acquire interleaved MRI and MEG with the same instrument at the same time.
- SQUID sensors are broadband and consequently can be used to measure and image NMR signals from multiple nuclei in the same experiment.

- Lower-cost and lighter systems do not require specialized facilities.
- These innovations may allow bringing the MRI scanner to the subject, not the subject to the scanner, with important resulting applications in the trauma department and the intensive care unit, and in battlefield medicine to diagnose traumatic brain injury earlier.
- Generally greater contrast is available for some materials and tissue types.
- New methodologies can be used for measurements such as electrical impedance tomography.
- Susceptibility artifact caused by the coupling of the applied magnetic field and different materials in the sample can be dramatically reduced. These artifacts broaden resonance lines due to the local inhomogeneities produced.
- *J*-coupling may provide a powerful tool for molecular structure determination because of the sharp line widths attainable at ULF.
- The extraordinarily sharp line widths attainable at ULF provide for enhanced SNR because of the narrow frequency bands in which the signal resides and over which the noise is integrated.
- AC fields (RF at high fields) are not necessary but may be used (additional versatility).
- The much lower frequency of AC fields induce no neural stimulation due to the much smaller dB/dt used to drive currents in tissue.
- The effect of conductors is significantly reduced in terms of image distortion, signal absorption, and heating.
- New physics will be attainable due to resonant interactions at a tremendous range of frequencies, from near DC to 1MHz. These include the prospect for direct neural current imaging.
- There is the potential to image subjects with medical implants.
- There is the potential to use ULF MRI intraoperatively.

While ULF MRI has many benefits, there is one overarching consideration that will determine the efficacy of the approach, and there are a few limitations. The proverbial "showstopper" for ULF MRI is signal. If insufficient NMR signal is available to reconstruct a useful image, then none of the benefits outlined above can overcome this basic drawback and attain a usable image. However, as we have shown in this chapter and will detail in later chapters, there are many approaches to increase signal and SNR at ULF. Finally, it is important to recognize that there are a few distinct limitations at ULF as compared to HF imaging. These include:

- The dramatically reduced susceptibility artifact at ULF nearly eliminates the BOLD effect upon which fMRI is based.
- The dramatically reduced chemical shift has a negative impact on molecular structure determination.

In conclusion, we believe that a wealth of benefits drive the investigation of ULF MRI and enhance prospects of use for various applications.

REFERENCES

1. Lauterbur PC (1973). Image formation by induced local interactions: Examples of employing nuclear magnetic resonance. *Nature 242*: 190–191.
2. Bandettini PA (2009). What's new in neuroimaging methods? *Annals of the New York Academy of Sciences*, pp. 260–293.

3. Kleinman A (1995). *Writing at the Margin: Discourse Between Anthropology and Medicine*. University of California Press.
4. Chhem RK, Brothwell DR (2008). *Paleoradiology: Imaging Mummies and Fossils*. Springer-Verlag.
5. Falk D, Gibson KR (2001). *Evolutionary Anatomy of the Primate Cerebral Cortex*. Cambridge University Press.
6. Hopkins WD, Rilling JK (2000). A domparative MRI study of the relationship between neuroanatomical asymmetry and interhemispheric connectivity in primates: Implication for the evolution of functional asymmetries. *Behav Neurosci 114*(4): 739–748.
7. Hennessy MJ (2005). Industrial applications of magnetic resonance. *Materials Processing in Magnetic Fields*, pp. 347–351.
8. Leisen J, Märtin M, Schipotinin T, et al. (2005). A synergistic approach by MRI and CFD for the study of micro-flow in textiles. Presented at ISC'2005: 3RD Industrial Simulation Conf. 2005.
9. Hills B (1995). Food processing—an MRI perspective. *Trends in Food Science & Technology* 6(4): 111–117.
10. Li Y, Szlachetka K, Lin X et al. (2009). Application of NMR & MRI in food process, quality control and shelf stability improvement. Presented at 5th Intl Technical Symposium on Food Processing, Monitoring Technology in Bioprocesses and Food Quality Management, pp. 1086–1089.
11. Veliyulin E, Aursand IG, Erikson U (2005). Study of fat and water in Atlantic salmon muscle (Salmo salar) by low-held NMR and MRI. In *Magnetic Resonance In Food Science: The Multivariate Challenge*, pp. 148–155.
12. See, for example, Buxton RB (2002). *Introduction to Functional Magnetic Resonance Imaging* (Cambridge University Press) and Moonen CTW, Bandettini PA (Eds.) (2000). *Functional MRI* (Springer-Verlag).
13. Hashemi RH, Bradley WG, Lisanti CJ (2010). *MRI: The Basics*. Lippincott Williams & Wilkins.
14. Hendee WR, Morgan CJ (1984). Magnetic resonance imaging part I—physical principles. *West J Med* (4): 491–500.
15. Hayashi N, Watanabe YW, Masumoto T, et al. (2004). Utilization of low-field MR scanners. *Magn Resn Med Sci* 3: 27–38.
16. Blanco RT, Ojala R, Kariniemi J, et al. (2005). Interventional and intraoperative MRI at low field scanner—a review. *Eur J Radiol* 56: 130–142.
17. De Salles AAF, Frighetto L, Behnke E, et al. (2004). Functional neurosurgery in the MRI environment. *Minim Invasive Neurosurg* 47: 284–289.
18. Tseng CH, Wong GP, Pomeroy VR, et al. (1998). Low-field MRI of laser polarized noble gas. *Phys Rev Lett 81*: 3785–3787.
19. Matlachov AN, Volegov PL, Espy MA, et al. (2004) SQUID detected NMR in microtesla magnetic fields. *J Magn Reson 170*: 1–7.
20. Mair RW, Hrovat MI, Patz S, et al. (2005). He-3 lung imaging in an open access, very-low field human magnetic resonance imaging system. *Magn Reson Med* 53: 745.
21. Mößle M, Myers WR, Lee S-K, et al. (2005). SQUID-detected in vivo MRI at microtesla magnetic fields. *IEEE T Appl Supercon* 15: 757.
22. Venook RD, Matter NI, Ramachandran M, et al. (2006). Prepolarized magnetic resonance imaging around metal orthopedic implants. *Magn Reson Med* 56: 177.
23. Planinsic G, Stepišnik J, Kos M (1994). Relaxation-time measurement and imaging in the Earth's magnetic field. *J Magn Resn A110*: 170–174.
24. Clarke J, Hatridge M, Mößle M (2007). SQUID-detected magnetic resonance imaging in microtesla fields. *Ann Rev Biomed Eng* 9: 389–413.
25. Lee S-K, Mößle M, Myers W, et al. (2005). SQUID-detected MRI at 132μT with T_1-weighted contrast established at 10 μT–300 μT. *Magn Reson Med* 53: 9.
26. Kraus RH Jr, Volegov P, Matlachov A, Espy M (2008). Toward direct neural current imaging by resonant mechanisms at ultra-low field. *Neuroimage* 39: 310–317.
27. Zotev VS, Matlachov AN, Volegov PL, et al. (2007). Multi-channel SQUID system for MEG and ultra-low-field MRI. *IEEE Trans Appl Supercond 17*: 839–842.

28. Albert MS, Cates GD, Driehuys B, et al. (1994). Biological magnetic resonance imaging using hyperpolarized. *Nature 370*: 199–201.
29. Albert MS, Balamore D (1997). Development of hyperpolarized noble gas MRI. *Nucl Instr and Meth*, pp. 441–453.
30. Cherubini A, Bifone A (2003). Hyperpolarized xenon in biology. *Prog Nucl Magn Reson Spectr 42*: 1–30.
31. Abragam A (1983). *Principles of Nuclear Magnetism*. Oxford University Press.
32. Hahn EL (1949). An accurate nuclear magnetic resonance method for measuring spin-lattice relaxation times. *Phys Rev 76*: 145–146.
33. Hahn EL (1950). Nuclear induction due to free Larmor precession. *Phys Rev 77*: 297–298.
34. Hahn EL (1950). Spin echos. *Phys Rev 80*: 580–594.
35. Jaklevic JC, Lambe J, Silver AH, Mercereau JE (1964). Quantum interference from a static vector potential in a field-free region, *Phys Rev Lett 12*: 159.
36. Zimmerman JE, Thiene P, Harding JT (1970). Design and operation of stable rf biased superconducting point-contact quantum devices, *J Appl Phys 41*: 1572.
37. Clarke J (1986). SQUIDs, brains and gravity waves. *Phys Today 86*: 36–44.
38. Pruessmann KP, Weiger M, Scheidegger MB, Boesiger P (1999). SENSE: sensitivity encoding for fast MRI. *Magn Reson Med 42*: 952–962.
39. Zotev VS, Matlashov AN, Volegov PL, et al. (2008). Microtesla MRI of the human brain combined with MEG. *J Magn Resn 194*: 115–120.
40. Haacke EM, Brown RW, Thompson MR, Venkatesan R (1999). *Magnetic Resonance Imaging: Physical Principles and Sequence Design*. Wiley.
41. Volegov PL, Mosher JC, Espy MA, Kraus RH Jr (2005). On concomitant gradients in low-field MRI. *J Magn Resn 175*: 103–113.
42. Yablonskiy DA, Sukstanskii AL, Ackerman JJH (2005). Image artifacts in very low magnetic field MRI: The role of concomitant gradients. *J Magn Reson 174*: 279–286.
43. Myers WR, Mößle M, Clarke J (2005). Correction of concomitant gradient artifacts in experimental microtesla MRI. *J Magn Reson 177*: 174–184.
44. Lin F-H, Wald LL, Ahlfors SP, et al. (2006). Dynamic magnetic resonance inverse imaging of human brain function. *Magn Reson Med 56*: 787–802.
45. Sodickson DK, Manning WJ (1997). Simultaneous acquisition of spatial harmonics (SMASH): fast imaging with radiofrequency coil arrays. *Magn Reson Med 38*: 591–603.
46. Pruessmann KP, Weiger M, Scheidegger MB, Boesiger P (1999). SENSE: sensitivity encoding for fast MRI. *Magn Reson Med 42*: 952–962.
47. Zotev VS, Volegov PL, Matlashov AN, et al. (2008). Parallel MRI at microtesla fields. *J Magn Resn 192*: 197–208.
48. Hill HDW, Richards RE (1968). Limits of measurement in magnetic resonance. *J Phys E Ser 2* 1: 977.
49. Hoult DI, Richards RE (1976). The signal-to-noise ratio of the nuclear magnetic resonance experiment. *J Magn Resn 24*: 71–85.
50. Otazo R, Mueller B, Ugurbil K, et al. (2006). Signal-to-noise ratio and spectral linewidth improvements between 1.5 and 7 Tesla in proton echo-planar spectroscopic imaging. *Magn Resn Med 56*: 1200–1210.
51. Darrasse L, Ginefri J-C (2003). Perspectives with cryogenic RF probes in biomedical MRI. *Biochimie 85*: 915–937.
52. Ohliger MA, Grant AK, Sodickson DK (2003). Ultimate intrinsic signal-to-noise ratio for parallel MRI: Electromagnetic field considerations. *Magn Resn Med 50*: 1018–1030.
53. Rojas R, Rodriguez AO (2009). A simple numerical method to compute the signal-to-noise ratio of a magnetic resonance imaging surface coil. *Prog Electromag Res M 7*: 109–122.
54. Myers W, Slichter D, Hatridge M, et al. (2007). Calculated signal-to-noise ratio of MRI detected with SQUIDs and Faraday detectors in fields from 10 T to 1.5 T. *J Magn Resn 186*: 182–192.
55. Hendrick RE (1987). Sampling time effects on signal-to-noise and contrast-to-noise ratios in spin-echo MRI. *Magn Reson Imag 5*: 31–37.
56. Hendrick RE, Kneeland JB, Stark DD (1987). Maximizing signal-to-noise and contrast-to-noise in FLASH imaging. *Magn Resn Imag 5*: 117–127.

57. Hendrick RE, Raff U (1992). *Magnetic Resonance Imaging* (2nd ed.). Mosby, pp. 109–144.
58. Hendrick RE (1987). Sampling time effects on signal-to-noise and contrast-to-noise ratios in spin-echo MRI. *Magn Resn Imag 5*: 31–37.
59. Hendrick RE, Kneeland JB, Stark DD (1987). Maximizing signal-to-noise and contrast-to-noise in FLASH imaging. *Mag. Resn Imag 5*: 117–127.
60. Packard M, Varian R (1954). Free nuclear induction in the Earth's magnetic field. *Phys Rev 93*: 941.
61. Bloom A, Mansir D (1954). Measurement of nuclear induction relaxation times in weak magnetic fields. *Phys Rev 93*: 941.
62. Bloom AL (1956). Field-dependent proton relaxation times in solutions of Mn$^{\backslash+\backslash+}$. *J Chem Phys 25*: 793.
63. Waters GS (1955). A measurement of the earth's magnetic field by nuclear induction. *Nature 176*: 691
64. Bene GJ (1980). Nuclear magnetism of liquid systems in the Earth field range. *Phys Reports 58*: 213–267.
65. Lauterbur P (1973). Image formation by induced local interactions: Examples employing nuclear magnetic resonance. *Nature 242*: 191–192.
66. Damadian R (1971). Tumor detection by NMR. *Science 171*: 1151–1153.
67. Mansfield P (1977). Multi-planar image formation using NMR spin-echos. *J Phys C Solid State Physics 10*: L55–L58.
68. Stepišnik J, Eřzen V, Kos M (1990). NMR imaging in the Earth's magnetic field. *Magn Reson Med 15*: 386–391.
69. Macovski A, Conolly S (1993). Novel approaches to low-cost MRI. *Magn Reson Med 30*: 221–230.
70. Clarke J (1986). SQUIDs, brains and gravity waves. *Physics Today 39*: 36–44.
71. Greenberg Ya S (1998). Application of superconducting quantum interference devices to nuclear magnetic resonance. *Rev Mod Physics 70*: 175–222.
72. Seton HC, Bussell DM, Hutchison JMS, et al. (1992). DC SQUID-based NMR detection from room temperature samples. *Phys Med Biol 37*: 2133–2138.
73. Hilbert C, Clarke J (1985). Nuclear quadrupole resonance detected at 30 MHz with a DC-SQUID. *Appl Phys Lett 47*: 637–639.
74. Freeman MR, Germain RS, Richardson RC (1986). Low temperature nuclear magnetic resonance with a DC-SQUID amplifier. *Appl Phys Lett 48*: 300–302.
75. Clarke J (1989). SQUID concepts and systems. In Weinstock H, Nisenoff M (Eds.) *Superconducting Electronics.* Springer-Verlag, pp. 87–148.
76. Seton HC, Hutchison JMS, Bussell DM (1999). Gradiometer pick-up coil design for a low field SQUID-MRI system. *Magn Resn Mater in Phys Biol Medicine 8*: 116–120.
77. Kumar S, Thorson BD, Avrin WF (1995). Broadband SQUID NMR with room-temperature samples. *J Magn Reson B 107*: 252–259.
78. Kumar S, Avrin WF, Whitecotton BR (1996). NMR of room temperature samples with a flux-locked DC SQUID. *IEEE Trans Magn 32*: 5261–5264.
79. Schlenga K, McDermott R, Clarke J, et al. (1999). Low-field magnetic resonance imaging with a high-Tc DC superconducting quantum interference device. *Appl Phys Lett 75*: 3695–3698.
80. Seton HC, Bussell DM, Hutchison JMS, Lurie DJ (1995). Use of a DC SQUID receiver preamplifier in a low field MRI system. *IEEE Trans Appl Superconductivity 5*: 3218–3221.
81. Seton HC, Hutchison JMS, Bussell DM (1997). A tuned SQUID amplifier for MRI based on a DOIT flux locked loop. *IEEE Trans Appl Superconductivity 7*: 3213–3216.
82. Seton HC, Hutchison JMS, Bussell DM (1997). A 4.2K receiver coil and SQUID amplifier used to improve SNR of low-field magnetic resonance images of the human arm. *Meas Sci Technol 8*: 198–207.
83. Gold GE, Wren TAL, Nayak K, et al. (2001). In vivo short echo time imaging of Achilles tendon. *Proc Intl Soc Mag Reson Med 9*: 244.
84. McDermott R, Trabesinger AH, Muck M, et al. (2002). Liquid-state NMR and scalar couplings in microtesla magnetic fields. *Science 295*: 2247–2249.
85. Hämäläinen M, Hari R, Ilmoniemi RJ, et al. (1993). Magnetoencephalograph—theory, instrumentation, and applications to noninvasive studies of the working human brain. *Rev Mod Phys 65*: 413–497.

86. Kraus RH Jr, Volegov P, Maharajh K, et al. (2002) Performance of a novel SQUID-based superconducting imaging-surface magnetoencephalography system. *Physica C 368*: 18–23.
87. Volegov P, Matlachov AN, Mosher J, et al. (2004). Noise-free magnetoencephalography (MEG) recordings of brain function. *Phys Med Biol 49*: 2117–2128.
88. Matlachov AN, Volegov PL, Espy MA, et al. (2004). SQUID detected NMR in microtesla magnetic fields. *J Magn Resn 170*: 1–7.
89. Espy MA, Volegov PL, Matlachov AN, et al. (2004). Simultaneously detected biomagnetic signals and NMR. *Neurol Clin Neurophysiol 30*: 12.
90. Volegov P, Matlachov AN, Espy MA, et al. (2004). Simultaneous magnetoencephalography and SQUID detected nuclear magnetic resonance in microtesla magnetic fields. *Magn Res Med 52*: 467–470.
91. Espy MA, Matlachov AN, Volegov PL, et al. (2005). SQUID-based simultaneous detection of NMR and biomagnetic signals at ultra-low magnetic fields. *IEEE Trans Superconductivity 15*: 635–639.
92. McDermott R, Kelso N, Lee S-K, et al. (2004). SQUID-detected magnetic resonance imaging in microtesla magnetic fields. *J Low Temp Phys 135*: 793–821.
93. Seton HC, Bussell DM, Hutchison JMS (1997). Liquified gas cryostat. UK Patents GB2331798 (Aug 1997) and GB2351549 (Aug 1997).
94. Burghoff M, Hartwig S, Trahms L, Bernarding J (2005). Nuclear magnetic resonance in the nanoTesla range. *Appl Phys Lett 87*: 054103.
95. Smythe WR (1989). Eddy currents. In: *Static and Dynamic Electricity*, 3rd ed. Hemisphere Pub. Co.
96. Vander Vorst A, Rosen A, Kotsuka Y (2006). *RF/Microwave Interaction with Biological Tissues.* Wiley-IEEE Press.
97. Matlachov AM, Volegov PL, Espy MA, et al. (2004). SQUID detected NMR in microtesla magnetic fields. *J Magn Reson 170*: 1–7.
98. Custo A, Wells WM III, Barnett AH, et al. (2006). Effective scattering coefficient of the cerebral spinal fluid in adult head models for diffuse optical imaging. *Appl Optics 45*: 4747–4755.
99. Shellock FG, Crues JV (1988). Corneal temperature changes associated with high-field MR imaging using a head coil. *Radiology 167*: 809–811.
100. Thompson SP (1910). A physiological effect of an alternating magnetic field. *Proc R Soc Biol 82*: 396–398.
101. Budinger TF, et al. (1991). Physiological effects of fast oscillating magnetic field gradients. *J Computer Assist Tomog 15*: 609–614.
102. Bourland JD, Nyenhuis JA, Schaefer DJ (1999). Physiologic effects of intense MRI gradient fields. *Neuroimaging Clin North Am 9*: 363–377.
103. Schaefer DJ, Bourland JD, Nyenhuis JA (2000). Review of patient safety in time-varying gradient fields. *J Magn Reson Imag 12*: 20–29.
104. Bencsik M, Bowtell R, Bowley R (2007). Electric fields induced in the human body by time-varying magnetic field gradients in MRI: numerical calculations and correlation analysis. *Phys Med Biol 52*: 2337–2353.
105. U.S. Food and Drug Administration, Center for Devices and Radiological Health, "Guidance for Industry and FDA Staff. Criteria for Significant Risk Investigations of Magnetic Resonance Diagnostic Devices," Issue date: July 14, 2003, (available at www.fda.gov).
106. Hartwig V, Giovannetti G, Vanello N, et al. (2009). Biological effects and safety in magnetic resonance imaging: a review. *Intl J Environ Res Public Health 6*: 1778–1798.
107. de Vocht F, Liket L, De Vocht A, et al. (2007). Exposure to alternating electromagnetic fields and effects on the visual and visuomotor systems. *Br J Radiol 80*: 822–828.
108. International Commission on Non-Ionizing Radiation Protection (ICNIRP) Statement, "Medical magnetic resonance procedures: protection of patients." *Health Physics 87*: 197–216.
109. Shellock FG, Crues JV (2004). MR procedures: biologic effects, safety, and patient care. *Radiology 232*: 635–652.
110. Hämäläinen M, Hari R, Ilmoniemi RJ, et al. (1993). Magnetoencephalogray, theory, instrumentation, and applications to noninvasive studies of the working human brain. *Rev Mod Phys 65*: 413–497.

111. Kraus RH Jr, Volegov P, Matlachov A, Espy M (2007). Toward direct neural current imaging by resonant mechanisms at ultra-low field. *Neuroimage 39*: 310–317.
112. Henrie JA, Shapley R (2005). LFP power spectra in V1 cortex: the graded effect of stimulus contrast. *J Neurophysiol 94*: 479–490.
113. Logothetis NK, Pfeuffer J (2004). On the nature of the BOLD fMRI contrast mechanism. *MRI 22*: 1517–1531.
114. Ramadan UA, Markkola AT, Halavaara J, et al. (1998). On- and off resonance spin-lock MT imaging of normal human brain at 0.1 T: possibilities to modify image contrast. *Magn Reson Imag 16*: 1191–1199.
115. Emsley J (1991). *The Elements*, 2nd ed. Oxford University Press.
116. Glover TJ (Comp.) (2003). *Pocket Ref*, 3rd ed., p. 324 (LCCN 2002-91021).

CHAPTER 2

NUTS AND BOLTS OF ULF MRI

2.1 INTRODUCTION

The primary focus of this chapter is to discuss hardware used for ULF MRI. We will discuss both the benefits of working at ultra-low fields and the limitations imposed by practical hardware. While most of our discussion is broadly applicable to ULF MRI, the reader should be aware that our primary driver for developing the hardware has been the goal of imaging the human brain and performing relaxometry used in differentiating materials. While most overviews of new technologies will place the hardware discussion near or at the end of the work (if at all), we have chosen to place the hardware discussion near the beginning because of the importance hardware plays in the practical implementation of ULF MRI. Chapter 1 presented many aspects of ULF MRI that simplify the practical realization of the technique over HF approaches and also alluded to the limitations imposed by hardware. We will endeavor to present the lessons we have learned thus far and discuss possible improvements we are considering. This should provide the reader with many avenues to explore for improving the current state-of-the-art of ULF MRI.

We begin the chapter by discussing the issues and methods surrounding magnetic field and gradient generation. Then, we move on to describe how the NMR signal is acquired, primarily by pickups coupled to SQUID sensors, but also briefly acknowledging a few other sensing techniques that have shown promise, either in our own group or elsewhere. Finally, we present a brief discussion of magnetic shielding. While HF MRI utilizes magnetic shielding to minimize the impact of the stray fields from the primary field on people and equipment in the vicinity of the machine, the exceedingly small fields used in ULF MRI require that we minimize the impact of ambient fields (from the Earth, equipment, and human activity) on ULF MRI.

One of the primary areas of interest and work of our research group has been imaging the function and anatomy of the human brain. Consequently, this will flavor much of the discussion about the instrumentation we have developed. MRI (whether it be at ULF or HF) provides images of brain structure and anatomy and, with the possible exception of direct neuronal imaging (DNI), does not directly provide information about neural activity and brain function. Even fMRI, widely practiced at high fields, is not a *direct* measure of brain function but rather a measure of hemodynamic and anatomical changes that are coupled to neural activity. MEG, on the other hand, is a technique that measures the magnetic fields that are a direct result of neural activity in the brain. Our group was historically motivated to develop ULF MRI because of its compatibility with MEG and the possibility of measuring both brain function and anatomy at the same time and with the same instrument. While most of the discussion about the "nuts and bolts" of ULF MRI is generally relevant to any application, we will repeatedly comment on limitations and constraints imposed by combining the technique with MEG.

2.1.1 Implications of ULF Compared to HF MRI

The measurement field, B_m, is usually of the same order as the Earth's magnetic field. While other investigators have acquired data using the ambient Earth's field as the measurement field (see, for example, reference [1]), medical imaging in an environment with appreciable human activity requires that we shield the ULF MRI instrumentation from the ambient field or otherwise compensate for that field. We have found this to be the only realistic approach to allow precise control over the measurement field in anything but a remote location. It is also important to note that for acquiring combined ULF MRI and MEG data, it is necessary to shield the Earth's magnetic field, as the MEG signals are many orders of magnitude smaller. As we saw in Chapter 1, combining conventional MRI and MEG is impossible because the SQUID sensors simply cannot function in that HF environment.

One benefit of ULF MRI that we have already seen is that the requirements on field homogeneity are much lower than in HF MRI, since the homogeneity scales with the absolute field (Chapter 1, Eqn. 1.20). One result of this scaling is that, at least in liquids, the measured NMR line-widths decrease with field and are now of the order of Hz instead of kHz. Also, the small-magnitude magnetic fields and gradient fields can be readily changed (in magnitude and direction) or turned on and off. While our hardware is largely limited to a single orientation of B_m, it is straightforward to add more coils to enable measurement fields that can be oriented in different directions and even altered in real time during an acquisition. These features enable new pulse sequences that may lead to new applications.

Switching the gradients in HF MRI induces massive magnetically induced mechanical forces on the hardware, which results in acoustic noise that is sufficiently loud to require patients and subjects to wear ear protection during a scan. In ULF MRI, the magnetic and mechanical forces are dramatically reduced to the point that the acoustic noise is typically barely perceptible, and the only sound typically heard by patients and subjects originates from switching the larger B_p field. In addition to the mechanical forces induced on the ULF MRI hardware, the same is true for conductors and ferromagnetic materials that may be in or on a patient or subject. The forces scale with the field gradient (which typically scales with the absolute field) and consequently do not pose a safety problem in ULF MRI. It is hoped that this will enable people with metallic implants and/or metal shrapnel to be safely scanned in ULF MRI systems.

Finally, the coils required to generate all of the fields needed in ULF MRI are relatively simple and light, especially in comparison to those required by superconducting HF systems. In addition to the massive coils required by the large superconducting magnets of HF MRI, those coils must also be submerged in an appropriate cryogen (typically liquid helium) in order to maintain the material in a superconducting state. The vessel, or cryostat, that contains the cryogen and magnetic field coil is typically a large cylindrical structure that is both mechanically robust and superbly thermally insulated. HF MRI cryostats, while being marvelous pieces of engineering, severely restrict the space and visibility for the subject being scanned. The simplicity and modest engineering requirements of the ULF MRI coils are far easier to construct in such a fashion as to provide easy access for subjects and operators and to leave a largely open vista for the subject. While some HF MRI systems are advertised as being "open" magnets, the access and visibility of such systems remain limited.

2.1.2 Signal, Noise, and SNR

Both SNR and CNR, the two most important metrics for MRI quality, depend directly on the measured signal (see Chapter 1, Eqns. 1.22 and 1.23). Thus, the most important and challenging aspect of ULF MRI is to obtain NMR signals that are sufficiently strong (while not increasing the noise) to achieve a desired SNR in the MR images. Key to maximizing SNR and obtaining the highest-quality ULF MR images is to apply the largest possible pre-polarizing field to maximize signal while minimizing noise. This will be a major discussion point in the following section. Moreover, at least two magnetic/gradient fields must be applied during the time the sensors acquire signal, which puts very demanding constraints on the fields (and the hardware used to generate those fields) to ensure the utmost stability without introducing additional measurement noise.

A key metric for judging MRI quality, if not the foremost metric, is the image resolution. As the spatial resolution is increased, the voxel size becomes smaller and smaller and the volume from which the signal is derived decreases geometrically with the voxel size. To maintain a constant SNR as we decrease voxel size, there must be a commensurate increase in signal, most obviously (though not necessarily *easily*) attained by increasing the pre-polarizing field, as was mentioned in Chapter 1. While this reality is essential to achieve clinically relevant ULF MR images, the hardware designer is faced with a coupled triple challenge: increase B_p without a commensurate increase of noise and without preventing signal acquisition by SQUID sensors.

2.1.3 Compatibility with Other Imaging Modalities

ULF MRI is compatible with several brain imaging modalities, including EEG, MEG, and near-infrared spectroscopy (NIRS). ULF MRI is the MRI method most readily compatible with MEG since any approach that utilizes higher fields (during the readout) would simply render the SQUID sensors, necessary to acquire the MEG signal, useless (if not destroyed) due to very large induced currents and trapped flux in the superconducting material. Moreover, isolating the system inside a (minimally) double-layer magnetically shielded room (MSR) is a prerequisite for MEG measurements, as the low-frequency ambient magnetic field noise would completely dominate over the miniscule neuromagnetic signals in the open environment. This environment is impractical if not impossible for HF MRI systems, due to the magnetization of the MSR by the HF magnet. This reality does not even address the fact that the magnetic field for the vast majority of HF MRI systems cannot be easily "turned off."

2.1.4 System Overview

In the most general sense, ULF MRI systems require hardware that is basically similar to conventional MRI: (1) the sample must be polarized by a magnetic field, B_p; (2) a measurement field, B_m, and gradient fields, $G_{x,y,z}$, are needed for the precession of the spins and spatial encoding of the NMR signals; (3) fields used to manipulate the orientation of the spin population (such as spin-flip fields, B_1) can be used to induce precession and to invert the spins to create echoes; and (4) the signal must be recorded by a sensor or an array of sensors. Figure 2.1 shows two typical pulse sequences, the spin-echo and field-/gradient-echo sequences, for ULF MRI, illustrating the interleaving of various magnetic field and gradient pulses and signal acquisition as a function of time. It is also important to note that combinations of spin- and field-/gradient-echo sequences are also possible.

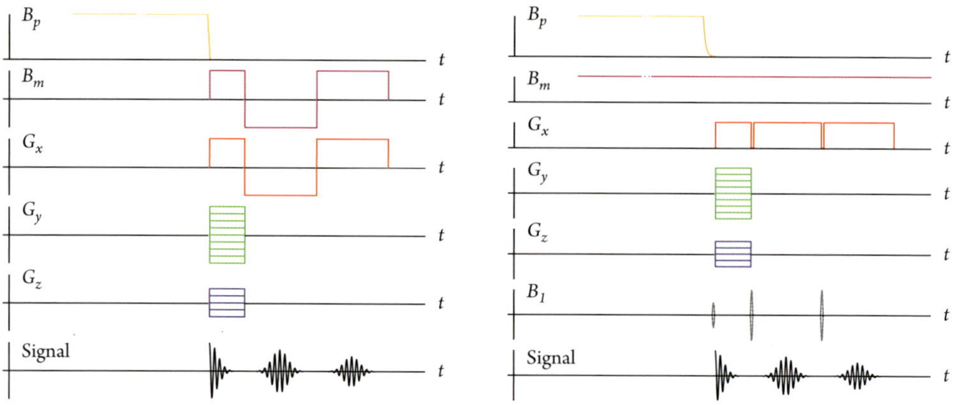

FIGURE 2.1 Pulse sequences for ULF MRI. (Left) Gradient and measurement field echo sequence. (Right) Spin-echo sequence.

While the components of ULF and HF MRI are in a general sense similar, the actual components in ULF MRI differ substantially from the HF MRI counterparts. One example of an ULF MRI system our team built is shown in Figure 2.2. The supporting structures and the coil formers are constructed out of nonmetallic materials such as wood or plastic. We intentionally keep the amount of conducting parts to a minimum to reduce the effect of eddy currents induced in such materials when fields and gradients are pulsed. The effect of such conductors on the noise and overall image quality is proportional to the field and gradient strengths; consequently it is particularly important to minimize the use of any conductors close to the imaging volume. Clearly, an MSR introduces a massive amount of conducting and ferromagnetic material in the vicinity of the imaging system. While not ideal, it becomes an optimization challenge: minimizing the ambient magnetic field while not introducing eddy current or remnant magnetic field artifacts at an affordable cost-point.

We will now describe the different parts of the ULF MRI system in greater detail.

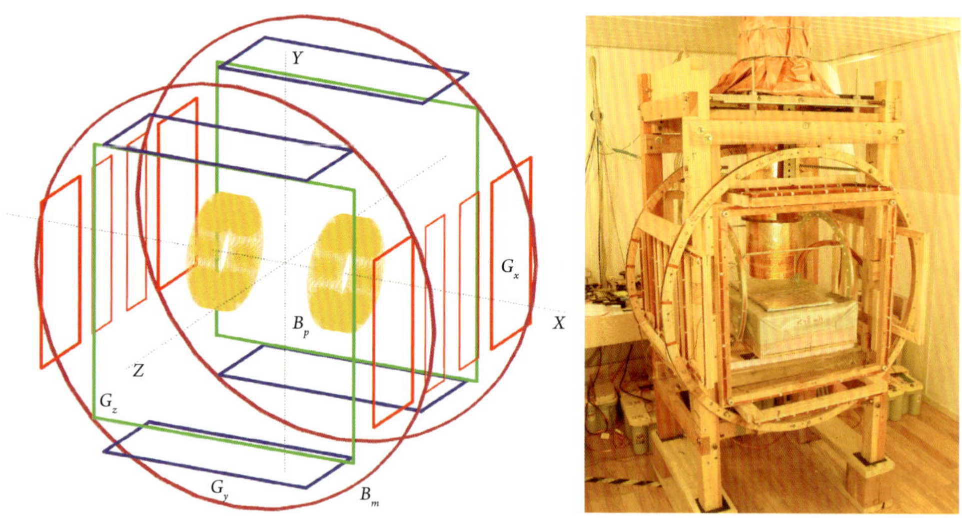

FIGURE 2.2 (Left) Schematic of our first-generation ULF MRI system with orthogonal B_p and B_m fields. (Right) Photograph of the same system, but with a single, vertical B_p coil and B_1 coils.

2.2 GENERAL CONCEPTS OF PRE-POLARIZATION FIELD GENERATION

A recurring theme for successful ULF MRI has been the need for more signal, and the seemingly easiest path to that end is to simply increase the magnitude of the pre-polarizing field, B_p. While we will not discuss magnet or coil design in any detail (there are numerous excellent references available, such as references [2] and [3]), we will examine a few of the tradeoffs facing the ULF MRI system designer. Let us assume we wish to use ULF MRI to image the physical anatomy of the human brain. In this case, the pre-polarizing field should cover the head volume, which can be approximated as a 20cm-diameter sphere. We have shown that a great benefit to ULF MRI is that the field uniformity requirement is far more relaxed than at high fields. In practice, the B_p uniformity over this volume can, for example, be as poor as 10%, especially when an adiabatic ramp-down is used to align the spins with the much more uniform B_m field. Note that the resulting variability in SNR over the imaging volume due to B_p non-uniformity can be corrected for by calibration on uniform phantoms. However, we believe that a reduction in SNR of 10% or less in some parts of the imaging volume is in many cases acceptable even without correction. This relatively low uniformity requirement results in much simpler and less expensive B_p coils than in any conventional MRI, where great pains and expense are invested to ensure field uniformity of 1 part per million (ppm) or better.

A major challenge for acquiring MEG-MRI is that switching any magnetic fields inside the MSR both induces eddy currents in the walls of the MSR (which results in transients that can saturate the sensors) and can magnetize the ferromagnetic μ-metal component of such rooms (resulting in image distortions due to the additional gradients). One can reduce the eddy currents by implementing a so-called self-shielded coil, which cancels the lower-order (dipole and quadrupole) moments of the B_p field [4]. This dramatically reduces the field at the walls of the MSR, consequently minimizing the artifact fields produced by the walls. A dynamic shielding method has recently been suggested to cancel the eddy-current modes more efficiently by using a shaped shielding pulse [5]. Our group noticed this problem with our unshielded B_p coil during the acquisition of interleaved MEG-MRI measurements [6], where we had to introduce a rather long delay between the MRI pulses and the MEG stimulation and readout. It is also important to note that, as illustrated in Figure 2.1, while B_p is not the only field that is switched during the MRI protocol, it is by far the largest field with also the largest dB/dt.

2.2.1 Maximizing B_p to Increase SNR

We showed with Eqn. 1.9 in Chapter 1 that the amplitude of the measured NMR signal scales directly with B_p. We therefore conclude that a primary focus of the instrumentation development should be to maximize the pre-polarization field while taking limiting factors such as dB/dt, drive voltage, cooling capacity, and noise into account.

In the following discussions we will neglect the aforementioned eddy-current effects since they are specific to the installation and cannot be easily generalized for a discussion. However, another aspect of an increased B_p field is that dB/dt is likely to increase and will at some point start to activate neurons or other cells, such as muscle cells. Such neuronal activation spans the range from simple retinal activation that induces perceived light flashes to significantly altering normal brain activity, as in transcranial magnetic stimulation (TMS). This is typically not a problem in ULF MRI, but as we strive toward larger and larger B_p fields, the dB/dt during switching the polarizing field (especially in non-adiabatic sequences) may become significant and must be taken into account. FDA guidelines state that the field changes should be sufficiently small that they do not produce significant discomfort or painful nerve stimulation [7]. Older FDA guidelines stated that dB/dt should be below 20T/s [8], but this value was removed in the latest guidance. At field changes above the threshold (which varies between individuals), peripheral nerves can cause visual artifacts (such as flashes of light), perceptible tingling, or a sensation of tapping. Discomfort has been reported for amplitudes 50% to 100% above the perception threshold [9]. When imaging the head, stimulation of the optical nerve and/or the retina could introduce light flashes, often long before other sensory nerve stimulation is perceptible. A proposed estimate of a threshold of the field changes is given by

(Eqn. 2.1)

$$\frac{dB}{dt} = 54 \cdot \left(1 + \frac{138 \cdot 10^{-6}}{t_d}\right) \left[\frac{T}{s}\right],$$

where t_d is the pulse duration in seconds [9]. These values were obtained by using statistics for the most sensitive 1% of the population.

In general, for normal conducting coils (e.g., not superconducting and without a ferromagnetic core), the magnetic field produced by a given coil scales with the number of conductor turns in the coil. While this rule of thumb provides general guidance, it does not take into account factors such as volume of interest, field uniformity, and the physical dimensions of the coil package. However, the reality is that generating larger B_p requires larger (more turns) coils. The inductance, L, for such a coil also generally increases with coil size. This is particularly important for magnetic field coils where one wishes to rapidly change (ramp) the field. The voltage required to drive the field produced by a coil (either increasing or decreasing) at some desired rate is roughly

(Eqn. 2.2)

$$V = L\frac{dI}{dt},$$

where I is the current and t is the time; note that $dI/dt \propto dB/dt$. This holds for both ramping the current up or down; however, in practice it is typically less important how quickly the field is ramped up (tending to affect only scan time), while a rapid ramp-down of the field is often desirable (directly affecting the behavior of the spin population). On the other side of the large-coil/small-coil "equation" is the power dissipation in the coil. The power dissipation for a current passing through a coil of given resistance, R, is given by $P = R{\cdot}I^2$. Since the magnetic field magnitude, B, scales roughly linearly with the number of turns in a coil, we can say that the coil resistance scales roughly linearly with the desired B at a given I. Thus it is easy to see that if we double the number of turns in a coil (which doubles R), we can halve the current to attain the same B, and the resulting larger coil will roughly reduce the total power by a factor of two. Larger coils reduce the requirements not only on the power supply end but also on the thermal management and cooling end of the system. The only caveats we would add here are to note that as the cross-sectional area of the coil increases, the challenge to remove thermal energy from the center of the coil bundle increases, and that a coil with more turns has a larger inductance and thus requires more voltage for the current (field) to be ramped up and down. Finally, it is a greater challenge to find exceptionally low-noise high-current power supplies, which again pushes one toward the larger coil side of the optimization equation.

A novel approach for generating the pre-polarizing field incorporates a superconducting B_p coil built into the same cryostat as the sensor array [4,10]. This is an attractive solution that enables a compact system in which the same cryogen reservoir is used to cool both sensors and B_p coil while dramatically reducing both power and thermal dissipation requirements. However, the group at Aalto University has reported problems with remnant magnetization of the B_p coil for currents higher than 12A, which corresponds to 22mT in their system. They fabricated their B_p coil with a Nb wire in a bronze matrix coupled to leads consisting of high-T_c rare-earth-barium-copper-oxide (REBCO). The high-T_c conductor is an elegant solution that allows the material to remain superconducting in the helium vapor all the way up to the neck of the cryostat. While this approach is intriguing and provides a nice solution to the B_p coil design challenge, the remnant magnetization remains a problem that must be solved.

2.2.2 Power Handling and Coil Cooling

While magnet design has innumerable parameters to optimize, the rule of thumb in our group and that of most other groups pursuing ULF MRI is that the current in the B_p coil is typically in the range of tens to hundreds of amperes to generate the field strength required in most ULF MRI applications. This assumes a simple air-core magnet since the use of ferromagnetic materials in a core would produce unacceptable levels of noise. There are a variety of options for powering the B_p coils that span the range from power amplifiers to batteries. The choice will depend on factors such as acceptable noise level, system stability and flexibility, available "wall power," system configuration, and desired pulse sequences, to name a few. A typical system configuration and pulse sequence described in Chapter 1 utilizes orthogonal B_p and B_m fields in which one ramps down the B_p field non-adiabatically and retains B_m. The orthogonality of B_p and B_m provides a simple system with which to induce precession of the spins. In such a system (with orthogonal B_p and B_m coils), it is possible to use lead-acid batteries to power the B_p coil. This method provides a simple solution with extraordinarily low noise; however, the drive voltage, and thus the B_p field, will drift with time (as the batteries discharge or if the resistance of the coil changes due to temperature drifts or insufficient cooling). A simple design using a battery bank of parallel batteries can mitigate the drift somewhat. While relatively bulky, batteries have some advantages, including zero noise and not needing "wall power." On the other hand, power amplifiers provide great flexibility and a relatively small footprint.

When an adiabatic (precisely controlled) ramp-down is required, one has to shape the ramp-down profile to fulfill $dB_p/dt \ll \gamma B_m^2$ (for a derivation of this expression see Chapter 3). Many power amplifiers (such as those used in conventional MR gradient generation and pulsed magnet control) can be employed for this purpose. There are many commercial power amplifiers available that are stable over time; however, the noise performance must be carefully scrutinized to ensure they will meet the performance required by ULF MRI. In addition, these amplifiers may limit the scan time due to their maximum duty cycle over long runs. Many such amplifiers, because of the large drive voltages required, are high-voltage amplifiers, so necessary safety precautions should be taken.

While the measurement magnetic field and gradient coils used in ULF MRI systems are typically low power and do not require any active cooling, this is rarely true for the B_p coils. The most common method of cooling high-power magnets, namely using hollow-core conductors, has recently been used also in ULF MRI applications [5,11]. One common type of conductor used in ULF MRI applications is a stranded, separately insulated conductor such as Litz wire. Active cooling of the ULF MRI B_p coils is most commonly accomplished by circulating a coolant at or near room temperature through a bath in which the coil is submerged (e.g., water or fluorinert [12]). More efficient extraction of heat can be accomplished by designing a coil into which coolant channels are incorporated. Alternatively, the B_p coil can be submerged in liquid nitrogen (~77K), which greatly enhances coil cooling by reducing coil resistance by a factor of about eight (thereby reducing the power dissipated in the coil). Cooling copper to 77K also increases the thermal conductivity, which enhances the cooling; however, this effect is relatively small. A practical issue associated with using cryogenic cooling is the required thermal insulation, which adds distance between the coil and the imaging volume (which reduces the effective field in the volume of interest). In addition, the cryogen gas must be carefully exhausted from the area around the subject to prevent frostbite and low-oxygen conditions (primarily a concern in an MSR).

2.2.3 Current Switching and Control

We have seen that two different regimes for the switching or ramping down of the pre-polarization field are commonly used in ULF MRI: the non-adiabatic (or fast) switching and the adiabatic (or slow) switching. In addition, the ideal adiabatic field ramping for some ULF MRI applications may require a shaped (programmed) nonlinear ramp.

Our group has widely used solid-state switches for fast non-adiabatic ramp-down. These switches can be operated in parallel and/or in series to accommodate the required current and voltage, respectively. In addition, ULF MRI applications require complete isolation of the coil from the power supply to prevent any noise leakage into the coil. We have used solid-state switches (MOSFETs, IGBTs) combined with mechanical relays for galvanic disconnection of the drive supply. Depending on the voltage of the drive supply and the inductance of the coil, we have routinely observed ramp-down times as fast as a few ms.

Adiabatic ramp-down is most easily accomplished by employing amplifiers capable of generating shaped current waveforms. Such waveforms can also be generated by custom-designed lumped element circuits; however, they must be designed with the power-handling requirements in mind.

A general feature that our group has found to be extremely important is to incorporate a damping resistor in parallel with the coil, especially in the case of non-adiabatic switching, to prevent "ringing" of the coil after ramping the current down. While such a damping resistor is less important for adiabatic switching, it still helps to provide a smooth transition of the circuit without ringing.

The current switching approaches we have described (and most commonly employ ourselves) are very simple, with an overarching focus on simplicity and low noise. There is a variety of other approaches that can be used, such as those developed for field-cycling NMR, where elaborate electrical schemes are used to provide the different fields and/or to transfer the energy in the coil to capacitors [13–15]. Many of these ideas have been implemented in pulsed ULF MR. However, there is probably still significant room for improvement and innovation. Regardless of the technical approach, the most important performance specification for generating and switching the B_p field is the field noise and residual coil noise that can affect the measurement of the NMR signal.

2.2.4 B_p Coil Coupling with the Sensor System

Following the admonition immediately above, all aspects of the ULF MRI system must strive to minimize noise in every way possible. The pre-polarization coil can be viewed as a very large antenna; as such, it is essential to galvanically disconnect it from any and all circuitry immediately after the pre-polarization period and before the signal-acquisition period. This is especially true if a drive source that is outside the shielded environment (such as power amplifiers) is used. Any unshielded part of the circuit that remains coupled to the B_p coil will pick up the local electromagnetic fields and couple that noise directly into the vicinity of the ULF MRI sensors. In addition to noise that is picked up from the environment, a resistive coil also introduces a noise that results from the random *thermal* fluctuations of currents within any resistor, called "Johnson noise." The Johnson noise power spectral density can be described by the simple relation

(Eqn. 2.3)
$$V_n^2 = 4k_B TR,$$

where V_n^2 is the mean square voltage noise per Hz of bandwidth, k_B is Boltzmann's constant, R is the coil resistance, and T is the absolute temperature (in kelvins). The RMS voltage noise measured in a resistor is given by

(Eqn. 2.4)
$$V_n = \sqrt{V_n^2}\sqrt{\Delta f} = \sqrt{4k_B TR}\sqrt{\Delta f}.$$

where Δf is the measurement bandwidth. It is immediately clear that the Johnson noise scales with the coil resistance. Consequently, in addition to using the lowest-resistance material available (typically high-purity copper), one can also reduce the Johnson noise by cooling the coil, the more the better.

Finally, the Johnson noise generated by any coil and measured by the ULF MRI sensors falls off with distance according to the size of the cross-sectional area of the conductor (e.g., resistor) that generates the noise [8,16]:

(Eqn. 2.5)
$$V_n \propto d_w^2,$$

where d_w is the diameter of the conductor. Therefore, building the B_p coil (and other field coils) using multistranded, individually insulated Litz wire can significantly reduce the noise at the sensors.

2.3 GENERATION OF MEASUREMENT FIELD, GRADIENTS, AND SPIN-FLIP

ULF MRI utilizes a number of magnetic fields and gradients to manipulate the spin population prior to and during the NMR signal measurement. While none of the fields and gradients used are anywhere near as large as the B_p field, most of the other fields are turned on during some part of the signal measurement. Consequently, we must pay careful attention to how these fields and gradients are generated, because any noise produced in these fields and gradients will increase noise and reduce the SNR and CNR. In this section we discuss some of the requirements on those magnetic fields and gradient pulses that are used to obtain a ULF MR image, apart from the pre-polarization field discussed in the previous section.

Our group and most practitioners of ULF MRI use coils for the generation of the measurement, gradient, and spin-flip fields that are almost universally fabricated by winding copper wire on nonmetallic (e.g., wood, plastic, or fiberglass) formers. We will assume this general type of construction of such room-temperature coils for the following discussions.

2.3.1 Measurement Field

The measurement field, B_m, is typically in the range of 1 to 100μT, and a common coil topology used to produce this field is the Helmholtz coil pair. While virtually any homogeneity requirement in a specified volume of interest can be realized with a Helmholtz pair, primarily by increasing the size of the coil set, at some point this solution becomes impractical. Another approach to improving the field quality in the volume of interest is by using tetra-coil [17] or other multi-coil topologies [18–20]. This can be especially important if the coil system is housed in a small MSR [21] where the size constraint is severe and the fringe field outside the coil set should be minimized to reduce eddy currents and magnetization induced in the MSR.

B_m is present during the entire signal readout period, and therefore it is essential to minimize the noise introduced by a nonstable B_m to the extent possible. Measures to minimize the B_m noise include using batteries or an exceptionally low-noise current supply to drive the coils. If the measurement field is constant this can be achieved readily with batteries or an amplifier coupled to filters and large capacitors to mitigate the noise. If a field- and gradient-echo sequence is needed where the polarity of the field must be changed for every other echo, our experience has been that it is extremely difficult to find an amplifier-based system that is both sufficiently fast and low-noise. We have found that in this case a drive circuit powered by lead-acid batteries coupled to an H-bridge can be used to meet both rise-time and noise requirements.

2.3.2 Readout Gradient

The readout gradient consists of a linear gradient (e.g., dB_z/dx) for a measurement field in the z direction. The strength (T/m) of the gradient is almost always the same during the imaging sequence (though it is pulsed on and off). A variety of coil configurations can be used to approximate a linear field gradient along a desired axis (with the caveat, as we saw in Chapter 1, that it is not possible to generate a linear gradient exclusively along one axis). One popular design is the Golay coil [22]. The readout gradient, as the name implies, is present during the readout period, just as B_m. Consequently, we again need to use low-noise power supplies to power these gradient coils. Furthermore, fast switching is typically required, especially if the bandwidth of the spin-flip pulses is too narrow to have the gradient on during the spin-flip, or if a field- and gradient-echo sequence is used (see the discussion of these pulse sequences and applications in Chapter 4). In the end, we have the same choices for powering the readout gradient coils as we do with the B_m coil, with the primary requirement being low noise.

2.3.3 Phase-Encoding Gradients

The phase-encoding gradient is a linear field gradient (such as dB_z/dz and dB_z/dy) applied by a coil that can be designed according to a handful of configurations, one of which is the Maxwell configuration [22]. If a Fourier imaging sequence is used, the phase-encoding gradient is applied to the spin population, thereby causing the phase of the spin population to vary spatially by an amount that is determined by the strength of the gradient and how long it is applied. The gradient strength is varied as we step through k-space (in the common language of Fourier imaging) and applied for a prescribed period of time, as described in Chapter 4, after which the phase-encoding gradient is turned off and the signal is acquired. In such a typical pulse sequence, the phase-encoding gradient is off during signal acquisition, and consequently the noise of the drive supply for this coil is less important. We learned that transient noise is an additional issue that we need to consider, especially (though not exclusively) when performing ULF MRI inside an MSR. We saw that transient noise is a major concern with the large fields and fast ramps used in application of the B_p field. While significantly smaller, the group at Aalto University has reported that even switching the gradient fields can cause harmful transients [10,23]. To solve this problem, they have implemented a short encoding period, but with stronger gradients, to let the transient from switching the gradient decay before the readout period.

2.3.4 Spin-Flip Pulses

The last coil set we will consider generates the spin-flip field. This field is used to rotate the spin population about an axis, which is typically perpendicular to the measurement field in order to produce a measurable periodic change of the magnetization. The π-pulse, described in Figure 1.3 of Chapter 1, is one example of a spin-flip pulse. In this application, the spin-flip pulse rotates the spin population, in-plane, by 180 degrees such that their relative position in the population becomes a mirror image (see discussion related to Fig. 1.3, Chapter 1). A spin-flip pulse is also necessary to observe any signal when an adiabatic ramp-down of the pre-polarization field is used, which induces the spin population to follow the ramp-down to eventually align the spin population with B_m. Unless the spin population is reoriented (flipped) into the transverse plane, no measurable signal is produced.

The needed duration of the spin-flip pulse depends on the desired flip angle and the frequency distribution of the spin population at the time it is applied. This is because the bandwidth of the spin-flip pulse is inversely proportional to the duration of the pulse. Hence, a short pulse has a larger bandwidth, affecting a spin population with a broader distribution of frequencies. For example, an ensemble of spins will have a relatively narrow frequency distribution (bandwidth) in the presence of a uniform measurement field, B_m, whereas the frequency distribution can be extraordinarily large in the presence of a gradient. The spin-flip pulse must be appropriately tuned for the given spin population being affected.

2.3.5 Final Words About Fields and Gradients

The application of conventional MRI to human subjects requires diligence to track the specific absorption rate (SAR), which describes the power absorption of tissue (or any material, for that matter) from the time-varying magnetic field. The SAR is a measure of how much energy resistive materials absorb from the time-varying magnetic field that induces heating. In some sense, the SAR is related to field variation, and while the instantaneous dB/dt can be a concern in ULF MRI (primarily due to fast ramp-down of the large B_p), the SAR, which is a time-averaged effect, is typically of little concern at ULF. SAR is commonly defined by

(Eqn. 2.6) $$\mathrm{SAR} \propto B_0^2 \theta^2 \Delta f,$$

where θ is the flip angle and Δf is the bandwidth of the pulse [24]. Both B_0 (B_m at ULF) and Δf are several orders of magnitude smaller in ULF MRI than in conventional HF MRI; therefore, the SAR is much smaller at ULF. In fact, not only is the SAR (and resultant heating) small for tissue at ULF, but it is also orders of magnitude smaller for other conducting materials that may be imbedded in or in close proximity to tissue. This is one of the primary reasons that it may be possible to image subjects and patients with or in the presence of metallic materials, pointed out in Chapter 1.

A final word about the specific coil design should be included here. While there are a number of different coil configurations that can generate each of the required fields and gradients, a major consideration for the system designer is how the various coils physically nest together. Designing a single Helmholtz or tetra-coil system that can generate a field of desired strength and uniformity over a given volume of interest is relatively straightforward. However, the design of a ULF MRI system requires numerous different field and gradient coil sets, all of which need to apply a field or gradient with certain strength and homogeneity requirements over the volume of interest. The number of coils becomes even larger if one desires to dynamically and incrementally manipulate the direction of fields during an experiment (e.g., rotating B_p or B_m around some axis). Optimizing the various parameters (including field or gradient strength, quality, size of the volume of interest, physical access, etc.) for such an ensemble of coils becomes a nontrivial challenge.

2.4 SENSING THE ULF MR SIGNALS

We defined the regime of ULF for the purposes of NMR and MRI a/the regime of measurement fields $B_m < 10$mT. This translates to proton Larmor frequencies in the range from DC (zero field) to $\omega_L(B) = 426$kHz at 10mT. Ideally, a ULF MRI sensor would be sensitive to this entire signal frequency range. We have seen the large penalty paid by Faraday-type pickups as the signal frequency decreases (Chapter 1, Eqn. 1.17ff), with an extreme sensitivity of zero at zero-field (DC). Furthermore, the same detector needs to have an instantaneous bandwidth that would allow signal acquisition across the entire frequency range of a sample in B_m and gradients, ideally with equal sensitivity.

There are a few types of magnetic field sensors that have been used for ULF MRI. These include low-T_c (T_c is the superconducting transition temperature) SQUIDs, high-T_c SQUIDs, atomic magnetometers, hybrid GMR, and Faraday coils. Regardless of which sensor is used, the essential common quality is that it has the lowest possible noise contribution to the measured signal, especially when the necessary fields are applied. Furthermore, in pre-polarized ULF MRI, the sensor and associated circuitry must survive the pre-polarization field and switching and, assuming the sensor circuit is held in an insensitive state during application and switching of B_p, must become operational quickly after the large field is turned off.

In most cases, as the magnetic field and signal frequency decrease, it is more advantageous for the sensor to detect the field directly instead of changes in the field. Sensors that derive the signal from a change in the magnetic field, most commonly the Faraday coil, become less sensitive as the magnetic field and rate of change of the field decrease. For example, the Faraday coil generates a voltage signal based on Faraday's law: $V_{\text{Faraday}} \propto d\Phi/dt$ (where Φ is the magnetic flux threading a sensor loop, see Chapter 1, Eqn. 1.15ff). For ULF MRI measurements, the flux through the loop originates from the magnetic moment of the spin population, which is proportional to the polarization field, B_p, and the rate of change of that flux is proportional to the measurement field, B_m (recall $\omega = \gamma B_m$). Hence, a Faraday coil would produce a signal for ULF MRI experiments according to $V_{Faraday} \propto B_p \cdot B_m$, which is more commonly expressed for HF MRI as $V_{Faraday} \propto B^2$ since B_p and B_m are the same. In ULF MRI, B_p is typically two orders of magnitude smaller than the analogous field in HF MRI and B_m is four to six orders smaller, resulting in a total Faraday coil signal loss of 10^6 to 10^8 at ULF compared to HF MRI. On the other hand, the signal from a SQUID depends directly on the flux through its loop and thus depends only on B_p. However, it is also worth noting that the magnetic field noise generated by the conductivity of a human subject depends on the frequency ($\sim f^{0.2}$ [25]). Although the level of magnetic field noise from the body is negligible in ULF MRI, it becomes significant at HF.

Our team has used SQUID sensors as the primary tool for measuring ULF NMR and MRI signals because they are sensitive to only the absolute field being measured and have extraordinary bandwidth from DC to MHz. While SQUIDs are the mainstay for our ULF MRI work, members of our team have demonstrated that it is feasible to use atomic magnetometers (AM) to measure ULF MRI without the need for cryogens [26].

In the following sections, we will focus on SQUID sensors and describe how they work and how our team has used them to measure the signals for ULF MRI. We will briefly discuss other sensor types thereafter.

2.4.1 SQUID Basics

Our discussion of SQUIDs for the scope and purpose of this book will focus on how they work as magnetic field sensors. For further investigation of SQUID sensors, we refer the reader to several excellent references that describe the SQUID in great detail [27–29]. We will also limit our discussion to the DC SQUID, which is almost exclusively used in all applications today.

The DC SQUID consists of a superconducting loop that is interrupted by two Josephson junctions [30,31], which are weak links through which Cooper pairs (paired electrons that carry the current in superconductors) can tunnel. Two effects govern how a SQUID works: flux quantization in the superconducting loop and the Josephson effect of the weak links [32].

In principle, a SQUID transforms magnetic flux changes (the input) through its loop into voltage changes (output). SQUIDs are used for precision measurements of a vast array of physical values or signals (such as electric voltage or current, mechanical displacement or rotation, gravity waves, pressure, temperature, etc.)—indeed, anything that can be effectively transformed into magnetic flux. The functional characteristics of the SQUID are illustrated in Figure 2.3, where the two extrema of the current-voltage characteristic are shown ($n\Phi_0$ and $(n + 1/2)\Phi_0$, where Φ_0 is the flux quantum; $\Phi_0 = h/2e = 2.07 \cdot 10^{-15}$ Wb, where h is Planck's constant and $2e$ is the elementary charge of the Cooper pair). The DC SQUID is most often current biased (that is, a steady current is applied to the SQUID such that the Josephson junctions are driven into the normal regime). Biasing the SQUID causes the circuit to generate an output voltage that varies periodically with the flux that threads through the loop, with a period of one flux quantum. Since the voltage-to-flux ($V\Phi$) response is multivalued, it is most common to linearize the response by using readout electronics that employ a feedback circuit with an integrator and a resistor that feed flux into the SQUID loop to maintain the circuit at a fixed working point. Another common description for this type of circuit is a "null detector," where the feedback signal required to maintain a "null" is precisely measured and provides the output signal. The sensitivity of the basic SQUID is enhanced by incorporating it into an appropriately designed circuit that maximizes the

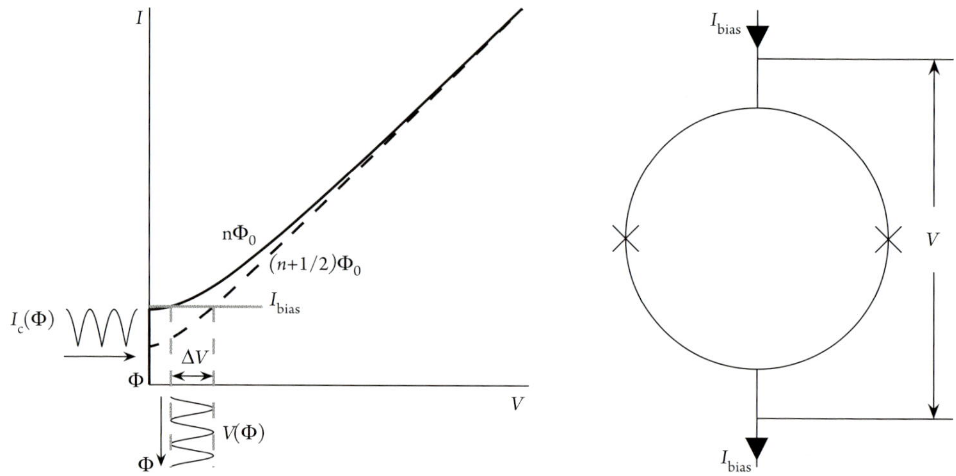

FIGURE 2.3 Illustration of how the SQUID works as a magnetic field sensor. (Left) The SQUID's current-voltage characteristics for the two extrema of the flux penetrating the SQUID: $n\Phi_0$ and $(n+1/2)\Phi_0$. The SQUID is current biased at I_{bias} and as the flux through the SQUID changes the voltage changes sinusoidally. (Right) A schematic representation of the SQUID with its superconducting loop with two Josephson junctions.

slope at the inflection point of the initially simple sinusoidal SQUID response. The working point at which the null-detector circuit is tuned (e.g., centered) is the steepest point of the $V\Phi$ curve, thereby generating the largest voltage change per unit flux change. A schematic of a simple feedback circuit is shown in Figure 2.4.

The SQUID itself is relatively small (sub-mm). The flux threading the SQUID loop is given by $\Phi = B \cdot A$, where B is the magnetic field at the SQUID and A is the area of the SQUID loop. Hence, a bare SQUID chip is quite insensitive to magnetic fields. The flux noise of a SQUID is typically a few $\mu\Phi_0/\text{Hz}^{1/2}$, but to translate this into a low magnetic field noise the size of the pickup coil has to be increased.

To improve the sensitivity of the sensor, a larger pickup coil can be coupled to the SQUID. The coil can have different configurations, as shown in Figure 2.5. A clear advantage of gradiometric coils is their insensitivity to distant sources. First- and second-order wire-wound axial gradiometers can readily be wound on glass-fiber formers and can achieve

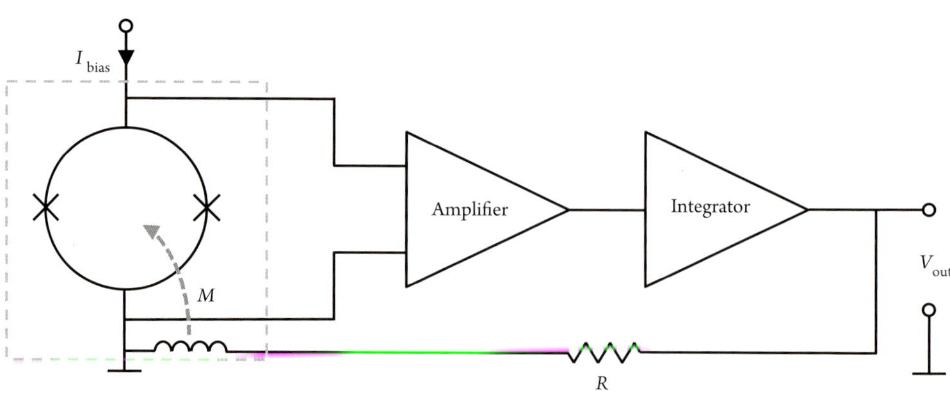

FIGURE 2.4 SQUID feedback circuit with the feedback-resistor, R.

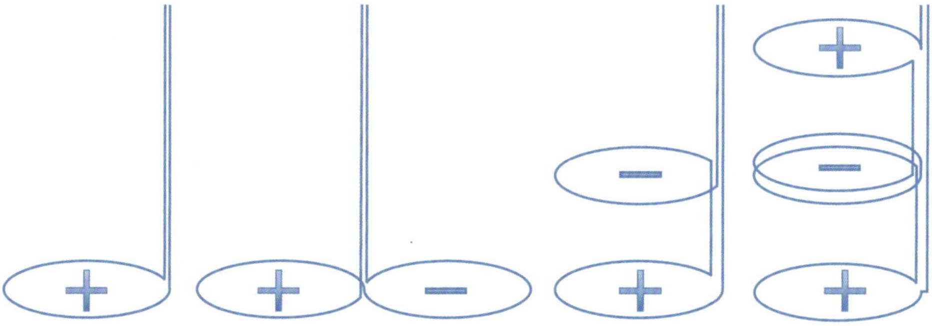

FIGURE 2.5 SQUID pickup coil and different coil configurations. From left: magnetometer, first-order planar gradiometer, first-order axial gradiometer, and second-order axial gradiometer. The plus and minus signs indicate the winding directions of the wire loops.

a balance of ~1,000, which is a measure of their insensitivity to homogenous fields or distant sources. When choosing a pickup coil, its field sensitivity, depth sensitivity, spatial sensitivity, and noise-rejection capability should be optimized for the specific application. Design aspects of SQUID sensor arrays are described in detail in reference [33], where MEG sensor arrays are considered.

An example of a noise spectrum of a wire-wound second-order axial gradiometer with 37mm-diameter loops and 60mm baseline measured inside a shielded room is shown in Figure 2.6. The gradiometer noise is shown as the corresponding magnetic field noise with respect to the bottom loop. The noise is flat (or white) down to a few Hz, where the $1/f$ or Flicker noise starts to dominate. The roll-off at a few kHz is due to a low-pass filter on the SQUID output. This particular SQUID gradiometer showed a corresponding magnetic field white noise of ~1.9fT/Hz$^{1/2}$.

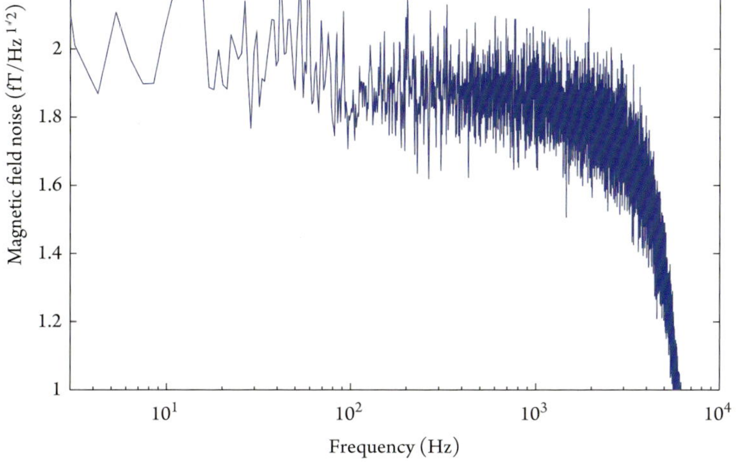

FIGURE 2.6 Noise spectrum of a SQUID with a 6kHz low-pass filter present. The spectrum is very flat down to a few Hz. The white noise of this SQUID is about 1.9fT/Hz$^{1/2}$.

The SQUID sensors can represent a significant fraction of the overall ULF MRI system cost, especially for multisensor systems. If the MRI modality is combined in a large-array MEG/ULF MRI system, then the SQUID sensors represent the major system cost because typically 200 to 300 sensors are desired. While SQUID-sensor fabrication technology for low-T_c SQUIDs is well established, the per-sensor cost remains exceptionally high due to the relatively small worldwide market. SQUID-sensor technology is based on thin-film techniques similar to the semiconducting fabrication with deposition and patterning of relatively simple materials; however, those materials are superconducting at liquid helium temperature, ~4K. Our focus on low-T_c SQUIDs is driven by the fact they are lower-noise devices, less expensive, and more robust. The cost and reliability of high-T_c SQUIDs is largely driven by the production technology, which involves exotic materials with complex stoichiometries that significantly complicate the fabrication. There are very few places in the world that produce any significant quantities of SQUID sensors for a reasonable price. The current worldwide demand for SQUIDs cannot support large-scale mass production that would drive the price point toward typical semiconductor components. Our current best estimate of the world market for SQUIDs is between 1,000 and 10,000 sensors per year (in 2011). The major companies that have commercialized SQUID sensors and SQUID-based instrumentation on a modest to moderately large scale include Quantum Design [34], Star Cryoelectronics [35], and Tristan Technologies [36] in the United States; Supracon [37] and Magnicon [38] in Germany; Elekta Neuromag [39] in Finland; and Cryoton [40] in Russia. The current price for SQUID chips ranges from roughly US$1,000 for off-the-shelf devices to US$3,000 or more for custom sensors.

2.4.2 SQUID Operation After Exposure to Large Pre-polarization Field

Until recently, SQUID sensors have not been able to operate or in many cases even tolerate magnetic fields significantly above the Earth's field of 50μT. This imposes an unacceptable limitation for ULF MRI applications, and a significant effort has been devoted to developing technologies that enable SQUIDs to operate in stronger fields with large dB/dt. The most common technique has been to develop circuits and technology that protect the SQUID chip from the (from the SQUID's perspective) strong fields involved in ULF MRI. One approach that has been used for years has been to shield SQUIDs with superconductors that exclude external fields. For example, SQUID chips can be encapsulated in lead boxes (lead is a superconductor at liquid helium temperatures) that have a critical field of about 80mT [41]. Recently, Luomahaara et al. [42] have reported locally shielded SQUID chips where niobium plates shield the sensitive SQUID while the pickup coils are protruding outside the shields and sense the magnetic fields generated by the spin population (for MRI) or the neurons in the brain (for MEG).

While we can easily shield the SQUID itself from strong magnetic fields used in ULF MRI, it defeats the purpose of measuring the external spin precession magnetic field to shield the pickup coil that is coupled to the SQUID. This leads to the obvious question: how does one prevent the large fields and dB/dt used in ULF MRI that couple into the pickup coils from damaging the SQUID? A common approach is to use circuits or technologies that limit or exclude the current produced in a pickup coil from reaching the SQUID. Our team has successfully used externally controlled superconducting switches containing a small superconducting element that is heated above its critical temperature. When the "switch" is turned on, it becomes resistive, thereby drastically reducing the current that reaches the SQUID. The effect is to protect the SQUID by making the circuit much less sensitive to magnetic fields. Other groups have used arrays of Josephson junctions [43] or

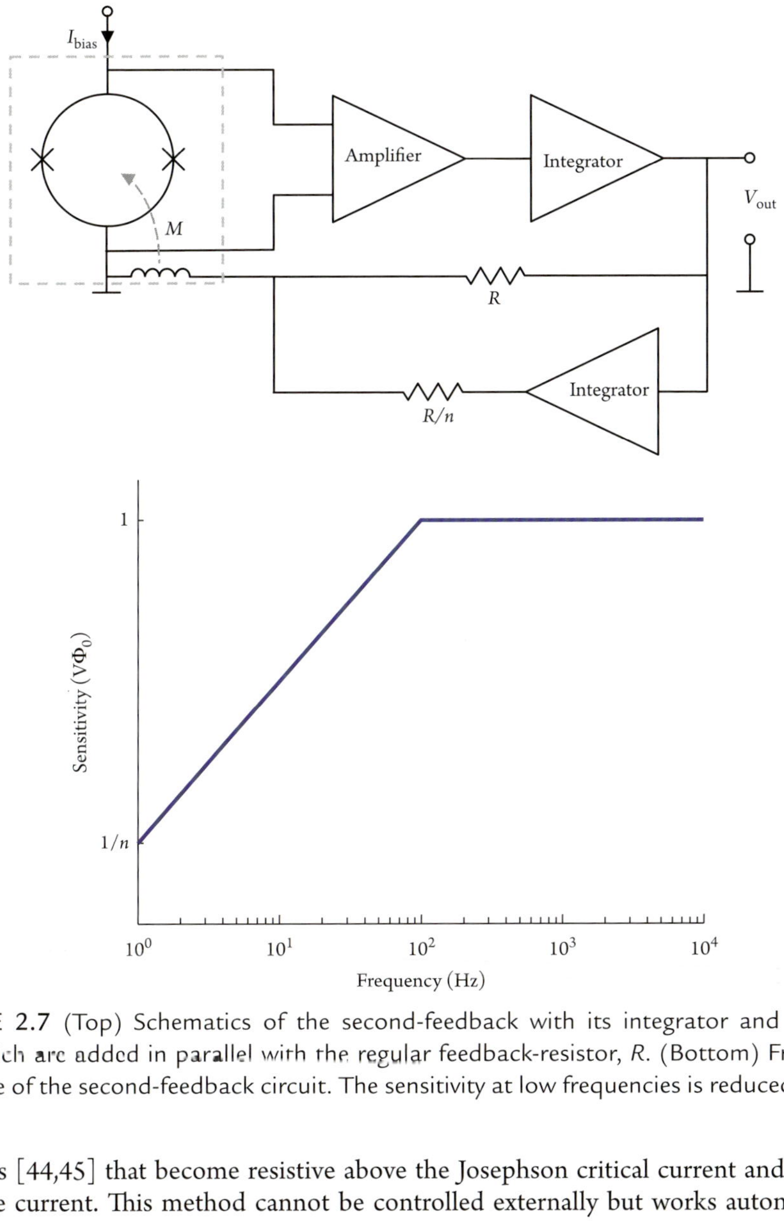

FIGURE 2.7 (Top) Schematics of the second-feedback with its integrator and resistor, R/n, which are added in parallel with the regular feedback-resistor, R. (Bottom) Frequency response of the second-feedback circuit. The sensitivity at low frequencies is reduced.

SQUIDs [44,45] that become resistive above the Josephson critical current and thereby limit the current. This method cannot be controlled externally but works automatically. Each approach has some benefits and drawbacks, including the response and reset times.

When performing ULF MRI inside a small MSR or when using very large fields, it is difficult to fully compensate for transients induced by eddy currents (and other effects). The long decay time for some eddy-current effects can delay NMR signal acquisition for prohibitively long times. To address this and other problems, our group has successfully implemented a second-feedback [46] technique that reduces sensitivity to low-frequency signals (see Figure 2.7) while retaining the sensitivity to the NMR signal (recall the Larmor frequency, ω_L, is typically on the order of kHz). The practical result is that the SQUID sensor will maintain a high sensitivity for the NMR signal while having a reduced sensitivity at low frequencies that prevents the slow decay of eddy currents induced by the large pulsed fields from driving the SQUID sensor outside the operating dynamic range. This technique will also be useful for screening the SQUID sensor from large slow transients caused by things like vehicle movement, gurneys being pushed down the hallway, and other common magnetic "noise" sources.

2.4.3 SQUID Pickup Coil Size Optimization

The maximum MRI resolution is set by the applied gradients and the pulse-sequence parameters and not by the size of the pickup coil; however, the pickup coil has to be sensitive enough to detect the signal of the voxel of interest to achieve the desired resolution (sufficient SNR). The SQUID pickup coil plays a complex role in realizing a specific resolution through the effective SNR for a pickup coil of specific size and design when measuring the signal from a given voxel. The situation in MEG is different because the pickup coil size (and thus the number of sensors) determines the spatial resolution. The MEG pickup coil size should be small enough to prevent smoothing of magnetic field patterns with high spatial frequency. This typically leads to MEG pickup coil sizes in the 5mm to 20mm range and a full helmet-shaped array with several hundred channels. ULF MRI, on the other hand, benefits from larger and more sensitive pickup coils and fewer channels than MEG.

A method to calculate the flux, which originates from a given voxel (or unit volume), threading the SQUID loop for a wire-wound magnetometer is described in reference [46]. The described method consists of numerically solving the Bloch equation of a single magnetic moment and then integrating and averaging across the volume to get the magnetization of an entire voxel. In the example cited, the flux threading the SQUID loop is calculated for a voxel that was pre-polarized by a 200mT field for a time sufficient to reach equilibrium. A hypothetical ULF MRI experiment was modeled in which the diameter of the pickup loop and the depth of the 1mm^3 water voxel were varied. The results are summarized in Figure 2.8. We found, as one might expect, that the pickup coil for deep voxels (those relatively far from the pickup) should be as large as reasonably possible, whereas smaller pickup loops are more sensitive to shallow voxels. Sadly, there is no "one-size-fits-all" solution, so if one is limited to a single sensor size in a multisensor system, it should be designed to have reasonable sensitivity for both shallow and deep voxels within the volume of interest—which leads to the obvious conclusion that an intermediate-size pickup coil provides the best compromise. Alternatively, one could design a more complex multichannel system that incorporates both small and large pickups, for which the ideal configuration would require optimization modeling that takes into account the volume of interest, source distribution, desired resolution, and other factors.

Our group recently modeled the SNR performance of pickup coils as a function of pickup loop size and voxel (source) depth for SQUID-based ULF MRI systems in preparation for building a new system. Figure 2.8 presents a summary of that modeling study that provides a most interesting basis from which we can compare pickup sensitivity to the noise level of the system to obtain the SNR performance of a given coil configuration. As an example, we compared the performance of three pickup coil sizes for different noise environments. We assumed an intrinsic noise of the SQUID to be $3\mu\Phi_0/\text{Hz}^{1/2}$, and the uncorrelated background noise was $1\text{fT/Hz}^{1/2}$. The three pickup coil configurations studied were (1) a single 40mm-diameter coil, (2) a single 60mm-diameter coil, and (3) seven 20mm-diameter coils that cover almost the same area as the single 60mm-diameter coil. When only the intrinsic noise is considered, the seven 20mm-diameter coils provide the lowest SNR (i.e., are the worst); because the intrinsic noise in the separate channels is additive, the resulting noise is therefore a factor of $\sqrt{7}$ higher than for a single coil. However, when the $1\text{fT/Hz}^{1/2}$ uncorrelated

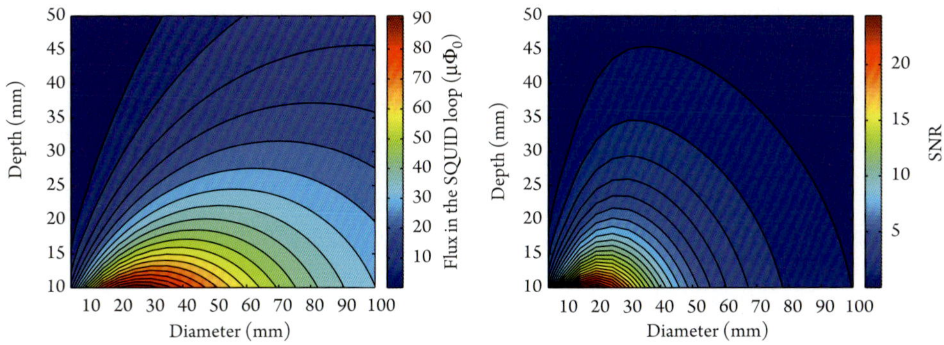

FIGURE 2.8 (Left) Flux in the SQUID as function of the diameter of the pickup loop and the depth of the 1mm^3 voxel. (Right) SNR when the SQUID has an intrinsic flux noise of $3\mu\Phi_0/Hz^{1/2}$ and an external field noise of $1fT/Hz^{1/2}$. Note that the larger pickup loops couple more of the external noise, and thus the SNR is reduced.

background noise is added, the smaller coils couple less flux noise to the SQUID and the increased noise for the seven 20mm-diameter pickups is the smallest of the three configurations. Conversely, the largest coil couples the most noise (i.e., is the worst) in terms of the amount of background noise. While the left panel of Figure 2.8 would tell us that a pickup coil configuration of at least 60mm in diameter provides the optimal signal for voxels located at depths larger than ~22mm, it does not inform us about the noise or optimal SNR. Optimizing the pickup coil configuration is clearly complicated by the fact that ULF MRI systems are rarely designed for one specific depth or simple noise profile (as we have assumed). The SNR for $3\mu\Phi_0/Hz^{1/2}$ intrinsic SQUID flux noise and an external noise of $1fT/Hz^{1/2}$ is shown in the right panel of Figure 2.8. By comparing the panels of Figure 2.8, the effect of larger coils picking up more of the external noise can be seen, as the SNR for larger coils is largely reduced.

The design goal for our group's new hybrid MEG/ULF MRI system is to provide whole-brain sensitivity, not just the shallow cortical region. This goal, together with an expected system background noise level of at least $1fT/Hz^{1/2}$, led us to choose 40mm-diameter coils as the best compromise between depth sensitivity and noise contribution. The added flux noise from the background is expected to be $7.1\mu\Phi_0/Hz^{1/2}$ for the 40mm-diameter pickup coil. Ultimately, we hope to implement multiple pickup coil sizes to truly optimize the SNR for the entire volume of interest; however, this would add too much complexity in the initial system design.

The use of large arrays of sensors is necessary for MEG and also provides benefits for ULF MRI over single-sensor systems, including enlarging the imaging field of view (FOV), increasing the SNR and image quality by simultaneously measuring the signal from a given voxel with multiple sensors, and accelerating the imaging. Parallel MRI is a technique that simultaneously acquires MR signals from multiple receiver coils, each with a characteristic spatial sensitivity. Parallel MRI had been used primarily for FOV and SNR improvement at high fields (see, e.g., [47–49]) until recently, when image acceleration became the primary driver. Accelerated image acquisition in parallel MRI is achieved at the expense of reduced imaging SNR.

Exploring parallel MRI for hybrid MEG/ULF MRI systems is clearly warranted and may also provide benefits for systems designed exclusively for ULF MRI. The first exploration of parallel ULF MRI was published by our group [50]. We found that, as expected, increased imaging speed is feasible only when the SNR is sufficiently large to obtain an image of desired quality in a single average. Therefore, in practice, each application must determine whether image acceleration or improved image SNR is preferable. We find that when acquiring ULF MRI (especially in brain imaging, where the SNR is relatively low), multisensor acquisition is most effective to increase the SNR and/or to increase the FOV. Recently, the effect of image acceleration was modeled for the Finnish MEG-MRI system [51]. It was shown that a moderate acceleration of two or three times in each direction results in a very limited reduction in the relative SNR efficiency. One possibility is that a shorter acquisition time to reduce the influence of subject motion can outweigh the reduction in SNR [51].

Coupling between individual (neighboring) sensors that results from the mutual inductance between pickup coils is an important consideration any time sensor arrays are used. The geometry of the array is the primary factor that determines the coupling between the channels. The SNR for parallel MRI depends on the channel sensitivities and the noise covariance matrix and is discussed further in Section 4.3.4. Finally, it is important to note that the real-world SNR will depend also on the specifics of the MRI pulse sequence used.

2.4.4 SQUID Cryostats and RF Interference Shielding

Every SQUID-based system (both high T_c and low T_c) requires a cryostat to maintain the sensor in the superconducting state. For the vast majority of systems we have used, that implies keeping the sensor in a bath of liquid helium (LHe). While a liquid nitrogen (LN) cryostat is little more than a high-quality Thermos bottle, the lower temperature and dramatically lower heat of vaporization for LHe requires a more sophisticated cryostat that incorporates not only vacuum isolation but additional components such as thermal reflective layers (superinsulation) and a thermal shield. Each component of the LHe cryostat affects the performance of the SQUID sensor in different ways and we will briefly touch on those that are most important. We include this brief discussion about LHe cryostats for SQUID applications not expecting that you, the typical reader, will build your own, but rather to point out design considerations if you contract with a vendor to build a custom cryostat. Another driver for including this section is to make the ULF MRI practitioner aware of the most common components of an LHe cryostat that our experience has shown can be sources of unexpected noise (e.g., eddy current and Johnson noise) that originate from the cryostat.

The LHe cryostat consists of an inner vessel surrounded by an outer vessel, with a vacuum space between the two. An obvious consideration is that the vessel material should not be metal (stainless steel being the most common low-temperature cryostat material) because of the massive amount of noise such materials will produce. Another obvious point is that the vessel material should be compatible with the low temperatures and large temperature fluctuations to which it will be exposed. For example, there are innumerable forms of fiberglass available, but very few are designed for cryogenic applications; additionally, the glues used to bond the fiberglass components must also be cryogenically rated. Finally, our group almost exclusively measures ULF MRI for samples at or near room temperature; consequently, the sample volume is outside the cryostat. We showed that regardless of the sensor chosen, the measured signal in a single sensor from a voxel drops off with distance as $1/d^3$ (as pointed out in Eqn. 1.9 in Chapter 1). This factor drives the design consideration to enable placing the sample volume as close to the sensors as possible by minimizing both the vessel wall thickness and vacuum space. Obvious tradeoff considerations are vessel strength (or fragility) and efficiency of thermal isolation.

In addition to the vacuum vessel that is a component of any cryostat, low-temperature (LHe) cryostats must also incorporate other components to further isolate the cryogenic space from the room-temperature (laboratory) environment. The most important component further minimizes heat transfer between inner and outer vessels primarily by reflecting infrared radiation away from the interior vessel. This is accomplished by adding infrared reflecting layers made of aluminized Mylar (commonly called superinsulation) to the vacuum space of the cryostat. While the reduction in heat transfer is important for a system to minimize LHe use (long LHe hold time) and minimize the mechanical noise cause by rapid LHe boil-off, the superinsulation can also be a significant source of eddy-current noise in ULF MRI. Seton et al. [52] and later the Berkeley group [8,16], reported replacing the aluminized Mylar with aluminized polyester fabric, which eliminates continuous conducting paths and thereby reduces the magnetic field noise. We have found that an extraordinarily simple (and low-cost) method to break up the conduction paths in the aluminized Mylar is to crinkle it. This method has been implemented by Cryoton, one of the companies that custom fabricates LHe cryostats for SQUID applications.

Another component that is often incorporated in LHe cryostats is a thermal shield. The purpose of the shield is to divert thermal energy from the region of the cryostat near the SQUIDs (typically the bottom) to a region of the cryostat near where the He exhaust gas exits. The thermal shield must be a good thermal conductor and has traditionally consisted of a moderately thick (substantial fraction of a millimeter) layer of copper that surrounds the inner cryostat vessel and is physically attached to the inner vessel near the top. Our team, while building the first SIS-MEG system [53], found that the thermal shield produced an intolerable level of Johnson noise. Our solution was to etch polyimide-backed copper into long strips to minimize the effective conductor size and significantly reduce (though not eliminate) the noise. In addition to Johnson noise, eddy-current transients would plague a ULF MRI system that uses a thermal shield in the cryostat. Better superinsulation and methods to incorporate more layers between vessels have obviated the need for this noise source.

Finally, any SQUID, regardless of application, is extraordinarily sensitive to interference from RF signals such as those that emanate from cellphones, microwave ovens, etc. The effect of the RF interference (RFI) on the SQUID sensors is to decrease the slope at the working point (and also the voltage swing) of the SQUID, thus making them less sensitive. To shield our SQUID sensors from this ubiquitous noise, we routinely wrap our cryostats with gold-plated Mylar [54] (single-sided 90nm-thick gold) to minimize RFI while adding as little Johnson noise as possible. The goldized Mylar is used primarily to surround the bottom parts of the cryostat, while for the upper part of the cryostat (further from the SQUID sensors) one can use thicker and more durable copper-plated polyester fabric [55] because the Johnson noise falls off rapidly with distance for such materials. Finally, when fabricating an RFI shield, it is crucial to have a low-ohmic connection between the RFI shield and the SQUID electronics. These materials and methods are designed to minimize noise, but there will always be a tradeoff between better shielding (thermal and RFI) and more noise generated by the shielding. The noise contribution from conducting sheets, such as the superinsulation and RFI shield, can be estimated using the method described in reference [56].

2.4.5 Other Sensors

Thus far we have focused on low-T_c SQUID sensors for acquisition of the ULF MR signals. However, several other types of sensors have been and could be used to detect and measure the ULF MR signals. Different sensors have different pros and cons, and in the end there is a tradeoff between the many different factors (e.g., sensitivity, ease of use, and price) when deciding what type of sensor to use. We present here a few of the possible alternatives to SQUID sensors for ULF MRI. We do not include a separate discussion of high-T_c SQUID sensors because they are essentially similar to low-T_c SQUIDs. They both require cryogenic cooling, and modern high-T_c SQUID sensors are only slightly less sensitive than their low-T_c counterparts. Our group has chosen to stick with low-T_c SQUID sensors because it has been our experience that they are more robust and they cost less.

The cheapest and simplest MR sensor is the room-temperature Faraday coil. Such coils are used in conventional MR as their sensitivity scales quadratically with the static field strength present in conventional MR systems. At low fields, however, the high Johnson noise reduces the SNR drastically. Reference [25] compares the noise of a single-turn Faraday coil (65mm in diameter, 6.5-mm wire diameter, and 25mm from the sample) to the noise of tuned and untuned SQUID magnetometers and gradiometers (of 65mm diameter and the same separation to the sample). At ~25MHz the noise of the Faraday coil becomes lower than that of the untuned SQUID gradiometer. We also presented a detailed analysis of Faraday coil performance for ULF MR signal acquisition in Chapter 1.

While Faraday coils may not compete head to head with SQUIDs in sensitivity, they are far less expensive and do not have the complications of requiring cryogenic cooling. Our team demonstrated a ULF MR system that included a multiturn Faraday coil (90mm outer diameter, 20mm inner diameter, and 14mm height) consisting of 1,400 turns of AWG24 (0.51mm) copper wire for which a noise of $20\text{fT/Hz}^{1/2}$ has been measured at 3.3kHz [57]. The coil was coupled to an amplifier with INA217 instrumentation amplifiers in the first stage; the resulting voltage and current noise were $1.2\text{nV/Hz}^{1/2}$, and $0.8\text{pA/Hz}^{1/2}$, respectively. These multiturn coils have successfully been used for MR detection of liquid explosives [57] but are not sensitive enough for brain imaging.

An *atomic magnetometer* (AM) consists of a gas cell filled with a vapor of alkali or other atoms in which measuring the Larmor spin precession frequency of the optically pumped vapor yields the magnetic field; thus, AMs measure the absolute magnetic field. Spin-exchange-relaxation-free (SERF) AMs have high atomic densities and reach a higher sensitivity than older cesium vapor-type AMs. Modern SERF AMs have extraordinarily low noise and are becoming competitive with SQUIDs in terms of sensitivity. The first demonstration of NMR detection using atomic magnetometers was reported in 2005 [58], and the first MRI was realized a year afterward [59].[1] Noise levels as low as $0.24\text{fT/Hz}^{1/2}$ have been demonstrated at 423kHz [60]. For the ULF regime, $12\text{fT/Hz}^{1/2}$ was reported at 3.2kHz [61] when used for MRI by members of our group at Los Alamos National Laboratory (LANL). To spatially separate the AM from the MR fields and gradients, a room-temperature copper-wire air-core transformer was used to sense the NMR signal and transfer the signal to the AM. Recently, the LANL team moved the AM-MRI system out of the shielded room and increased the Larmor frequency to 85kHz to be able to use simple copper magnetic shielding. We successfully demonstrated anatomical imaging of the hand [26] with this "lightly" shielded AM.

About a decade ago researchers at the National Institute of Standards and Technology (NIST) developed a chip-scale AM (CSAM) [62]. The CSAMs enable highly scalable multichannel systems. Both magnetocardiographic (MCG) measurements [63] and MEG [64]

---

[1] Note that both these experiments were carried out on flowing water that was polarized externally and then transferred into the measurement chamber.

have been demonstrated with these sensors. An initial noise level of ~200fT/Hz$^{1/2}$ was reported when used for MEG [64], which is at least two orders of magnitude worse than SQUIDs. However, the NIST group recently reported a noise level of 10 to 20fT/Hz$^{1/2}$ [65]. While microfabricated atomic magnetometers have the potential of scaling for low-cost manufacturing, the small size sacrifices sensitivity.

Other groups are also working on multichannel AM systems for MCG and MEG, for example, using small, but not chip-scale, gas cells [66–68]. At the BIOMAG 2012 conference the Jena group showed plans for a 57-channel MEG system [69] and the Princeton group presented a design for a 32-channel MEG system [70]. While AMs can be placed closer to the skin than cryogenic sensors, they still need to be heated to above 100°C and thus need some insulation in order to be placed onto the surface of the body/head.

A giant magnetoresistance (*GMR*) sensor consists of (1) a hard magnetic thin-film layer, in which the orientation of the magnetization is fixed; (2) a spacer material; and (3) a free magnetic thin film whose orientation of the magnetization changes when small magnetic fields are applied. In 2004 scientists at CEA-Saclay improved the field sensitivity by several orders of magnitude by using a large superconducting flux-transformer that concentrates the induced circulating current in one place where the GMR sensor is placed in close proximity [71]. These *hybrid GMR* sensors (also called *mixed sensors*) can improve the field sensitivity from ~1pT/Hz$^{1/2}$ for a bare GMR sensor down to ~30fT/Hz$^{1/2}$ for a high-T_c flux-transformer at 4K. These hybrid sensors have been used in the European Union-funded MEGMRI program as MR sensors [72,73]. The hybrid sensors can tolerate relatively high fields and have been used for MRI in a 10mT static field (i.e., no pre-polarization as is typically used in ULF MR). We note that SQUID sensors would not work in such a strong static field.

A comparison of sensor noise of several types of magnetic field sensors is shown in Figure 2.9. The lines show the white noise-dominated regions (horizontal portions of each line at higher frequencies) and the Flicker or $1/f$ noise that begin to dominate at different frequencies for different sensors. The low noise and wide bandwidth of low-T_c SQUID sensors are clearly evident and serve as the motivation for our choice of these sensors. Note that at higher frequencies (≥200kHz) the simple Faraday pickup coil produces less noise than the SQUID. Included in the graph are also two noise levels reported by our group for a multiturn Faraday coil [57] and AM [61]. This graph is highly generalized and provides only an overall guide to the different sensor types discussed in this section.

In some cases it can be beneficial to combine different sensor types or at least different pickup coil configurations. If a helmet-shaped array is used and one measurement field orientation, different types of sensors/pickup coils are preferably used to maximize the measurement sensitivity of the precessing spins all around the head. The group at Aalto University has solved this by using sensor modules with a magnetometer and two orthogonal planar gradiometers [10]. Furthermore, a different kind of sensor than the primary MR sensors in the system can be used as reference sensors for field and/or noise cancellation, as will be discussed further in Section 2.5.

In terms of sensitivity and bandwidth, it is hard for any other sensors to compete with low-T_c SQUID sensors. The requirement that SQUID sensors be placed within a cryostat results in an effective reduction of sensitivity in comparison to most sensors that can be operated at room temperature because the large temperature gradient between LHe and room temperature effectively puts the sensors farther away from the spins (volume of interest). Nonetheless, the SQUID sensitivity, even located slightly farther away from the sources, is typically greater than that of any other sensor. The need for LHe to cool the sensors can be a limiting factor due to the price and also the decreasing availability.

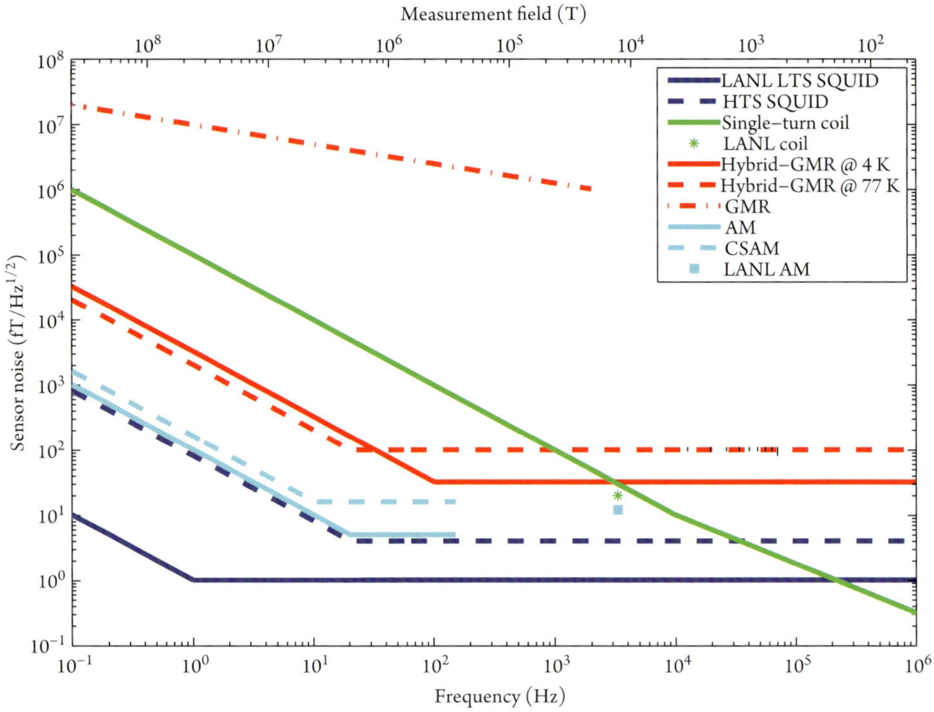

FIGURE 2.9 Comparison of sensor noise as function of frequency for a few different types of sensors: SQUIDs (blue), Faraday coils (green), GMRs (red), and AMs (cyan).

The system cryostat has to be refilled with LHe regularly, which could be inconvenient in a clinical setting. It is worth noting that this operational requirement has not presented a significant impediment for MEG systems that have the same requirement and are used in several clinical settings. If the use of LHe presents an unacceptable operational requirement or if LHe costs skyrocket, there are alternatives available. Currently, various SQUID applications use cryocoolers to directly cool the SQUIDs in LHe-free systems. Alternatively, the LHe bath can be cooled by a cryocooler (dramatically reducing the frequency of LHe fills), or a helium capture and reliquification system can be employed. While these options are currently technologically feasible, they are costly. Finally, we note that conventional MEG systems that use large arrays of SQUID sensors are not suitable for acquiring ULF MR data, either separately or in combination with MEG. This is because the SQUID sensors used in conventional MEG systems are not designed to cope with the MR fields.

2.4.6 Data Acquisition

Data acquisition is a subject that is both broad and deep, with entire books written on the subject. A good reference to start with, specifically for SQUID-sensor data acquisition, is reference [27]. Consequently, we present only a brief summary of the major considerations in designing such systems specific to SQUID-based ULF MRI. In most SQUID systems, the output is an analog voltage signal (see Fig. 2.4). For the information to be stored on digital media, an analog-to-digital converter (ADC) interfaces the SQUID electronics and the computer. The dynamic range of the ADC is limited and is commonly matched to the output range of the SQUID electronics. It is important that the resolution of the ADC is exceeded by the voltage noise of the SQUID output by several least significant bits (LSBs) for the overall noise to be dominated by the SQUID and not the ADC [27]. The ADCs also have noise of a few LSBs for up to 20 bits [27]. This internal noise increases for higher resolution. According to the Nyquist sampling theorem, the maximum frequency that an ADC can resolve is half of its sampling rate. It is important to avoid aliasing of noise down into the recorded bandwidth. Low-pass filters take care of this "anti-aliasing" filtering. However, the low-pass filters introduce phase-shifts in the signals even at frequencies far below the cutoff frequency. If the timing of the different channels has to be precise (as for MR and MEG applications), the low-pass filters should be meticulously matched. A common problem with ADCs is that they introduce noise from the digital electronics back into the SQUID electronics. RF filters on the lines connecting the SQUID outputs and the ADC can remove this noise. Also, if the cables between the SQUID electronics and the ADC are long, balanced differential and shielded wire pairs should be implemented to reduce interference picked up by the wires. Once the data have been digitized, it is crucial that the data are still continuous without time gaps. If the SQUID system is placed inside an MSR, there is a clear advantage of using a data acquisition system with optical fibers connecting the ADC and the computer to galvanically separate the instrumentation from the outside.

2.5 MAGNETIC SHIELDING

The environment in which the vast majority of people live and, perhaps even more so, work is teaming with electromagnetic noise. Everything—from cellphones and microwave ovens to subways and trains to vehicles—produces large amounts of magnetic field noise that can disturb sensitive measurements such as ULF MR. Examples of other common noise sources are fluorescent lights, computers, power cables, permanent magnets, motors, transformers, trams, and any moving ferromagnetic object, such as sliding an office chair from one desk to another. Also, the Earth's magnetic field varies diurnally on the order of 20 to 40nT per day, and magnetic storms can cause fluctuations up to 10% of the total magnitude [27]. These countless sources vary not only in the magnitude of the magnetic field noise they produce, but also in the frequency spectrum they affect. The electromagnetic noise produced by cellphones and microwave ovens is largely in the high MHz to GHz range, while moving vehicles and chairs produce magnetic noise in the low to very low (sub-kHz) frequency regime. Motors, computers, and fluorescent lights (especially the newer compact fluorescent bulbs) produce a noise typically somewhere in between.

Background electromagnetic noise in almost every modern environment affects ULF MR measurements in two primary ways: (1) the magnetic background is superposed on top of the ULF MR signal of interest (and may bury it) and (2) the background signal directly interferes with the sensor (e.g., electromagnetic noise in the RF regime directly interferes with the performance of a SQUID sensor). With all this magnetic noise in the typical workplace or medical environment, it becomes necessary to shield sensors measuring ULF MR signals from the electromagnetic background that interferes with the measurement. There is no "one-size-fits-all" approach to electromagnetic shielding for ULF MRI. There are a variety of requirements and tradeoffs that must be examined, including the power spectral density (PSD) of the noise in the environment, details of the ULF MRI methods being employed (e.g., amplitude of pulsed fields and range of ω_L being measured, to name but two), and the goals of the measurement.

The efficiency of magnetic shielding depends strongly on the frequency of the fields. It is relatively straightforward to shield high-frequency fields (10kHz to GHz) and more cumbersome to shield static (DC) and low-frequency fields (<10kHz). In principle, there are three categories of shielding approaches for ULF MRI: (1) passive shielding of both high- and low-frequency fields inside high-permeability MSRs, (2) passive high-frequency shielding by a highly conducting shield combined with static compensation of the local fields and gradients, and (3) active shielding of high-and low-frequency fields. It is important to note that the first method of passive shielding has been demonstrated for combined MEG and ULF MRI. While various groups have used combined passive and active shielding for MEG, it has not yet been demonstrated in combination with ULF MRI, where the pulsed fields used to produce the MRI will present challenges for the active-shield sensors.

In this section, we will examine some of the shielding options and tradeoffs to be considered for ULF MRI applications.

2.5.1 Shielding of External Fields

There are two mechanism of passive shielding: absorption and reflection. In addition, there are two approaches to absorptive shielding: eddy-current shielding [74] and magnetic (high-permeability) shielding. Absorptive eddy-current shielding is based on the principle of image currents, where (*very* simply stated) a time-varying field outside the shield induces currents in the shield (a conductor) that produce fields in opposition to the external field. As a result, as the electromagnetic wave penetrates the shield material, the amplitude decays exponentially in the material, $\exp(-\alpha x)$, where x is the position inside the material, and $\alpha = \sqrt{\pi f \mu \sigma}$ is the attenuation constant (Np/m);[2] μ is the permeability of the material, σ is the electrical conductivity, and f is the frequency of the wave [75]. The total absorption, S_A, for a sheet of metal of thickness, t_m, can be approximated by [27,76–78]:

(Eqn. 2.7) $$S_A = 20 \log_{10} e^{t_m/\delta} = 8.69 \frac{t_m}{\delta} \quad [\mathrm{dB}],$$

where t_m and the skin depth, $\delta = 1/\alpha$, have to be expressed in the same length units. This is the same effect we discussed in the section on skin depth in Chapter 1. The efficacy and ease of shielding by absorption depend strongly on the frequency. Shielding by absorption at noise frequencies above about 1MHz is relatively straightforward, since a millimeter-thick layer of copper ($t_m/\delta \approx 15$ at 1MHz) will reduce the noise by at least 130dB (more as the frequency increases). As the noise frequency decreases, the tradeoff is increasing shielding thickness (and weight and expense) to maintain the shielding level or allow more low-frequency noise to penetrate the shield.

A passive magnetic shield that is effective at low frequency consists of a material with large permeability (e.g., μ-metal, which is a trade name for one particular high-permeability nickel–iron alloy). A key consideration when designing passive magnetic shielding is to ensure that the magnetic induction level in the shielding material is kept well below its saturation level for the shield. For ULF MRI applications, this design consideration must include both fields from external noise sources *and* the magnetic field produced by the ULF MRI coils, particularly the B_p coil. In practice, multiple shield layers are more efficient in increasing the shielding factor than increased material thickness. Using multiple layers also allows the designer to more easily separate modeling of saturation from noise sources outside the shield from saturation induced by the ULF MRI coils. A practical aspect of using magnetic shields to provide the lowest-possible-level field inside the shield is the need to periodically implement a demagnetizing procedure for the material. The demagnetization procedure includes magnetically saturating the material, followed by slowly decreasing the

[2] Neper, Np, is dimensionless. 1 Np/m = 8.69 dB/m.

time-varying field (commonly powered by directly coupling the field coils to the power-line frequency) to zero. For investigators with limitless resources, the ideal passive electromagnetic shield would be a superconducting enclosure that excludes all field from the volume of interest [79]. Two examples of passive magnetically shielded structures are shown in Figure 2.10: one larger room designed for MEG and more recently also used for ULF MRI, and one smaller enclosure specifically designed to house a ULF MR relaxometer system for liquid explosives detection.

An important question to consider when designing shielding for ULF MRI is: "How good does the shielding need to be?" It may be sufficient for some applications simply to ensure that the sensors will work and that the magnetic noise is sufficiently low that it will not saturate the sensor. If we assume that our sensors are SQUIDs, these two requirements translate to reducing RF interference sufficiently that SQUID sensors will perform to specification and the magnetic noise does not exceed the dynamic range of the SQUID electronics.

MSRs that reduce magnetic noise across the entire frequency range down to pT amplitudes or less are relatively costly, heavy, and large. Nonetheless, measuring combined MEG and ULF MRI requires the very best MSR affordable. The shielding factor for a typical MEG-type MSR with one aluminum layer and two μ-metal layers exceeds 10^3 between 1Hz and 10Hz and exceeds 10^4 at frequencies above 10Hz [80]. In principle, the MSR works as a low-pass filter with a cutoff frequency around 1Hz because of the frequency dependence of the permeability of the nickel–iron alloy [81]. The shielding factor of a (passive) MSR can be enhanced further by adding active compensation of the ambient field, which is particularly effective at lower frequencies (<kHz). Active compensation reduces noise by both directly cancelling noise fields and reducing the saturation of the MSR magnetic material to levels where the maximum permeability is obtained. Also, "shaking" of the MSR [82] at a frequency of ~50Hz (typical power-line frequency) improves the shielding factor. The effect is described by the constant motion of the magnetic domains, which prevents the domains from becoming trapped at lattice defects in the material [82]. The same setup can be used to demagnetize the shield.

Reflective shielding results from the effect at the interface between air and the shielding material where a part of the incoming electromagnetic wave energy is reflected due to the mismatched impedance the wave experiences at the interface. The reflection coefficient

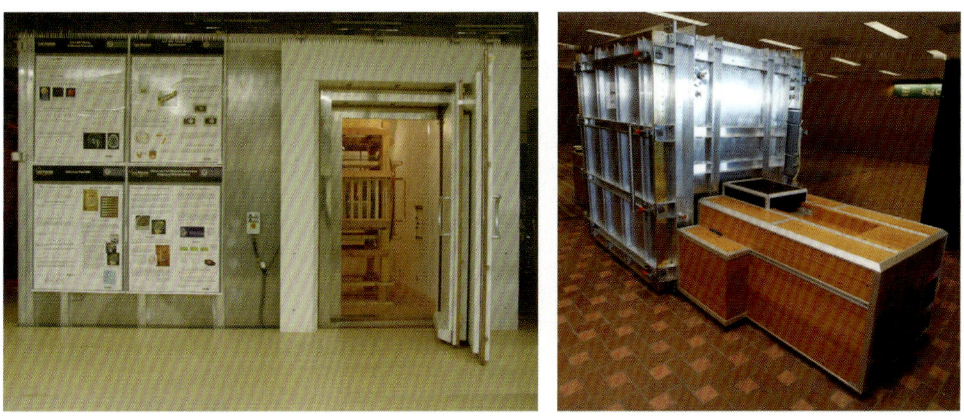

FIGURE 2.10 (Left) MSR originally built for MEG. Our first MRI coil setup has been moved from the center of the MSR to show the scale. The size of the interior volume of the MSR is $4.0 \times 3.0 \times 2.4\text{m}^3$. (Right) Magnetically shielded enclosure used for ULF MR relaxometry of liquids for explosives detection. The size of the mobile enclosure is $\sim 2 \times 2 \times 2\text{m}^3$.

at different interfaces can be determined from the wave impedances in the air and in the shielding material from which the amplitude reduction due to reflection can be calculated. However, the impedance of the incident wave, Z_W, depends on the type of electromagnetic source and also the distance between the source and the shield, which complicates accurate impedance estimations. Moreover, the impedance levels for incident electrical fields and magnetic fields are very different close to the source (near field) but approach the intrinsic impedance of free space ($Z_0 = 377\Omega$) far from the source (far field) [27]. The impedance of the shield material, on the other hand, is given by [75]

(Eqn. 2.8)
$$Z_S = \sqrt{\frac{2\pi f \mu}{\sigma}} \quad [\Omega],$$

which is very small ($\gg 1\Omega$) for high-conductivity materials up to even GHz frequencies, at least for materials with moderate permeability. The attenuation from reflection can be expressed as

(Eqn. 2.9)
$$S_R = 20 \log_{10} \frac{(Z_W + Z_S)^2}{4 Z_S Z_W} \quad [\text{dB}],$$

where the effect of multiple reflections within the shielding material has been neglected. For shielding materials with high permeability, $S_R > S_A$ at low frequencies (of the order of the line-frequency). For RF shields with low permeability, $S_R > S_A$ at much higher frequencies (e.g., ~0.1–1MHz for 1mm-thick copper for both magnetic and electrical dipole sources). For near-field (low-impedance) magnetic sources, a correction factor due to the multiple reflections has to be taken into account. The correction factor is given by

(Eqn. 2.10)
$$S_C = 20 \log_{10} \left(1 - e^{-2t_m/\delta}\right) \quad [\text{dB}],$$

and the total shielding is thus expressed as $S_A + S_R + S_C$, where S_C is negative and hence reduces the total shielding efficiency. If $S_A \geq 15$ dB ($t_m/\delta \geq 1.73$), the correction factor is small enough to be neglected [27].

Active shielding can be used either in combination with passive shielded rooms [83–86] or as the only shielding mechanism in otherwise unshielded systems [87–90]. In unshielded environments, the power-line noise at frequencies from the primary up to rather high harmonics can have significant amplitude that the active compensation system must cancel. The usually large inductance of the compensation coils can limit the frequency range of the active shielding due to the introduced phase shifts [27]. Also, the frequency response of the reference sensor (especially for flux-gates) and the feedback circuitry can be limiting factors. The best active shielding is obtained when the reference sensors are placed relatively close to the measurement sensors because the active field compensation need only correct for field and gradient variations within the imaging volume. However, reference sensors that contain ferromagnetic material and/or emit fields cannot be positioned close to a sensitive MR pickup coil as it will couple additional noise/field into the pickup coil.

Acquisition of ULF MRI requires that the measurement field and the imaging gradients are stable and known to a certain precision. A variety of factors contribute to adding poorly understood fields and gradients to the imaging environment, including any ferromagnetic or conducting materials (including shielding) in the vicinity of the imaging volume. Magnetic materials and conductors induce fields and gradients in response to both external sources and the fields and gradients generated by the ULF MRI instrumentation. The level of precision for which the fields and gradients in the imaging volume must be known and stable can be deduced by determining the allowable error at each point in k-space. The important factors are that the actual points must be positioned within the set area/volume in k-space and that the discrepancy from the desired gradient strengths is measured. If Fourier imaging is considered, the encoding time is used to move to a starting point in k-space and then a line is acquired during the readout period. The time for imaging one line is usually of the order of a hundred milliseconds (approximately two times the encoding time). Changes in the fields and gradients during the encoding period will change the position of the starting point, and the trajectory during the readout is altered by changes during the readout period.

Another key function of active field compensation is to ensure that the minimum imaging requirements are met. Therefore, active magnetic field compensation systems should keep the MR sensors within their dynamic range, with sufficient headroom to acquire the ULF MR signals of interest during the acquisition time. Such active compensation systems for magnetic field disturbances are commonly implemented for electron microscopes, ion beam experiments, and conventional MRI systems, for example, to eliminate interference from noisy environments in urban locations (see, e.g., references [91] and [92]). For an active compensation system for ULF MRI the full tensor of the ambient fields should ultimately be considered. In total, three magnetic field components, $\mathbf{B} = (B_x, B_y, B_z)$, and at least five independent first-order gradient tensor components should be measured and compensated for:

(Eqn. 2.11)
$$\begin{pmatrix} B_{xx} & B_{xy} & B_{xz} \\ B_{yx} & B_{yy} & B_{yz} \\ B_{zx} & B_{zy} & B_{zz} \end{pmatrix} = \begin{pmatrix} \frac{\partial B_x}{\partial x} & \frac{\partial B_x}{\partial y} & \frac{\partial B_x}{\partial z} \\ \frac{\partial B_y}{\partial x} & \frac{\partial B_y}{\partial y} & \frac{\partial B_y}{\partial z} \\ \frac{\partial B_z}{\partial x} & \frac{\partial B_z}{\partial y} & \frac{\partial B_z}{\partial z} \end{pmatrix} \Rightarrow \begin{pmatrix} \frac{\partial B_{x'}}{\partial x'} & & \\ \frac{\partial B_{y'}}{\partial x'} & \frac{\partial B_{y'}}{\partial y'} & \\ \frac{\partial B_{z'}}{\partial x'} & \frac{\partial B_{z'}}{\partial y'} & \end{pmatrix},$$

where the five independent elements out of the nine follow from Maxwell's equations. However, the cross-interference between the different gradient compensation coils has to be characterized carefully, as all gradient coils have non-negligible concomitant gradient components, which follow from Maxwell's equations. Moreover, even magnetic field coils, such as Helmholtz coils, produce undesired gradient, the effect of which can be reduced by using concentric multicoil setups [17,19,20]. Some multicoil setups can, however, limit the ease of access to the imaging volume. Note that three of the gradients are used for 3D imaging (B_{zx}, B_{zy}, B_{zz}), while the other gradients are reducing the image quality and the apparent transverse relaxation time, T_2^*. For more detail, the reader is referred to the discussion of concomitant gradients in Chapter 4.

Effects of low-frequency disturbance fields (noise) and gradients on LF NMR have been investigated in reference [93]. The same Shanghai group has built an active magnetic field- and (linear) gradient-compensated NMR system that uses a flux-gate magnetometer spatially separated from the measurement volume to provide an input signal for the custom-built proportional-integral-differential (PID) controller that drives the compensation coils [90]. To our knowledge, no active full-tensor-compensated ULF MR imaging system has been reported yet, but the Shanghai group has implemented a system with static compensation of six of the first-order gradients [94]. The vertical direction was left out due to geometrical limitations. Their gradient tensor remained constant over more than a week, which suggests that the environmental gradients they observed and corrected were mainly produced by stationary magnetic sources. They reported that gradient compensation reduced the NMR line width from 1.6Hz to 0.76Hz [94]. Our team and the wider MEG community have a vast amount of experience with low-frequency field and gradient noise, which is rarely stable over more than a few minutes or hours at the most. The most significant sources of such noise are movement of vehicles, gurneys, equipment, furniture, etc.

2.5.2 Interactions with Fields Produced by ULF Instrumentation

In the design of MSRs for MEG the only concerns are external fields, while in ULF MRI fields and gradients are also generated and switched within the MSR. We have already examined the need for ULF MR sensors to survive the pre-polarization pulse and to be able to work while the measurement field and the readout gradient are applied. However, in addition to the fields and gradients produced by the coils themselves, the switching of gradients and/or fields during the pulse sequence introduces transients in the walls of the MSR and in conducting parts of the system. Furthermore, each individual transient has a different characteristic spatial distribution and decay time that depends on the material in which the transient is generated. One simple way to minimize the influence of the transients is to place the system at the center of the MSR to both maximize the distance from the nearest transient-producing material and to allow symmetry to potentially cancel some of the effects [95]. We also mentioned at the beginning of Section 2.2 that a self-shielded polarization coil is desirable, especially for strong pre-polarization fields, to minimize the transient fields in any material outside the coils after turning off the pre-polarization field.

2.5.3 Noise Issues

We have discussed various approaches to shield the ULF MR measurement system from environmental magnetic noise with passive constructs consisting of ferromagnetic and/or conducting materials. We also briefly mentioned how these shielding materials can interact with the ULF MR system to induce sources of undesirable magnetic fields. In addition to the sources created directly by the induced fields of the ULF MR system, when large B_p fields are used, the magnetic flux level inside the shield can cause saturation of the magnetic material. The saturation of the MSR magnetic material reduces the shielding factor, which leads to increased external noise "leaking" into the MSR. Such saturation effects are greatly reduced with the aforementioned self-shielded B_p coil, arguing yet again for such coil designs.

Sadly, the shielding materials contribute still other sources of noise: conductors generate Johnson noise and magnetic domains generate Barkhausen noise. Both Johnson and Barkhausen noise fall off rapidly with distance, especially if the conductors (responsible for Johnson noise) do not represent large volumes. Eddy-current shields integral with MSRs may represent significant conductor volumes, but the typical installation locates such shields a meter or more from the imaging volume to reduce the Johnson noise effect. At the other extreme, extremely thin (sub-micron thickness) goldized Mylar serves as an extremely effective RF shield for the SQUID sensors without significant conductor volume. While one must be vigilant to maintain a separation between ferromagnetic materials and ULF MR sensors, Barkhausen noise results from the thermal flipping of magnetic domains in ferromagnetic materials and is a significant concern only in close proximity to the magnetic material. Typical MSR design locates the magnetic materials far from the ULF MR sensors.

The noise generated by active shielding systems depends largely on the kind of reference sensors (and associated electronics) that are used for the compensation, as the feedback signal is generated by the reference sensors and electronics to process the measured signals. When active shielding is combined with passive magnetic shielding, it may be possible to utilize reference sensors consisting of low-noise sensors with limited dynamic range, as they are placed inside the MSR and measure only the residual field. The tradeoff for ULF MR systems is, of course, the dynamic range of the fields produced by the field and gradient coils used during acquisition times (the periods of time during which compensation is most important). In contrast, systems that rely entirely on active shielding must guarantee that the dynamic range of the reference sensors is sufficient to measure the ambient fields, which limits the possible sensor types to ones with higher noise.

Finally, we reiterate a point made in Section 2.5.1 that any active field compensation system can cancel noise only up to a certain frequency due to the inherent lag of the feedback system, which is most commonly limited by the inductance of the compensation coils. In other words, the noise cancellation is low-pass-filtered, with the cutoff frequency determined by the inductance of the compensation coils.

2.5.4 Possible Alternatives

The minimum requirement for performing ULF MR, as noted in Section 2.5.1, is that the sensors (presumably SQUIDs) will perform to specification and with sufficient dynamic range above the noise to enable acquisition of the ULF MR signal. A magnetically unshielded ULF MR system is plausible but must rely on high-quality RF shielding to enable the SQUID sensors to operate in a typical environment and hardware noise cancellation through higher-order gradiometer pickups to reduce the dynamic range of the noise coupled into the electronics. A useful "trick" for acquiring ULF NMR or simple ULF MR signals in a noisy environment (assuming the SQUID sensors function with sufficient dynamic range above the noise) is to select a Larmor frequency (B_m) that is at a minimum in the background noise PSD. Depending on the ambient fields and gradients, a static compensation system might be sufficient for simple NMR systems (i.e., no imaging) for material and/or phantom studies. The complexities of a medical imaging system (e.g., long sampling times over broad frequency ranges required to reconstruct gradient and phase encoding) would require a sophisticated field- and gradient-cancellation system that has yet to be implemented. In reference [27], the authors state that active shielding is effective only for magnetometers that lack noise cancellation. Moreover, they claim that the active shielding degrades the noise attenuation of second- or higher-order gradiometers, as the cancellation coils introduce higher-order gradients that are larger than that of the ambient noise. These are challenges that have yet to be overcome to realize clinically relevant images with unshielded or lightly shielded ULF MRI systems.

Acquisition of MEG signals using high-order gradiometers and specialized signal processing has been demonstrated in unshielded environments [96]. Similar techniques can be applied to acquisition of ULF MR signals; however, the sensitivity of high-order gradiometers falls off rapidly with distance, and thus such sensors mainly detect shallow MEG sources that are at or near the surface of the cortex. Early SQUID-based biomagnetic experiments were performed in rural areas, sometimes even in cabins located in a field or meadow, where the electromagnetic noise was far lower than in urban areas. While rural areas have much less magnetic field noise, the ever-present power-line noise transmitted through ground currents [27] is observed at even the most remote locations.

Consequently, it may be plausible to operate unshielded or lightly shielded ULF MRI systems away from urban disturbances as a cost-effective solution to a low-noise environment.

Finally, we note that a wide variety of noise-cancellation methods are commonly employed as methods in MEG, where reference sensors in the cryostat, placed farther from the head, are used to reduce the noise picked up by the MEG sensors [53]. Similar methods can be adapted to ULF MRI; however, the reference SQUID sensors must tolerate the pulsed fields and also function in the presence of the required MR fields and gradients. As with the MR sensors, they must be disconnected or have current limiters in their input circuit to survive the pre-polarization field. Moreover, in MEG one can use the multitude of sensors and implement signal space projection (SSP) [33,97], which reduces the environmental noise by projecting out from the measurement the spatial vectors along which the noise components are oriented. SSP works well if the noise components are orthogonal and stationary compared to the signal components. ULF MRI systems have only recently begun to have a large number of sensors, but SSP has, to our knowledge, not yet been implemented in ULF MRI. Moreover, in multichannel ULF MRI systems, the fact that the signals from the precessing spins are circularly polarized could possibly be used to filter out only one of the circular polarization orientations [98].

2.6 SUMMARY

Building the hardware for ULF MRI is relatively straightforward if one is aware of the pitfalls (e.g., noise sources) and strives, as much as possible, to avoid them. The required imaging coils can consist of simple coil configurations wound on square or round formers and rarely require special cooling. Pre-polarization is typically used to increase the SNR and is the one magnetic field coil that may require care to properly engineer. One avenue to maximizing the SNR for ULF MRI is to build a pre-polarization coil capable of delivering the largest possible B_p within the constraints of the available power and cooling capacities. Ultrasensitive magnetic field sensors are also used to increase the SNR. The sensors used to acquire the NMR signal (or the associated electronics) are typically turned off during the pre-polarization and must be operational as soon after the pre-polarization as possible. The sensors must also have sufficient dynamic range and be sufficiently robust to work in the presence of the measurement field and readout gradient. Our group has mainly used wire-wound Nb pickup coils coupled to low-T_c SQUIDs that are protected by superconducting switches in the input circuitry. However, other types of sensors have also been used by our group and others and offer a variety of tradeoffs. Finally, the requirements for magnetic shielding depend on the particular application, but in the combination of ULF MRI and MEG a multilayered magnetically shielded rooms is virtually required, especially in any typical urban environment.

REFERENCES

1. Stepišnik J, Eržen V, Kos M (1990) NMR imaging in the earth's magnetic field. *Magn Reson Med* *15*(3): 386–39.
2. Mansfield AN (1901). *Electromagnets: Their Design, and Construction.* D. Van Nostrand Company.
3. Montgomery TB (1948). *Design of Magnets and Electromagnets.* Lindsay Publications.
4. Nieminen JO, Vesanen PT, Zevenhoven KCJ, et al. (2011). Avoiding eddy-current problems in ultra-low-field MRI with self-shielded polarizing coils. *J Magn Reson 212*(1): 154–160.
5. Zevenhoven KCJ (2011). *Solving transient problems in ultra-low-field MRI.* M.Sc. thesis, Aalto University, Helsinki, Finland.

6. Magnelind PE, Gomez JJ, Matlashov AN, et al. (2011). Co-registration of interleaved MEG and ULF MRI using a 7 channel low-T_c SQUID system. *IEEE Trans Appl Supercond 21*(3): 456–460.
7. Criteria for significant risk investigations of magnetic resonance diagnostic devices. *Food and Drug Administration, U.S. Dept. of Health and Human Services*, 2003.
8. Myers WR (2006). *Potential applications of microtesla magnetic resonance imaging detected using a superconducting quantum interference device*. Ph.D. thesis, University of California, Berkeley.
9. Schaefer DJ, Bourland JD, Nyenhuis JA (2000). Review of patient safety in time-varying gradient fields. *J Magn Reson Imaging 12*: 20–29.
10. Vesanen PT, Nieminen JO, Zevenhoven KCJ, et al. (2013). Hybrid ultra-low-field MRI and magnetoencephalography system based on a commercial whole-head neuromagnetometer. *Magn Reson Med 69*(6): 1795–1804.
11. Hatridge MJ (2010). *SQUID magnetometry from nanometer to centimeter length scales*. Ph.D. thesis, University of California, Berkeley.
12. Sims JR, Schillig JB, Swenson CA, et al. (2010). Low-noise pulsed pre-polarization magnet systems for ultra-low field NMR. *IEEE Trans Appl Supercond 20*(3): 752–755.
13. Job C, Zajicek J, Brown MF (1996). Fast field-cycling nuclear magnetic resonance spectrometer. *Rev Sci Instrum 67*(6): 2113–2122.
14. Kimmich R, Anoardo E (2004). Field-cycling NMR relaxometry. *Prog Nucl Magn Reson Spectr 44*: 257–320.
15. Matter NI, Scott GC, Grafendorfer T, et al. (2006). Rapid polarizing field cycling in magnetic resonance imaging. *IEEE Trans Med Imaging 25*(1): 84–93.
16. Clarke J, Hatridge M, MÖssle M (2007). SQUID-detected magnetic resonance imaging in microtesla fields. *Annu Rev Biomed Eng 9*: 389–413.
17. Gottardi G, Mesirca P, Agostini C, et al. (2003). A four coil exposure system (Tetracoil) producing a highly uniform magnetic field. *Bioelectromagnetics 24*: 125–133.
18. Kirschvink JL (1992). Uniform magnetic fields and double-wrapped coil systems: improved techniques for the design of bioelectromagnetic experiments. *Bioelectromagnetics 13*: 401–411.
19. Tsai LL, Mair RW, Rosen MS, et al. (2008). An open-access, very-low-field MRI system for posture-dependent ^{3}He human lung imaging. *J Magn Reson 93*(2): 274–285.
20. Morgan P, Conolly S, Macovski A (1997). Design of uniform field biplanar magnets. *Proceedings of the 5th ISMRM*, Vancouver, Canada.
21. Espy M, Flynn M, Gomez J, et al. (2010) Ultra-low-field MRI for the detection of liquid explosives. *Supercond Sci Technol 23*: 034023.
22. Jin JM (1999). *Electromagnetic Analysis and Design in Magnetic Resonance Imaging.* CRC Press.
23. Zevenhoven KCJ, Dabek J, Nieminen JO, et al. (2012). *Multi-channel SQUID system for hybrid magnetic resonance imaging and magnetoencephalography.* Presented at the Applied Superconductivity Conference in Portland, Oregon.
24. Bernstein MA, King KF, Zhou XJ (2004). *Handbook of MRI Pulse Sequences.* Elsevier Academic Press.
25. Myers W, Slichter D, Hatridge M, et al. (2007). Calculated signal-to-noise ratio of MRI detected with SQUIDs and Faraday detectors in fields from 10 T to 1.5 T. *J Magn Reson 186*: 182–192.
26. Savukov I, Karaulanov T, Castro A, et al. (2011). Non-cryogenic anatomical imaging in ultra-low field regime: Hand MRI demonstration. *J Magn Reson 211*(2): 101–108.
27. Clarke J, Braginski AI (Eds.) (2004). *The SQUID Handbook: Fundamentals and Technology of SQUIDs and SQUID Systems, vol. I.* Weinheim, Germany: Wiley-VCH Verlag GmbH & Co. KGaA.
28. Clarke J, Braginski AI (Eds.) (2006). *The SQUID Handbook: Applications of SQUIDs and SQUID Systems, vol. II.* Weinheim, Germany: Wiley-VCH Verlag GmbH & Co. KGaA.
29. Pizzella V, Della Penna S, Del Gratta C, Romani GL (2001). SQUID systems for biomagnetic imaging. *Supercond Sci Technol 14*: R79–R114.
30. Josephson BD (1962). Possible new effects in superconductive tunnelling. *Phys Lett 1*: 251–253.
31. Anderson PW, Rowell JM (1963). Probable observation of the Josephson superconducting tunneling effect. *Phys Rev Lett 10*(6): 230–232.

32. Castellano MG (2003). Macroscopic quantum behavior of superconducting quantum interference devices. *Fortschr Phys 51*(4–5): 288–294.
33. Vrba J, Robinson SE (2002). SQUID sensor array configurations for magnetoencephalography applications. *Supercond Sci Technol 15*(9): R51–R89.
34. Quantum Design, Inc. [Online]. Available: www.qdusa.com.
35. Star Cryoelectronics. [Online]. Available: www.starcryo.com.
36. Tristan Technologies, Inc. [Online]. Available: www.tristantech.com.
37. Supracon AG. [Online]. Available: www.supracon.com.
38. Magnicon, GmbH. [Online]. Available: www.magnicon.com.
39. Elekta Neuromag. [Online]. Available: www.elekta.com.
40. Cryoton Co. Ltd. [Online]. Available: www.cryoton.ru/eng/.
41. Decker DL, Mapother DE, Shaw RW (1958). Critical field measurements on superconducting lead isotopes. *Phys Rev 112*(6): 1888–1898.
42. Luomahaara J, Vesanen PT, Penttilä J, et al. (2011). All-planar SQUIDs and pickup coils for combined MEG and MRI. *Supercond Sci Technol 24*: 075020.
43. Hilbert C, Clarke J, Sleator T, Hahn EL (1985). Nuclear quadrupole resonance detected at 30 MHz with a dc superconducting quantum interference device. *Appl Phys Lett 47*(6): 637–639.
44. Hilschenz I, Körber R, Scheer H-J, et al. (2013). Magnetic resonance imaging at frequencies below 1 kHz. *Magn Reson Imaging 31*(2): 171–177.
45. Drung D, Assmann C, Beyer J, et al. (2007). Highly sensitive and easy-to-use SQUID sensors. *IEEE Trans Appl Supercond 17*(2): 699–704.
46. Matlashov AN, Burmistrov E, Magnelind PE, et al. (2012). SQUID-based systems for co-registration of ultra-low field nuclear magnetic resonance images and magnetoencephalography. *Physica C 482*: 19–26.
47. Hyde JS, Jesmanowicz A, Froncisz W, et al. (1986). Parallel image acquisition from noninteracting local coils. *J Magn Reson 70*(3): 512–517.
48. Roemer PB, Edelstein WA, Hayes CE, et al. (1990). The NMR phased array. *Magn Reson Med 16*(2): 192–225.
49. Wald LL, Carvajal L, Moyher SE, et al. (1995). Phased array detectors and an automated intensity-correction algorithm for high-resolution MR imaging of the human brain. *Magn Reson Med 34*(3): 433–439.
50. Zotev VS, Volegov PL, Matlachov AN, et al. (2008). Parallel MRI at microtesla fields. *J Magn Reson 192*(2): 197–208.
51. Lin F-H, Vesanen PT, Nieminen JO, et al. (in press). Noise amplification in parallel whole-head ultra-low-field magnetic resonance imaging using 306 detectors. *Magn Reson Med,* doi: 10.1002/mrm.24479.
52. Seton HC, Hutchison JM, Bussell DM (1997). A 4.2 K receiver coil and SQUID amplifier used to improve the SNR of low-field magnetic resonance images of the human arm. *Meas Sci Technol 8*(2): 198–207.
53. Kraus RH Jr, Volegov P, Maharajh K, et al. (2002). Performance of a novel SQUID-based superconducting imaging-surface magnetoencephalography system. *Physica C 368*(1-4): 18–23.
54. Sheldahl. [Online]. Available: www.sheldahl.com.
55. Less EMF Inc. [Online]. Available: www.lessemf.com.
56. Sandin HJ, Volegov PL, Espy MA, et al. (2011). Noise modeling from conductive shields using Kirchhoff equations. *IEEE Trans Appl Supercond 21*(3): 489–492.
57. Matlashov AN, Schultz LJ, Espy MA, et al. (2011). SQUIDs vs. induction coils for ultra-low field nuclear magnetic resonance: experimental and simulation comparison. *IEEE Trans Appl Supercond 21*(3): 465–468.
58. Savukov IM, Romalis MV (2005). NMR detection with an atomic magnetometer. *Phys Rev Lett 94*(12): 123001.
59. Xu S, Yashchuk VV, Donaldson MH, et al. (2006). Magnetic resonance imaging with an optical atomic magnetometer. *Proc Natl Acad Sci USA 103*(34): 12668–12671.

60. Lee S-K, Sauer KL, Seltzer SJ, et al. (2006). Subfemtotesla radio-frequency atomic magnetometer for detection of nuclear quadrupole resonance. *Appl Phys Lett 89*(21): 214106.
61. Savukov IM, Zotev VS, Volegov PL, et al. (2009). MRI with an atomic magnetometer suitable for practical imaging applications. *J Magn Reson 199*(2): 188–191.
62. Schwindt PD, Knappe S, Shah V, et al. (2004). Chip-scale atomic magnetometer. *Appl Phys Lett 85*(26): 6409–6411.
63. Knappe S, Sander TH, Kosch O, et al. (2010). Cross-validation of microfabricated atomic magnetometers with superconducting quantum interference devices for biomagnetic applications. *Appl Phys Lett 97*(13): 133703.
64. Sander TH, Preusser J, Mhaskar R, et al. (2012). Magnetoencephalography with a chip-scale atomic magnetometer. *Biomed Opt Express 3*(5): 981–990.
65. Mhaskar R, Knappe S, Kitching J (2012). A low-power, high-sensitivity micromachined optical magnetometer. *Appl Phys Lett 101*(24): 241105.
66. Bison G, Castagna N, Hofer A, et al. (2009). A room temperature 19-channel magnetic field mapping device for cardiac signals. *Appl Phys Lett 95*(17): 173701.
67. Shah V, Romalis MV (2009). Spin-exchange relaxation-free magnetometry using elliptically polarized light. *Phys Rev A 80*(1): 013416.
68. Johnson C, Schwindt PD, Weisend M (2010). Magnetoencephalography with a two-color pump-probe, fiber-coupled atomic magnetometer. *Appl Phys Lett 97*(24): 243703.
69. Bison G (2012). *Clinical MCG with optical room-temperature sensors.* Presented at the BIOMAG conference in Paris.
70. Romalis M (2012). *Atomic magnetometers for biomagnetic measurements—from first principles to off-the-shelf sensors.* Presented at the BIOMAG conference in Paris.
71. Pannetier M, Fermon C, Le Goff G, et al. (2004). Femtotesla magnetic field measurement with magnetoresistive sensors. *Science 304*(5677): 1648–1650.
72. Dyvorne H, Fermon C, Pannetier-Lecoeur M, et al. (2009). NMR with superconducting-GMR mixed sensors. *IEEE Trans Appl Supercond 19*(3): 819–822.
73. Sergeeva-Chollet N, Dyvorne H, Dabek J, et al. (2011). Low field MRI with magnetoresistive mixed sensors. *J Phys Conf Ser 303*(1): 012055.
74. Zimmerman JE (1977). SQUID instruments and shielding for low-level magnetic measurements. *J Appl Phys 48*(2): 702–710.
75. Cheng DK (1993). *Fundamentals of Engineering Electromagnetics*. Addison-Wesley.
76. Chatterton PA, Houlden MA (1992). *EMC: Electromagnetic Theory to Practical Design*. John Wiley & Sons.
77. Mills JP (1993). *Electromagnetic Interference Reduction in Electronics Systems.* Prentice Hall, pp. 42–71.
78. Ott HW (1988). *Noise Reduction in Electronic Systems*, 2nd ed. Wiley.
79. Matsuba H, Shintomi K, Yahara A, et al. (1995). Superconducting shield enclosing a human body for biomagnetic measurements. In *Biomagnetism: Fundamental Research and Clinical Applications*.
80. IMEDCO AG. [Online]. Available: www.imedco.ch.
81. Kandori A, Miyashita T, Tsukada K (2000). Cancellation technique of external noise inside a magnetically shielded room used for biomagnetic measurements. *Rev Sci Instrum 71*(5): 2184–2190.
82. Kelha V, Peltonen R, Rantala B (1980). The effect of shaking on magnetic shields. *IEEE Trans Magn 16*(4): 575–578.
83. Platzek D, Nowak H, Giessler F, et al. (1999). Active shielding to reduce low frequency disturbances in direct current near biomagnetic measurements. *Rev Sci Instrum 70*(5): 2465–2470.
84. ter Brake HJ, Huonker R, Rogalla H (1993). New results in active noise compensation for magnetically shielded rooms. *Meas Sci Technol 4*(12): 1370–1375.
85. Malmivuo J, Lekkala J, Kontro P, et al. (1987). Improvement of the properties of an eddy current magnetic shield with active compensation. *J Phys E Sci Instrum 20*(2): 151–164.
86. Bork J, Hahlbohm HD, Klein R, Schnabel A (2001). The 8-layered magnetically shielded room of the PTB: design and construction. *Biomag2000 Proc.*, pp. 970–973.

87. Matsumoto K, Magishi Y, Wakusawa A, et al. (1992). SQUID-based active shield for biomagnetic measurements. *Biomagnetism: Clinical Aspects, Biomag 91*, pp. 506–509.
88. Skakala M, Zrubec V, Manka J (1993). Active compensation for ambient magnetic noise in the unshielded environment. *Meas Sci Technol 4*(4): 468–472.
89. Hilgenfeld B, Strähmel E, Nowak H, Haueisen J (2003). Active magnetic shielding for biomagnetic measurement using spatial gradient fields. *Physiol Meas 24*(3): 661–669.
90. Qiu L, Liu C, Dong H, et al. (2012). Magnetic field improved ULF-NMR measurement in an unshielded laboratory using a low-T_c SQUID. *Phys Procedia 36*: 388–393.
91. ETS-Lindgren. [Online]. Available: www.ets-lindgren.com.
92. Stefan Mayer Instruments. [Online]. Available: www.stefan-mayer.com.
93. Qiu L, Krause H-J, Zhang Y, et al. (2009). The effect of low frequency disturbance to SQUID based low field NMR. *IEEE Trans Appl Supercond 19*(3): 827–830.
94. Dong H, Qiu L, Shi W, et al. (2013). Ultra-low field magnetic resonance imaging detection with gradient compensation in urban unshielded environment. *Appl Phys Lett 102*(13): 102602.
95. Vesanen PT, Nieminen JO, Zevenhoven KC, et al. (2012). The spatial and temporal distortion of magnetic fields applied inside a magnetically shielded room. *IEEE Trans Magn 48*(1): 53–61.
96. Vrba J, Betts K, Burbank M, et al. (1995). Whole cortex 64 channel system for shielded and unshielded environments. In *Biomagnetism: Fundamental Research and Clinical Applications.*
97. Uusitalo MA, Ilmoniemi RJ (1997). Signal-space projection method for separating MEG or EEG into components. *Med Biol Eng Comput 35*(2): 135–140.
98. Volegov P. *Private communication.*

CHAPTER 3

MAGNETIC RESONANCE PHENOMENA AT ULF

The study of NMR phenomena in weak magnetic fields has attracted the attention of researchers since the discovery of NMR. Even though conducting nuclear resonance experiments in weak magnetic fields is difficult due to the very low strength of the NMR induction signal, numerous publications on the topic have continued since the earliest investigations of NMR. Because this chapter is mathematically intensive and we rely on numerous references to provide detail omitted in our discussion, we use B_0 to describe the magnetic polarizing field because it is consistent with most of the references cited. The reader is reminded that the polarizing magnetic field in ULF MRI is often specified as B_p and the magnetic field at which the signal is acquired is B_m.

Initially the interest in NMR phenomenon at low magnetic fields was driven by the question: Does the absolute amplitude of the applied field have an essential influence on the nature of the phenomenon? The first experiments were aimed at verifying the linearity of the dependence of Larmor frequency on the applied magnetic field. Bene et al. [1,2] determined the magnetogyric ratio of the proton and the fluorine nucleus for the fields on the order of a few tens millitesla. Brown [3] experimentally verified the linearity of the dependence of Larmor frequency on the applied magnetic field down to ~1mT with 100 part-per-million (ppm) precision. The hypothesis behind those experiments was that interactions *between* the nuclear magnetic moments or interactions between nuclear magnetic moments and electron magnetic moments will perturb this linear dependence. While this turned out not to be the case, it is interesting to start our discussion thinking about these interactions and why they are so interesting in the ultra-low magnetic field regime.

Conceptually, one can think about these phenomena (chemical shift, J-coupling, relaxation, etc.) as arising purely from nuclear magnetic moments interacting with the surroundings. A single spin in an applied field, while not a very interesting system, is the simplest to treat. To begin let us compare the energy of the NMR transitions with the potential energy of these perturbing interactions. As we saw in Chapter 1, the energy levels of a system of spin I with a magnetic moment μ described by quantum number $I_z = m$ $(m = -1,...,1)$ in the presence of the magnetic field B_0 is given by

(Eqn. 3.1) $$W_{\mathrm{m}} = -\boldsymbol{\mu} \cdot \boldsymbol{B}_0 = -\gamma \hbar m B_0$$

For a spin I = ½ there are two possible magnetic levels, corresponding to m = –½ and ½. Thus in this case the change of energy ΔE associated with a NMR transition (Fig. 3.1)

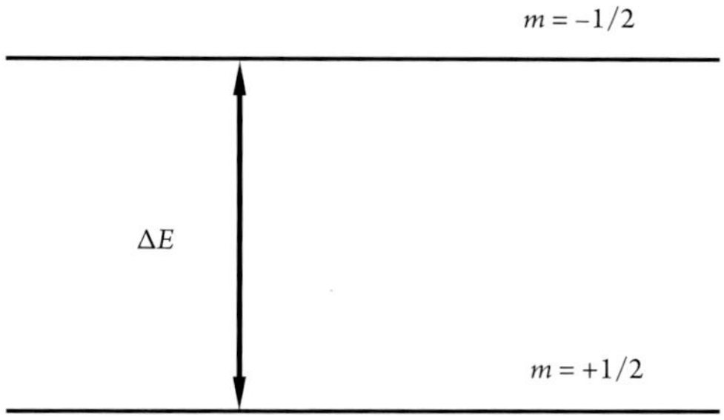

FIGURE 3.1 The magnetic levels for nuclei of spin ½.

is $\Delta E = \gamma\hbar B_0 = \hbar\omega_0$. Using the typical range of magnetic fields considered in this book, B_0~1..1000μT, and assuming that the spin system in question is a proton ($\gamma \approx 2.68\cdot10^8$ radian per Tesla), we will get change of energy range $\Delta E \sim 3\cdot10^{-32}\ldots3\cdot10^{-29}$ Joule or $1.8\cdot10^{-13}\ldots1.8\cdot10^{-10}$ electron-Volt per transition.

The main interaction between the spins of two nuclei is the dipole–dipole coupling between their magnetic moments. To estimate the magnitude of this effect, let's consider dipole–dipole interaction between two magnetic moments, $\mathbf{m}_1$ and $\mathbf{m}_2$ [4]. The potential energy of the interaction for this case is

(Eqn. 3.2)
$$W_{1,2} = \frac{\mu_0}{4\pi}\left\{\frac{\mathbf{m}_1\cdot\mathbf{m}_2}{r_{1,2}^3} - \frac{(\mathbf{m}_1\cdot\mathbf{r}_{1,2})(\mathbf{m}_2\cdot\mathbf{r}_{1,2})}{r_{1,2}^5}\right\}$$

where μ_0 is vacuum permeability, $W_{1,2}$ is the potential energy of the dipolar interaction, and $\mathbf{r}_{1,2}$ is a vector from position of the first magnetic moment to the second. Typically the strength of the nuclear magnetic moments is about a few nuclear magnetons[1] $\mu_{\mathrm{N}} = e\hbar/2m_{\mathrm{p}} \approx 5.051\cdot10^{-27}\ \mathrm{J}\cdot\mathrm{T}^{-1}$, where e is elementary charge and m_{p} is the proton mass. For example, the magnetic moment of the proton itself is $2.79\mu_{\mathrm{N}}$. Since the internuclear distances are on the order of a few Ångström (1Å = 10^{-10}m), the energy of the dipolar coupling will be about $2\cdot10^{-30}$ J or $1.4\cdot10^{-11}$ eV, exactly in the range of NMR transitions of ULF regime.

It may also be illuminating to compare NMR transitions with other interaction energies. This can be instructive in terms of what interactions might be probed by NMR in the ULF regime. We now write the potential energy of the interaction W_{i} as

(Eqn. 3.3)
$$W_{\mathrm{i}} = -\boldsymbol{\mu}\cdot\mathbf{B}_{\mathrm{local}} = -\gamma\hbar m B_{\mathrm{local}},$$

where $\mathbf{B}_{\mathrm{local}}$ is the local magnetic field at the spin position associated with the interaction in question. Assuming the typical potential energy of internuclear interactions ~$2\cdot10^{-30}$ J, we will estimate the strength of the local magnetic fields as $1.4\cdot10^{-4}$ T. The fact that local fields

[1] The nuclear magneton μ_N is used for reporting the magnetic moments of nuclei: $\mu = g_I\mu_N I$, where μ is the magnetic moment of nuclei, g_I is the nuclear g-factor, and I is the spin of nuclei. Nuclear g-factors are empirical parameters of the order of 1.

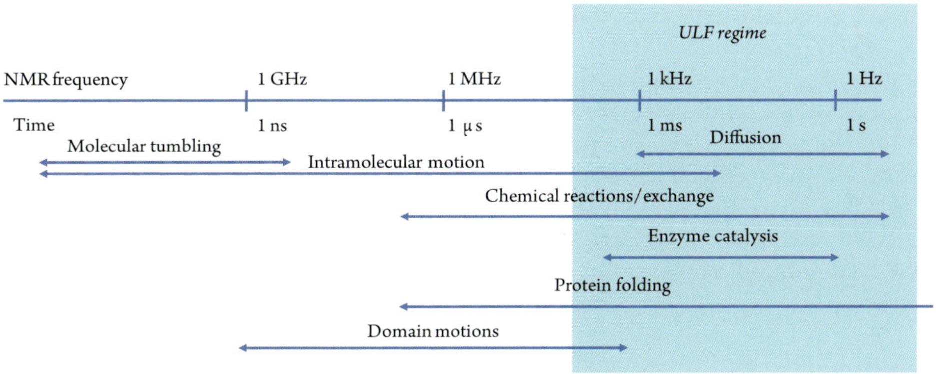

FIGURE 3.2 Timescales of ULF NMR and molecular processes.

(B_{local}) are comparable with the external magnetic field (B_0) under which the NMR signal is observed (i.e., the measurement field in the ULF regime) is a unique and fundamental feature of ULF NMR regime.

Thus, at ULF the local fields have a stronger and more direct effect on the spin evolution, and consequently on the NMR signal, than in traditional HF NMR experiments. On the one hand this direct coupling provides direct information about coupling between nuclei. On the other hand, effects of the local fields can lead to dramatic artifacts for NMR relaxation measurements in the kHz frequency range [5] and impede interpretation of the results, because a simple relaxation model—such as, for example, standard Bloch, Wangsness, and Redfield (BWR) theory [6]—is no longer adequate.

Here we would like to point out that as soon as we define the nuclei with which we are working—let it be protons—we can use frequency units to compare and discuss the strength of the interactions. For example the ULF NMR field range B_0 ~1..1000 μT translates to the Larmor frequency range of ~40..40000 Hz for protons. The potential energy of the internuclear dipole–dipole interaction of $2{\cdot}10^{-30}$ J translates to ~3000 Hz of dipolar broadening.

This frequency point of view leads us to another unique and important feature of NMR phenomenon at ultra-low fields, which originates from the fact that the Larmor frequency in the ULF regime overlaps (on a time scale of 10μs to 100ms) with the rate of molecular dynamic processes such as diffusion, intramolecular motion, chemical reactions, and biological processes (Fig. 3.2).[2] The general notion is that "in order to study atomic or molecular motions, one should employ a kind of spectroscopy involving a time scale comparable to the one under study" [7]. Indeed, local magnetic field fluctuations (e.g., due to particle motion) matching the spin Larmor frequency cause relaxation, so measurements of the magnetic field dependence of relaxation parameters—called the magnetic relaxation dispersion profile (MRD)—at low fields provides information about these "slow" processes, which is not revealed (to any appreciable extent) by conventional high-frequency techniques.

[2] Adapted from Michael Sattler, *Introduction to Biomolecular NMR Spectroscopy*, October 2002. Available at http://www.embl.de/nmr/sattler/teaching

Next, it should be pointed out that due to very low strength of the measurement field, effects proportional to the field strength—such as chemical shift and chemical shift anisotropy—are negligibly small. For example, the typical proton chemical shift of ~10 ppm would result in an absolute difference (or shift) in frequency at, say, 10kHz Larmor frequency of 0.1Hz. This magnitude of shift is typical of most substances and would be extraordinarily difficult to detect at ultra-low fields. That leaves most of the information obtainable with traditional HF NMR chemical shift spectroscopy outside the scope of ULF NMR. However, this shortcoming of the ULF NMR comes with a silver lining: the absence of the field-induced anisotropy in nuclear interactions allows us to study pure spin–spin interactions.

3.1 INTERACTION BETWEEN THE ELECTROMAGNETIC RADIATION AND THE NUCLEAR SPINS AT ULF

Now that we have established a conceptual picture of why NMR phenomena are so rich at ULF, let us move on to develop the formalism that describes the evolution of the spin system in an applied magnetic field. Here we need to mention that in the HF NMR regime, the change of the direction of the applied magnetic field generally occurs on a timescale much slower than the Larmor frequency, which significantly simplifies the analysis of the interaction of the nuclear spins and electromagnetic radiation. In ULF NMR this is generally not true, which opens the door for observing some phenomena that are not evident at high fields. So, when developing the formalism suitable for ULF NMR it may be important to provide the capability to change the magnetic field direction on the timescale comparable with spin precession. We shall explore the details of these interactions and the specific pulse sequences required to tease them out later.

The evolution of magnetic moment $\mathbf{m}$ in the applied magnetic field $\mathbf{B}(t)$ can be described in the frame of classical electrodynamics.

(Eqn. 3.4)
$$\frac{d\mathbf{m}}{dt} = \gamma[\mathbf{m} \times \mathbf{B}]$$

The description of the evolution of the spin system, using either classical electrodynamics or quantum mechanics approaches, is tightly related to the mathematical theory of rotations (rotation group); consequently, it is convenient to rewrite Eqn. 3.4 using matrix notation [8]:

(Eqn. 3.5)
$$\frac{d\mathbf{m}}{dt} + \mathbf{\Omega}^{\times} \cdot \mathbf{m} = \mathbf{0}.$$

It also worth noting that this approach helps to reveal and exploit the similarities in the classical and quantum mechanical description of the spin evolution.

The matrix in Eqn. 3.5 is defined by

(Eqn. 3.6)
$$\mathbf{\Omega}^{\times} \equiv \begin{bmatrix} 0 & -\gamma B_z & \gamma B_y \\ \gamma B_z & 0 & -\gamma B_x \\ -\gamma B_y & \gamma B_x & 0 \end{bmatrix}.$$

This skew-symmetric matrix (i.e., $\mathbf{\Omega}^\times = -\tilde{\mathbf{\Omega}}^\times$), defining the rotation about vector **B**, is called a rotation generator matrix (see, for example, [9,10]).[3] The cross notation, which denotes a rotation generator matrix associated with a vector—for example, $\mathbf{v}^\times$ (pronounced "vee-cross") associated with a vector **v**—is inspired by the relation $\mathbf{v}^\times \cdot \mathbf{a} \equiv [\mathbf{v} \times \mathbf{a}]$ and attributed to Prof. W. Kahan of the University of California at Berkeley [11]. A rotation generator matrix associated with a unit vector is called an *infinitesimal generator.*

The mathematical theory of rotations plays an extremely important role in the description of NMR phenomenon. We now present several practical results necessary for the discussion, but we encourage the reader to consult appropriate sources for a more complete treatment (see, for example, [12,13]).

It is useful to explicitly write out the infinitesimal generators associated with a rotation about the *x*-, *y*-, and *z*-axes (i.e., with rotations about unit vectors $\hat{\mathbf{e}}_1$, $\hat{\mathbf{e}}_2$, $\hat{\mathbf{e}}_3$), called *basic* rotations:

(Eqn. 3.7)
$$\boldsymbol{\alpha}_1 \equiv \hat{\mathbf{e}}_1^\times \equiv \begin{bmatrix} 0 & 0 & 0 \\ 0 & 0 & -1 \\ 0 & 1 & 0 \end{bmatrix}, \ \boldsymbol{\alpha}_2 \equiv \hat{\mathbf{e}}_2^\times \equiv \begin{bmatrix} 0 & 0 & 1 \\ 0 & 0 & 0 \\ -1 & 0 & 0 \end{bmatrix}, \ \boldsymbol{\alpha}_3 \equiv \hat{\mathbf{e}}_3^\times \equiv \begin{bmatrix} 0 & -1 & 0 \\ 1 & 0 & 0 \\ 0 & 1 & 0 \end{bmatrix}.$$

Using these definitions the rotation matrix $\mathbf{\Omega}^\times$ can be written in this basis as

(Eqn. 3.8)
$$\mathbf{\Omega}^\times = \gamma(B_x \boldsymbol{\alpha}_1 + B_y \boldsymbol{\alpha}_2 + B_z \boldsymbol{\alpha}_3).$$

In the simplest case where the applied magnetic field is constant, the solution of Eqn. 3.5 can be written as

(Eqn. 3.9)
$$\mathbf{m}(t) = e^{-\Omega^\times t} \cdot \mathbf{m}_0, \mathbf{m}_0 \equiv \mathbf{m}(t=0)$$

which is nothing but another way to write a clockwise rotation of vector $\mathbf{m}_0$ about the axis aligned with vector **B** with angular velocity $\omega = \gamma|\mathbf{B}|$.

Because matrix exponentials are so important in the description of rotation, we will spend some time explaining their properties. A matrix exponent is defined through the eigenvectors of the matrix as usual:

(Eqn. 3.10)
$$e^{\mathbf{A}} = \sum_k e^{\lambda_k} \mathbf{v}_k \tilde{\mathbf{v}}_k,$$

where $\{\mathbf{v}_k\}$ and $\{\lambda_k\}$ are eigenvectors and eigenvalues of the matrix $\mathbf{A}$(i.e., $\mathbf{A}\cdot\mathbf{v}_k = \lambda_k \mathbf{v}_k$).

Any skew-symmetric matrix $\mathbf{a}^\times$ of the third order (associated with a vector **a**) has the following eigenvalues [14]: $\lambda_k = ika, (k=-1,0,1), i=\sqrt{-1}, a=|\mathbf{a}|$. The eigenvectors $\{\mathbf{v}_k\}_{-1}^{1}$ are not uniquely defined; any complex multiples of these eigenvectors are also eigenvectors. One convenient way to select the eigenvectors of the matrix $\mathbf{a}^\times$ is

(Eqn. 3.11)
$$\mathbf{v}_0 = \hat{\mathbf{a}} \equiv \mathbf{a}/|\mathbf{a}|, \mathbf{v}_{\pm 1} = (\hat{\mathbf{b}} \pm i\hat{\mathbf{c}})/\sqrt{2},$$

---

[3] Here and afterward we use the following conventions: **bold** font denotes vectors and matrices, *italic*—scalars, a hat sign denotes a unit vector, a tilde sign or capital italic superscript *H* denotes a hermitian conjugate, a capital italic superscript *T* denotes a transposed matrix/vector, and the vectors are column vectors.

where $\hat{\mathbf{b}}$ is any unit vector orthogonal to $\hat{\mathbf{a}}$, $\hat{\mathbf{c}} = -\hat{\mathbf{a}}, \hat{\mathbf{b}}$ (i.e., $\{\hat{\mathbf{a}}, \hat{\mathbf{b}}, \hat{\mathbf{c}}\}$) is a right-handed set.

From this last statement it is easy to deduce that the matrix $e^{\phi \hat{\mathbf{a}}^{\times}}$ is nothing other than the matrix describing rotation about vector **a** by angle ϕ.

The eigenvectors of the basic rotations defined according to Eqn. 3.11 are tabulated in Table 3.1.

For convenience we list below, without the proof, useful relationships involving rotation generator matrices, which we will use throughout this book:

(Eqn. 3.12)

a. $\mathbf{a}^{\times} = -\tilde{\mathbf{a}}^{\times}$

b. $(\mathbf{a}+\mathbf{b})^{\times} = \mathbf{a}^{\times} + \mathbf{b}^{\times}$

c. $\mathbf{a}^{\times} \cdot (\mathbf{b}^{\times} \cdot \mathbf{v}) = (\mathbf{a}^{\times} \cdot \mathbf{b}^{\times}) \cdot \mathbf{v}$

d. $\mathbf{a}^{\times} \cdot \mathbf{v} = -\mathbf{v}^{\times} \cdot \mathbf{a}$

e. $\left(\mathbf{a}^{\times} \cdot \mathbf{v}\right)^{\times} = \mathbf{v} \cdot \tilde{\mathbf{a}} - \mathbf{a} \cdot \tilde{\mathbf{v}}$

f. $(\mathbf{Q} \cdot \mathbf{v})^{\times} = \mathbf{Q} \cdot \mathbf{v}^{\times} \cdot \tilde{\mathbf{Q}} \cdot \det(\mathbf{Q})$,

where $\mathbf{Q}$ is an orthogonal matrix (i.e., $\mathbf{Q}^{-1} = \tilde{\mathbf{Q}}$)

g. $\dfrac{d}{d\psi} e^{\psi \mathbf{a}^{\times}} = \mathbf{a}^{\times} \cdot e^{\psi \mathbf{a}^{\times}} = e^{\psi \mathbf{a}^{\times}} \cdot \mathbf{a}^{\times}$

h. $e^{\psi \mathbf{a}^{\times}} \cdot \mathbf{a} = \mathbf{a}$

i. $e^{\psi \mathbf{a}^{\times}} \cdot e^{\phi \mathbf{a}^{\times}} = e^{(\psi+\phi) \mathbf{a}^{\times}}$

j. $$e^{\psi \alpha_1} = \begin{bmatrix} 1 & 0 & 0 \\ 0 & \cos\psi & -\sin\psi \\ 0 & \sin\psi & \cos\psi \end{bmatrix}, e^{\psi \alpha_2} = \begin{bmatrix} \cos\psi & 0 & \sin\psi \\ 0 & 1 & 0 \\ -\sin\psi & 0 & \cos\psi \end{bmatrix},$$

$$e^{\psi \alpha_3} = \begin{bmatrix} \cos\psi & -\sin\psi & 0 \\ \sin\psi & \cos\psi & 0 \\ 0 & 0 & 1 \end{bmatrix}$$

TABLE 3.1 Eigenvectors of the Basic Rotations

	$\mathbf{V}_{-1}$	$\mathbf{V}_0$	$\mathbf{V}_{+1}$
α_1	$\frac{1}{\sqrt{2}}(\hat{\mathbf{e}}_2 + i\hat{\mathbf{e}}_3)$	$\hat{\mathbf{e}}_1$	$\frac{1}{\sqrt{2}}(\hat{\mathbf{e}}_2 - i\hat{\mathbf{e}}_3)$
α_2	$\frac{1}{\sqrt{2}}(\hat{\mathbf{e}}_1 + i\hat{\mathbf{e}}_3)$	$\hat{\mathbf{e}}_2$	$\frac{1}{\sqrt{2}}(\hat{\mathbf{e}}_1 - i\hat{\mathbf{e}}_3)$
α_3	$\frac{1}{\sqrt{2}}(\hat{\mathbf{e}}_1 + i\hat{\mathbf{e}}_2)$	$\hat{\mathbf{e}}_3$	$\frac{1}{\sqrt{2}}(\hat{\mathbf{e}}_1 - i\hat{\mathbf{e}}_2)$

Taking into account the properties of the rotation generator matrix, the matrix exponential in Eqn. 3.9 can be also written explicitly as

$$e^{\Omega^{\times}t} = \mathbf{I} + \hat{\mathbf{b}}^{\times} \cdot \sin(\omega t) + \left(1 - \cos(\omega t)\right) \cdot (\hat{\mathbf{b}}^{\times})^2, \tag{Eqn. 3.13}$$

where $\mathbf{I}$ is the identity matrix, $\hat{\mathbf{b}} = \mathbf{B}/|\mathbf{B}|$ is a unit vector in the direction of the magnetic field, $\hat{\mathbf{b}}^{\times}$ is infinitesimal generator associated with the vector $\hat{\mathbf{b}}$, and $\omega = \gamma|\mathbf{B}|$ is the precession frequency. The Eqn. 3.13 is known as *Rodrigues' identity*. This last formula can be also written as

$$e^{\Omega^{\times}t} = \mathbf{I}\cos(\omega t) + \hat{\mathbf{b}}^{\times} \cdot \sin(\omega t) + \left(1 - \cos(\omega t)\right) \cdot \hat{\mathbf{b}} \cdot \tilde{\hat{\mathbf{b}}}, \tag{Eqn. 3.14}$$

where we used the identity $(\hat{\mathbf{b}}^{\times})^2 = \hat{\mathbf{b}} \cdot \tilde{\hat{\mathbf{b}}} - \mathbf{I}$, and $\hat{\mathbf{b}} \cdot \tilde{\hat{\mathbf{b}}}$ is a projector on a vector $\hat{\mathbf{b}}$.

3.1.1 Adiabatic vs. Non-adiabatic Field Rotation

As we discussed in Chapter 1, it is not typical (and seldom possible) for the magnetic field in conventional MRI to change direction, but the direction of the magnetic field in the ULF NMR regime can easily change direction. In fact, reorientation of the magnetic field direction is an important and often-used feature in ULF MRI pulse sequences (see Chapter 4). Therefore it is important to develop a formalism that can take into account the change of the direction of the magnetic field. The change with time of the magnetic field $\mathbf{B}$ can be described quite generally by a rotation and a scaling:

$$\mathbf{B}(t) \equiv \mathbf{B} = \frac{\omega}{\gamma} \cdot \mathbf{R} \cdot \hat{\mathbf{b}}_0, \tag{Eqn. 3.15}$$

where $\omega \equiv \omega(t)$ is the instantaneous precession frequency; $\mathbf{R} \equiv \mathbf{R}(t)$ is a proper rotation matrix (i.e., rotation without a reflection), which has the following properties: $\tilde{\mathbf{R}} = \mathbf{R}^{-1}, \det(\mathbf{R}) = 1$; and $\hat{\mathbf{b}}_0$ is a constant unit vector.

In this case we can write

$$\frac{d\mathbf{m}}{dt} + \omega \cdot \left(\mathbf{R} \cdot \hat{\mathbf{b}}_0\right)^{\times} \cdot \mathbf{m} = 0, \tag{Eqn. 3.16}$$

where $(\mathbf{R} \cdot \hat{\mathbf{b}}_0)^{\times}$ denotes infinitesimal rotation generator associated with the vector $\mathbf{R} \cdot \hat{\mathbf{b}}_0$ (i.e., with the instantaneous direction of the magnetic field).

Let us consider Eqn. 3.16 in the rotating frame of reference, which continuously follows the rotation of the magnetic field as shown in Figure 3.3. As with any other vector, the magnetization vector in the laboratory frame of reference—$\mathbf{m}$—is related to the magnetization vector in this moving frame of reference the magnetization—$\mathbf{m}'$—by the following relation: $\mathbf{m} = \mathbf{R} \cdot \mathbf{m}'$. To obtain the equation for the magnetization vector in the moving frame we use the usual approach to change the frame of reference. Expressing the derivative of the

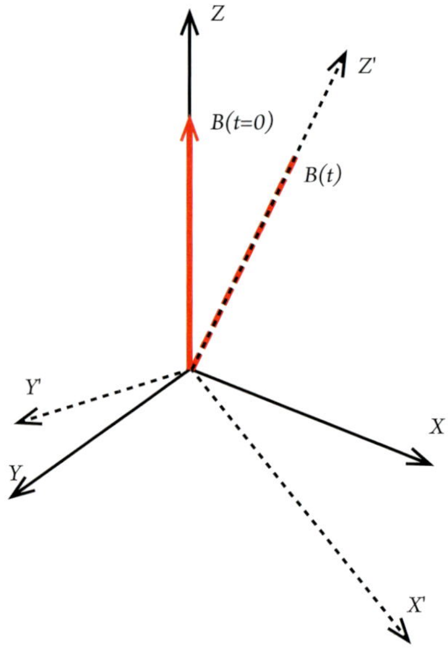

FIGURE 3.3 Moving reference frame.

magnetization vector in the laboratory frame through the derivative of the magnetization vector in the moving frame:

$$\frac{d}{dt}\mathbf{m} = \frac{d}{dt}(\mathbf{R}\cdot\mathbf{m}') = \frac{d\mathbf{R}}{dt}\cdot\mathbf{m}' + \mathbf{R}\cdot\frac{d}{dt}\mathbf{m}'$$

and using this last relation in Eqn. 3.16 we get the equation for the evolution of the magnetic moment in the moving reference frame:

(Eqn. 3.17)
$$\frac{d\mathbf{m}'}{dt} + \left(\omega\cdot\tilde{\mathbf{R}}\cdot\left(\mathbf{R}\cdot\hat{\mathbf{b}}_0\right)^{\times}\cdot\mathbf{R} + \tilde{\mathbf{R}}\cdot\frac{d\mathbf{R}}{dt}\right)\cdot\mathbf{m}' = 0.$$

The term $\tilde{\mathbf{R}}\cdot\frac{d\mathbf{R}}{dt}$ is usually referred to as "effective" magnetic field in the moving (rotating) frame of reference. Time derivative of any differentiable rotating matrix can be written as:

(Eqn. 3.18)
$$\frac{d\mathbf{R}}{dt} = \psi\cdot\mathbf{R}\cdot\hat{\mathbf{u}}^{\times} = \psi\cdot\hat{\mathbf{u}}^{\times}\cdot\mathbf{R}$$

where $\hat{\mathbf{u}}^{\times}$ is infinitesimal generator associated with the instantaneous rotation axis, defined by a unit vector $\hat{\mathbf{u}}$, and ψ is instantaneous angular velocity of rotation.

Using Eqn. 3.18, and the identity in Eqn. 12f, we can simplify Eqn. 3.17 and finally write the magnetization equation in the frame of reference following the magnetic field as

(Eqn. 3.19)
$$\frac{d\mathbf{m}'}{dt} + \left(\omega\cdot\hat{\mathbf{b}}_0^{\times} + \psi\cdot\hat{\mathbf{u}}^{\times}\right)\cdot\mathbf{m}' = 0,$$

where $\psi \cdot \hat{\mathbf{u}}^{\times}$ constitutes the effective magnetic field in the moving frame of reference. We can now see that the differential of magnetization (i.e., infinitesimal change of magnetization) in our moving reference frame is orthogonal to the magnetization and consists of two terms: $\omega \cdot \hat{\mathbf{b}}_0^{\times} \cdot \mathbf{m}' \cdot dt$ (rotation about the constant axis $\hat{\mathbf{b}}_0$ with angular velocity ω) and $\psi \cdot \hat{\mathbf{u}}^{\times} \cdot \mathbf{m}' \cdot dt$ (rotation about the instantaneous axis $\hat{\mathbf{u}}$ with angular velocity ψ, which, as we remember, is the instantaneous angular velocity of magnetic field rotation). Because we have $\left\|\hat{\mathbf{b}}_0^{\times}\right\| = \left\|\hat{\mathbf{u}}^{\times}\right\| = 1$, the relative contribution of these two terms is proportional to ω and ψ respectively. Here it is important to highlight two limiting cases: (a) when the spin precession frequency is much higher than the angular velocity of magnetic field rotation (i.e., $|\omega| \gg |\psi|$) and (b) when the spin precession rate is much lower than the rate of magnetic field rotation (i.e., $|\omega| \ll |\psi|$). It is easy to see that in the two cases presented, $|\omega| \gg |\psi|$ and $|\omega| \ll |\psi|$, we can safely neglect either the second or first term of Eqn. 3.19 respectively to solve the equation.

In the first case, where $|\omega| \gg |\psi|$, the magnetization simply precesses around the constant axis $\hat{\mathbf{b}}_0$ with variable angular velocity ω. So, in the moving frame of reference we have

(Eqn. 3.20) $$\mathbf{m}' = e^{-\phi(t)\hat{\mathbf{b}}_0^{\times}} \cdot \mathbf{m}_0', \mathbf{m}_0' \equiv \mathbf{m}'(t=0), \phi(t) = \int_0^t \omega(t')dt'.$$

Respectively in the laboratory frame we have:

(Eqn. 3.21) $$\mathbf{m} = \mathbf{R} \cdot e^{-\phi(t)\hat{\mathbf{b}}_0^{\times}} \cdot \mathbf{m}_0,$$

where we assume that $\mathbf{R}(t=0) = \mathbf{I}$.

So we can see that in this case, the magnetization precessing about the instantaneous magnetic field and follows the magnetic field, keeping the constant angle α with the magnetic field:

$$\cos(\alpha) = \frac{(\tilde{\mathbf{m}} \cdot \mathbf{B})}{|\mathbf{m}| \cdot |\mathbf{B}|} = \left(\mathbf{R} \cdot e^{-\phi(t)\hat{\mathbf{b}}_0^{\times}} \cdot \frac{\mathbf{m}_0}{|\mathbf{m}_0|}\right)^T \cdot (\mathbf{R} \cdot \hat{\mathbf{b}}_0) = \frac{\tilde{\mathbf{m}}_0 \cdot e^{\phi(t)\hat{\mathbf{b}}_0^{\times}} \cdot \tilde{\mathbf{R}} \cdot \mathbf{R} \cdot \hat{\mathbf{b}}_0}{|\mathbf{m}_0|} = \frac{(\tilde{\mathbf{m}}_0 \cdot \hat{\mathbf{b}}_0)}{|\mathbf{m}_0|} = const,$$

which constitutes the *adiabatic theorem* [5].

This slow (relative to the Larmor frequency) rotation of magnetic field is called an *adiabatic* rotation.

We now describe a practical example of an adiabatic rotation used in our ULF MRI systems. Initially the pre-polarization field B_p and magnetization are along an axis we define as $\hat{x}$. The measurement field B_m is oriented orthogonally along the $\hat{z}$ axis. The amplitude of the B_p field is typically ~30 to 100mT, whereas the amplitude of B_m field is approximately 100μT. If B_p is then removed such that the field rotates adiabatically, the magnetization will eventually end up aligned along B_m (i.e., the $\hat{z}$ axis). In this case there will be no precession until spin reorientation is induced (e.g., by a spin-flip pulse).

In the simplest case, one would remove B_p by ramping the field down linearly, requiring that the criteria $|\omega| \gg |\psi|$ be met during the entire ramp. There are applications and experiments in which it may useful to minimize the time required to ramp B_p down while still following the general criteria of adiabatic field rotation, $|\omega| \gg |\psi|$. So we ask: How fast can we remove B_p? As the measurement and polarization fields are orthogonal we have the following formula for the angular velocity of magnetic field rotation during polarization field removal:

$$\psi = \frac{d}{dt}\arctan\frac{B_p}{B_m} = \frac{1}{1+(B_p/B_m)}\cdot\frac{1}{B_m}\cdot\frac{dB_p}{dt}.$$

Requiring that this angular velocity were much less than the Larmor frequency, which is equal to $\omega = \gamma\sqrt{B_m^2 + B_p^2}$, we will get

(Eqn. 3.22)
$$\left|\frac{dB_p}{dt}\right| << \gamma B_m^2 \cdot \left(1+\frac{B_p^2}{B_m^2}\right)^{1/2} \cdot \left(1+\frac{|B_p|}{|B_m|}\right).$$

Because terms in brackets >1 in this inequality we can neglect them. This will give us the criteria of adiabatic removal of polarization field typically used in ULF NMR regime:

(Eqn. 3.23)
$$\left|\frac{dB_p}{dt}\right| << \gamma B_m^2.$$

We note that by solving the autonomous differential equation (Eqn. 22), we will get an implicit[4] formula defining the most efficient (i.e., fastest) way to switch off the polarization field:

(Eqn. 3.24)
$$t = -\frac{\alpha}{\gamma}\int_{B_p(t=0)}^{B_p(t)} \frac{d\xi}{(B_m^2+\xi^2)^{1/2}\cdot(B_m+\xi)},$$

where t is time, $B_p(t)$ is time dependence of the polarization field, and α is "how much less" is the angular frequency of magnetic field rotation compared to the Larmor frequency. The following equation defines the shortest time during which the polarization field can be removed adiabatically:

(Eqn. 3.25)
$$T_{off} = -\frac{\alpha}{\gamma B_m}\int_{B_p/B_m}^{0} \frac{d\xi}{(1+\xi^2)^{1/2}\cdot(1+\xi)}.$$

The adiabatic rotation can be quite beneficial for some pulse sequences, for example where a slowly changing B_p minimizes induced eddy currents in nearby conducting material. However, it has the disadvantage that it takes time (during which your spins are

[4] The explicit relation can be obtained using the following integral:

$$\int \frac{dx}{(x+b)\sqrt{x^2+a^2}} = \frac{1}{\sqrt{x^2+a^2}}\ln\left|\frac{a^2-bx-\sqrt{(a^2+b^2)(x^2+a^2)}}{x+b}\right|$$

undergoing T_1 relaxation). For example, to realize the adiabatic rotation in the example above, it takes about 230ms using linear ramp-down (i.e., the criteria in Eqn. 23), or 60ms using ramp-down waveform defined by Eqn. 3.24 (assuming $\alpha = 300$).

In the second case, where $|\omega| \ll |\psi|$, the solution of Eqn. 3.19 is simple:

(Eqn. 3.26) $$\mathbf{m}' = \tilde{\mathbf{R}} \cdot \mathbf{m}'_0.$$

In the rotating frame and in the laboratory frame we have

(Eqn. 3.27) $$\mathbf{m} = \mathbf{R} \cdot \tilde{\mathbf{R}} \cdot \mathbf{m}_0 = \mathbf{m}_0.$$

This last equation simply tells us that if the magnetic field rotates significantly faster than the Larmor frequency, then it has no effect on spin evolution. This fast (relative to the Larmor frequency) rotation of the magnetic field is called a *non-adiabatic* rotation.

At the other extreme is the non-adiabatic rotation that provides a different set of advantages that we apply to various imaging applications in our ULF MRI systems. In a non-adiabatic pulse sequence, the pre-polarization field B_p and magnetization are initially oriented along an axis we define as $\hat{x}$. The measurement field B_m is oriented orthogonally along the $\hat{z}$ axis. If we then remove B_p such that $|dB_p/dt| \gg \gamma B_m^2$ (non-adiabatically such that the orientation of the spin population does not have time to reorient), the magnetization will remain aligned along B_p (i.e., the $\hat{x}$ axis). In this case precession about $\hat{z}$ (B_m) will begin immediately, more precisely as soon as B_p becomes comparable with B_m. The non-adiabatic rotation has the benefit that no spin-flip pulse is needed to begin precession and is, in principle, the faster route to acquiring the precession signal. However, in practice we must often wait for induced transients to die down to a level that allows us to acquire usable NMR data, which imposes an effective hardware or signal dead time that can offset this benefit. Hardware dead time results when the SQUID sensors used to acquire the ULF MRI signal are unable to function properly due to the large transient. Signal dead time is when the ULF MRI signal is overwhelmed by the transient signal, even if the SQUID sensor is capable of accurately measuring the field.

The practical assumption in HF that the field doesn't change direction at all greatly simplifies the analysis. In ULF, however, the change of field direction has to be factored in. A further complication is in the regime where the rate at which the polarization field is removed is intermediate between the adiabatic and non-adiabatic case.

Let us illustrate the intermediate regime between adiabatic and non-adiabatic rotation of the magnetic field using a simple example themed after a geometrical phase phenomenon (Berry phase; see, for example, [15]). In this example, we start with a population of spins precessing about a magnetic field that we define to be aligned with the z-axis, then rotate the field clockwise first about the x-axis by $\pi/2$, then about the z-axis by $\pi/2$, and finally about the y-axis by $\pi/2$, as shown in Figure 3.4. We are interested in the difference in direction of the magnetization between the cases where the magnetic field changed orientation (as described previously) and where it remained static, assuming that the evolution time T is the same for static and rotating field cases.

In the static case, in the laboratory frame the magnetization vector just precesses about the z-axis, so at the end of evolution period, it will be

(Eqn. 3.28) $$\mathbf{m}(T) = e^{-\omega T \cdot \alpha_3} \mathbf{m}_0,$$

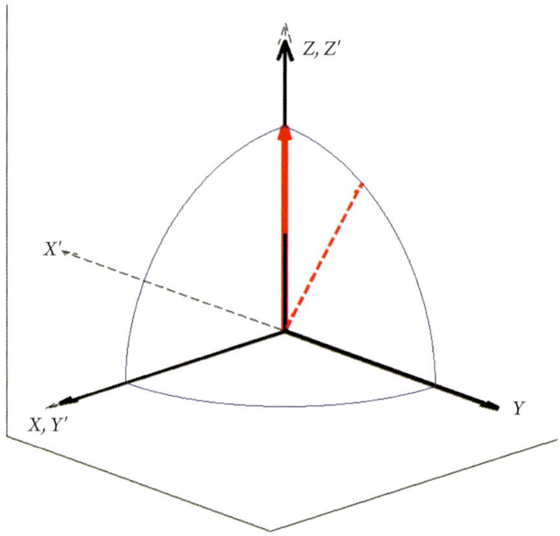

FIGURE 3.4 Geometric phase experiment field rotation.

where $\omega = \gamma\,|\mathbf{B}|$ is the Larmor frequency. Recall that the matrix $e^{-\omega T \cdot \alpha_3}$ is clockwise rotation about the z-axis by angle ωT.

In the case of the rotating field we will get the following equation for the magnetization in the reference frame aligned with the magnetic field:

(Eqn. 3.29)
$$\frac{d\mathbf{m}'}{dt} + \omega' \cdot \mathbf{u} \cdot \mathbf{m}' = 0$$

where $\omega' = \sqrt{\omega^2 + \psi^2}$ is an effective Larmor frequency, ψ is angular velocity of magnetic field rotation, and the matrix $\mathbf{u}$ is different for the three stages of our example rotations:

(a) magnetic field rotates about the x-axis: $\mathbf{u} = \mathbf{u}_a = (\omega \cdot \boldsymbol{\alpha}_3 - \psi \cdot \boldsymbol{\alpha}_1)/\omega'$,
(b) magnetic field rotates about the z-axis: $\mathbf{u} = \mathbf{u}_b = (\omega \cdot \boldsymbol{\alpha}_3 - \psi \cdot \boldsymbol{\alpha}_2)/\omega'$,
(c) magnetic field rotates about the y-axis: $\mathbf{u} = \mathbf{u}_c = (\omega \cdot \boldsymbol{\alpha}_3 + \psi \cdot \boldsymbol{\alpha}_1)/\omega'$.

Since during these three stages in the moving frame of reference we have precession about a static field, the resulting magnetization at the end of evolution period will be

$$\mathbf{m}'_{rotating} = e^{-\frac{\omega' T}{3} \cdot \mathbf{u}_c} \cdot e^{-\frac{\omega' T}{3} \cdot \mathbf{u}_b} \cdot e^{-\frac{\omega' T}{3} \cdot \mathbf{u}_a} \cdot \mathbf{m}'_0 .$$

Correspondently, in the laboratory frame we have

$$\mathbf{m}_{\text{rotating}} = \mathbf{R}(T) \cdot \mathbf{m}' = \mathbf{R}(T) \cdot e^{-\frac{\omega' T}{3} \cdot \mathbf{u}_c} \cdot e^{-\frac{\omega' T}{3} \cdot \mathbf{u}_b} \cdot e^{-\frac{\omega' T}{3} \cdot \mathbf{u}_a} \cdot \mathbf{m}_0 ,$$

where $\mathbf{R}(T) \equiv \mathbf{R}(t = T)$ is the matrix describing rotation of the magnetic field, so that $\mathbf{B}(t) = \mathbf{R}(t) \cdot \mathbf{B}(t = 0)$. Recalling the sequence of the field rotations, we see that at the end of the evolution period the matrix $\mathbf{R}(T)$ is nothing other than a rotation about the z-axis by $-\pi/2$:

$$\mathbf{R}(T)=e^{-\frac{\pi}{2}\alpha_1}\cdot e^{-\frac{\pi}{2}\alpha_3}\cdot e^{-\frac{\pi}{2}\alpha_2}=e^{-\frac{\pi}{2}\alpha_3}.$$

This is also illustrated in Figure 3.4, where we see that initially the moving frame coordinate axes, $\hat{\mathbf{x}}',\hat{\mathbf{y}}',\hat{\mathbf{z}}'$, were aligned with the laboratory coordinate system axes $\hat{\mathbf{x}}, \hat{\mathbf{y}}, \hat{\mathbf{z}}$, but at the end the moving frame axes are aligned with $-\hat{\mathbf{y}}, \hat{\mathbf{x}}, \hat{\mathbf{z}}$, axes. So in this case for the magnetization at the end of the evolution period we have

(Eqn. 3.30)
$$\mathbf{m}_{\text{rotating}}=e^{-\frac{\pi}{2}\alpha_3}\cdot e^{-\frac{\omega' T}{3}\mathbf{u}_c}\cdot e^{-\frac{\omega' T}{3}\mathbf{u}_b}\cdot e^{-\frac{\omega' T}{3}\mathbf{u}_a}\cdot\mathbf{m}_0.$$

In the case of adiabatic rotation (i.e., when $|\omega|\gg|\psi|$), we have $\omega'\approx\omega$ and $\mathbf{u}_a\approx\mathbf{u}_b\approx\mathbf{u}_c\,\boldsymbol{\alpha}_3$, and the solution of Eqn. 3.29 is simply

(Eqn. 3.31)
$$\mathbf{m}_{\text{adiabatic}}=e^{-\left(\omega T+\frac{\pi}{2}\right)\alpha_3}\mathbf{m}_0.$$

Consequently, the magnetization in our example three-step rotation at the end of the evolution period (where the total evolution time, T, consists of three $\pi/2$ rotations, each consuming $T/3$ time) is rotated by an additional $-\pi/2$ angle about the z-axis, compared with the static case (see Eqn. 3.28). This additional angle, or phase, exactly constitutes a geometric phase effect, which was described by Prof. Sir Michael Berry, the discoverer of this effect, as "remarkable and rather mysterious" [16].

In the case of non-adiabatic rotation (i.e., when $|\omega|\ll|\psi|$), we have $\omega'\approx\psi$ and $|\omega|T\ll 1$, resulting in

(Eqn. 3.32)
$$\mathbf{m}_{\text{non-adiabatic}}=\mathbf{m}_{\text{static}}=\mathbf{m}_0,$$

which tells us that in the non-adiabatic case field rotation does not introduce any additional phase shift. So, now we ask: What about when the rotation is intermediate? While it is straightforward to compute the end magnetization vector $\mathbf{m}_{\text{rotating}}$ for each specific case using Eqn. 3.30, in general this is quite tedious. To get an idea of what the effect of the magnetic field rotation may be when the adiabatic approximation cannot be used, we expand Eqn. 3.30 in Taylor series assuming $|\omega|>|\psi|$ and keeping only terms to the first order of ψ/ω:

(Eqn. 3.33)
$$\mathbf{m}_{\text{rotating}}=e^{-\left(\omega' T+\frac{\pi}{2}\right)\boldsymbol{\alpha}_3}\mathbf{m}_0+\left(\frac{\psi}{\omega}\right)e^{-\frac{\pi}{2}\boldsymbol{\alpha}_3}\left(p\boldsymbol{\alpha}_2+q(\boldsymbol{\alpha}_3\boldsymbol{\alpha}_2+\boldsymbol{\alpha}_2\boldsymbol{\alpha}_3)\right)\cdot\mathbf{m}_0+O\left(\left(\frac{\psi}{\omega}\right)^2|\mathbf{m}_0|\right),$$

where

$$p=\sin(\omega T)\cdot(2\cos(\omega T)-1)\cdot(2\sin(\omega T)-1);\text{ and}$$

$$q=-(\cos(\omega T)-1)\cdot(2\cos(\omega T)+1)\cdot(2\sin(\omega T)-1).$$

Comparing Eqns. 3.33 and 3.31, we see that violation of the adiabatic rotation condition results in an additional phase shift $\Delta\phi = (\omega' - \omega)T \approx 1/2 \cdot \psi^2 T / \omega$. In addition to this phase shift we see that the magnetization changes angle with magnetic field, as indicated by the second term in Eqn. 3.33, which is expected in the non-adiabatic case. The second term in Eqn. 3.33 can be explicitly written in vector components:

$$\frac{\psi}{\omega} e^{-\frac{\pi}{2}\alpha_3}(\ldots)\cdot \mathbf{m}_0 = \frac{\psi}{\omega} q(\hat{\mathbf{e}}_3^T \cdot \mathbf{m}_0)\hat{\mathbf{e}}_1 + \frac{\psi}{\omega} p(\hat{\mathbf{e}}_3^T \cdot \mathbf{m}_0)\hat{\mathbf{e}}_2 + \frac{\psi}{\omega}((q\hat{\mathbf{e}}_1^T + p\hat{\mathbf{e}}_2^T)\cdot \mathbf{m}_0)\hat{\mathbf{e}}_3 .$$

From this last relation we see that even if the magnetization vector was initially orthogonal to the magnetic field, after the field rotation we have a fraction of magnetization $\sim \psi|\mathbf{m}_0|/\omega$ aligned with the magnetic field, which is not the case for the adiabatic field rotation.

A practical example of this phenomenon can be observed during field-echo sequence. While this is discussed in detail in Chapter 4, we simply mention here that the field echo is generated by inverting the polarity of the total magnetic field in the system. This inversion of magnetic field is actually a rotation, and depending on the rate of the magnetic field change and the magnitude of the residual fields, which are invariably present in any practical system, it can be adiabatic, non-adiabatic, or anything in between. While it is commonly assumed that the field inversion during field-echo sequence is invoked non-adiabatically, the residual magnetic fields can lead to the violation of non-adiabatic condition, resulting in "ghost" artifact in the reconstructed image. While this artifact will appear much like an aliasing artifact, it has a rather different origin associated with the violation of the condition of non-adiabatic field rotation.

3.1.2 Interaction with an Alternating Magnetic Field

The traditional treatment of NMR (and MRI) describes the applied magnetic field as consisting of a constant field $\mathbf{B}_0$ and some variable field $\mathbf{B}_1(t)$, so that $\mathbf{B}(t) = \mathbf{B}_0 + \mathbf{B}_1(t)$. While in HF NMR experiments the variable field is usually much smaller than the static field, we find that in the ULF regime the $\mathbf{B}_1(t)$ is often not small relative to $\mathbf{B}_0$, which accounts for a number of effects usually not detectable at HF experiments. As an example let us consider the simple case when the spin population placed in the static magnetic field is irradiated by alternating magnetic field orthogonal to the static field.

So in our case we have

(Eqn. 3.34)
$$\frac{d\mathbf{m}}{dt} + (\mathbf{\Omega}_0 + \mathbf{\Omega}_1)\cdot \mathbf{m} = 0,$$

where $\mathbf{\Omega}_0$ and $\mathbf{\Omega}_1$ are rotation generators (see Eqn. 3.6) associated with fields $\mathbf{B}_0$ and $\mathbf{B}_1(t)$ respectively. It is convenient to transform the previous equation into rotating coordinates (i.e., to the frame of reference that continuously follows the rotation of the magnetic moment around the static field $\mathbf{B}_0$). The magnetic moment in the rotating frame of reference can be written as

(Eqn. 3.35)
$$\mathbf{m}' = e^{\Omega_0 t}\mathbf{m}.$$

Here the primed quantity denotes that the quantity in question belongs to the rotating frame of reference.

As usual, writing explicitly the derivative of the magnetization vector as

$$\mathbf{m} = e^{-\Omega_0 t}\mathbf{m}', \quad \text{and } \frac{d}{dt}\mathbf{m} = \frac{d}{dt}\left(e^{-\Omega_0 t}\mathbf{m}'\right) = -\mathbf{\Omega}_0 e^{-\Omega_0 t}\mathbf{m}' + e^{-\Omega_0 t}\frac{d}{dt}\mathbf{m}'$$

we will obtain the equation for the magnetic moment evolution in the rotating frame:

(Eqn. 3.36)
$$\frac{d\mathbf{m}'}{dt} + \mathbf{\Omega}_1' \cdot \mathbf{m}' = 0.$$

We now impose a typical change of the coordinate system by a similarity transformation:

(Eqn. 3.37)
$$\mathbf{\Omega}_1' = e^{\Omega_0 t}\mathbf{\Omega}_1 e^{-\Omega_0 t}.$$

Now, assume that the static field is aligned with the z-axis. In this case $\mathbf{\Omega}_0 = \omega_0 \boldsymbol{\alpha}_3$, where the $\omega_0 = \gamma|\mathbf{B}_0|$ is the frequency of precession around the static field and $\boldsymbol{\alpha}_3$ is the infinitesimal generator associated with rotation about the z-axis.

In the general case an alternating magnetic field with angular frequency ω orthogonal to the z-axis can be written as

(Eqn. 3.38)
$$\mathbf{B}_1(t) = B_x \cos(\omega t + \phi_x)\hat{\mathbf{e}}_1 + B_y \cos(\omega t + \phi_y)\hat{\mathbf{e}}_2.$$

It is convenient to write this field as a superposition of two circular polarized fields rotating in opposite directions about the z-axis:

(Eqn. 3.39)
$$\mathbf{B}_1(t) = \frac{\omega_+}{\gamma} e^{-\omega t \alpha_3} \cdot \hat{\mathbf{b}}_+ + \frac{\omega_-}{\gamma} e^{\omega t \alpha_3} \cdot \hat{\mathbf{b}}_-,$$

following the traditional NMR conventions where a positive subscript denotes clockwise rotation, so that ω_+ / γ and ω_- / γ are amplitudes of the fields rotating about the z-axis clockwise and counterclockwise respectively, and unit vectors $\hat{\mathbf{b}}_\pm$ define the phases of these rotating fields, so that

(Eqn. 3.40)
$$\frac{\omega_\pm}{\gamma} \cdot \hat{\mathbf{b}}_\pm = \frac{1}{2}\left(B_x \cos(\phi_x) \mp B_y \sin(\phi_y)\right) \cdot \hat{\mathbf{e}}_1 + \frac{1}{2}\left(B_y \cos(\phi_y) \pm B_x \sin(\phi_x)\right) \cdot \hat{\mathbf{e}}_2.$$

It is obvious that in the rotating frame of reference this field will consist of the "slow" field rotating with the angular frequency $\omega - \omega_0$ and the "fast" field rotating with the angular frequency $\omega + \omega_0$ in the opposite direction:

(Eqn. 3.41)
$$\mathbf{B}_1'(t) = \frac{\omega_+}{\gamma} \cdot e^{-(\omega-\omega_0)t\alpha_3} \cdot \hat{\mathbf{b}}_+ + \frac{\omega_-}{\gamma} \cdot e^{(\omega+\omega_0)t\alpha_3} \cdot \hat{\mathbf{b}}_-.$$

Correspondingly, the rotation generator matrix associated with this field (i.e., matrix $\mathbf{\Omega}_1'$) will be

(Eqn. 3.42)
$$\mathbf{\Omega}_1' = \omega_+ e^{-(\omega-\omega_0)t\alpha_3} \cdot \mathbf{u}_+ \cdot e^{(\omega-\omega_0)t\alpha_3} + \omega_- e^{(\omega+\omega_0)t\alpha_3} \cdot \mathbf{u}_- \cdot e^{-(\omega+\omega_0)t\pm_3}$$

where $\mathbf{u}_+$ and $\mathbf{u}_-$ are infinitesimal rotation generators associated with unit vectors $\hat{\mathbf{b}}_+$ and $\hat{\mathbf{b}}_-$ respectively.

Under the resonant conditions (i.e., $\omega = \omega_0$) we have

(Eqn. 3.43)
$$\mathbf{B}_1'(t) = \frac{\omega_+}{\gamma}\cdot\hat{\mathbf{b}}_+ + \frac{\omega_-}{\gamma}\cdot e^{2\omega_0 t\alpha_3}\cdot\hat{\mathbf{b}}_-$$

(Eqn. 3.44)
$$\mathbf{\Omega}_1' = \omega_+\mathbf{u}_+ + \omega_- e^{2\omega_0 t\alpha_3}\cdot\mathbf{u}_-\cdot e^{-2\omega_0 t\alpha_3}$$

which yields a static field $\mathbf{B}_+' = \omega_+/\gamma\cdot\hat{\mathbf{b}}_+$ and alternating field $\mathbf{B}_-'(t) = \omega_-/\gamma\cdot e^{2\omega_0 t\alpha_3}\cdot\hat{\mathbf{b}}_-$.

Transforming Eqn. 3.36 into the rotating frame of reference associated with the precession about $\mathbf{B}_+'$ we will get

(Eqn. 3.45)
$$\mathbf{m}'' = e^{\omega_+ t\cdot\mathbf{u}_+}\cdot\mathbf{m}' = e^{\omega_+ t\cdot\mathbf{u}_+}\cdot e^{\omega_0 t\cdot\alpha_3}\cdot\mathbf{m}$$

and

(Eqn. 3.46)
$$\frac{d\mathbf{m}''}{dt} + \omega_-\cdot\mathbf{u}_-''\cdot\mathbf{m}'' = 0$$
$$\mathbf{u}_-'' = e^{\omega_+ t\cdot\mathbf{u}_+}\cdot e^{2\omega_0 t\cdot\alpha_3}\cdot\mathbf{u}_-\cdot e^{-2\omega_0 t\cdot\alpha_3}\cdot e^{-\omega_+ t\cdot\mathbf{u}_+}.$$

Here a double-primed quantity denotes that the quantity in question belongs to this new rotating frame of reference.

Eqn. 3.46 describes evolution of magnetization in the presence of a rotating field of constant magnitude. As we saw earlier (see Eqn. 3.19 and discussion about adiabatic and non-adiabatic field rotation), to qualitatively understand the effects of this field we need to compare the field magnitude (which defines the Larmor frequency) to the rotational angular velocity. That means we need to compare ω_- with $2\omega_0$ (or with ω_+, whichever is larger).

If the magnitude of the counter-rotating field is much less than the magnitude of the static field (i.e., $\omega_- \ll 2\omega_0$), this field rotates non-adiabatically and, as we have seen before (Eqn. 3.27), has no effect on spin evolution.

So in the rotating frame of reference, defined by Eqn. 3.35, we have

(Eqn. 3.47)
$$\mathbf{m}' = e^{-\omega_+\mathbf{u}_+}\cdot\mathbf{m}_0',\ \mathbf{m}_0' \equiv \mathbf{m}'(t=0).$$

That is simply rotation about axis $\hat{\mathbf{b}}_+$, lying in the x-y plane, with angular frequency ω_+. This frequency is known as Rabi frequency, and in the context of NMR, the Rabi frequency is the nutation frequency of a sample's net nuclear magnetization vector about a radiofrequency field.

Now, if we shift our view to the laboratory frame of reference on the top of this precession in the rotating frame, we have rotation about the z-axis with angular frequency ω_0:

(Eqn. 3.48)
$$\mathbf{m} = e^{-\omega_0 t\cdot\alpha_3}\cdot e^{-\omega_+ t\cdot\mathbf{u}_+}\cdot\mathbf{m}_0,\quad \mathbf{m}_0 \equiv \mathbf{m}(t=0).$$

As we pointed out earlier, we find that $|\mathbf{B}_0| \gg |\mathbf{B}_1(t)|$, is typical in HF NMR; consequently one can usually neglect the counter-rotating component of an alternating field in the context of the HF NMR experiments. Such an assumption (approximation) is called the *rotating-wave approximation* (RWA).

In the opposite case, where the amplitude of the counter-rotating field is much larger than the amplitude of the static field (i.e., $\omega_- \gg 2\omega_0$), this counter-rotating field rotates adiabatically and, as we have discussed previously (Eqn. 3.21), the sample's magnetization follows the magnetic field precessing about the instantaneous magnetic field. So in the rotating frame defined by Eqn. 3.45 (i.e., the frame of reference associated with magnetization evolution under rotating-wave approximation), we have

(Eqn. 3.49) $$\mathbf{m}'' = e^{2\omega_0 t \cdot \alpha_3} \cdot e^{-\omega_- t \cdot \mathbf{u}_-} \cdot \mathbf{m}''_0, \quad \mathbf{m}''_0 \equiv \mathbf{m}''(t=0).$$

Correspondingly, in the laboratory frame of reference we have

(Eqn. 3.50) $$\mathbf{m} = e^{-\omega_0 t \cdot \alpha_3} \cdot e^{-\omega_+ t \cdot \mathbf{u}_+} \cdot e^{+2\omega_0 t \cdot \alpha_3} \cdot e^{-\omega_- t \cdot \mathbf{u}_-} \cdot \mathbf{m}_0, \quad \mathbf{m}_0 \equiv \mathbf{m}(t=0).$$

If we further assume that $|\omega_+| t \ll 1$, then we see that the sample magnetization adiabatically follows the counter-rotating field:

(Eqn. 3.51) $$\mathbf{m} = e^{-\omega_0 t \cdot \alpha_3} \cdot e^{\omega_- t \cdot \mathbf{u}_-} \cdot \mathbf{m}_0, \quad \mathbf{m}_0 \equiv \mathbf{m}(t=0).$$

Now let's apply this formalism to analyze the ULF NMR regime. In this regime we typically have $|\mathbf{B}_0| \cong |\mathbf{B}_1(t)|$, so the two limiting cases considered above are not applicable, and we need to estimate effects of the counter-rotating field.

3.1.3 Nonlinear Effects in NMR

To illustrate the effects of the counter-rotating magnetic fields, let's consider the simplest case of an alternating magnetic field: a field oscillating along the x-axis with angular frequency ω:

(Eqn. 3.52) $$\mathbf{B}_1(t) = B_1 \cos(\omega t)\hat{\mathbf{e}}_1.$$

This field, of course, can be presented as a sum of two circular polarized fields rotating in the opposite directions about the z-axis:

(Eqn. 3.53) $$\mathbf{B}_1(t) = \frac{\omega_1}{\gamma} e^{-\omega t \alpha_3} \cdot \hat{\mathbf{e}}_1 + \frac{\omega_1}{\gamma} e^{\omega t \alpha_3} \cdot \hat{\mathbf{e}}_1$$

where $\omega_1 = B_1 / 2\gamma$ is the Rabi frequency.

Before we attempt a formal solution of the evolution equation, let us qualitatively analyze the magnetization evolution under presence of those two fields. Following [5] we consider the case in the reference frame that follows the counter-rotating component. In this coordinate system we will have a large effective static field:

$$\mathbf{B}_{\text{eff}} = \frac{\omega_1}{\gamma}\cdot\hat{\mathbf{e}}_1 + \frac{(\omega_0+\omega)}{\gamma}\cdot\hat{\mathbf{e}}_3 = \frac{\omega_{\text{eff}}}{\gamma}\hat{\mathbf{b}}_{\text{eff}},\, \omega_{\text{eff}} = \sqrt{(\omega_0+\omega)^2+\omega_1^2},\, \hat{\mathbf{b}}_{\text{eff}} = \frac{\omega_1}{\omega_{\text{eff}}}\cdot\hat{\mathbf{e}}_1 + \frac{(\omega_0+\omega)}{\omega_{\text{eff}}}\cdot\hat{\mathbf{e}}_3$$

and three alternating fields: (a) a field parallel to $\mathbf{B}_{\text{eff}}$ oscillating with angular frequency 2ω, (b) a very small field orthogonal to $\mathbf{B}_{\text{eff}}$ rotating counter-clockwise with angular frequency 2ω, and (c) a field orthogonal to $\mathbf{B}_{\text{eff}}$ rotating clockwise with angular frequency 2ω. This can be obtained by formally applying the transformation $e^{-\omega t\alpha_3}$ to the total magnetic field.

The resonance condition requires, of course, that the precession frequency corresponds to the field rotation frequency, so the resonance conditions for the rotating fields are $(2\omega)^2 = \omega_{\text{eff}}^2$ or

$$(\omega-\omega_0)(3\omega+\omega_0)=\omega_1^2.$$

This equation has two solutions:

$$\omega=\frac{\omega_0 \pm \sqrt{4\omega_0^2+3\omega_1^2}}{3}.$$

The first solution (+) corresponds to the clockwise rotating field:

(Eqn. 3.54)

$$\omega=\frac{\omega_0 + \sqrt{4\omega_0^2+3\omega_1^2}}{3} \approx \omega_0\left(1+\frac{\omega_1^2}{4\omega_0^2}\right).$$

We see that the resonance is shifted by relative amount $\omega_1^2/4\omega_0^2$. This shift was discovered theoretically by F. Bloch and A. Siegert in 1940 [17] and has been known since then as *Bloch-Siegert shift*.

The second (–) solution:

$$\omega=\frac{\omega_0 - \sqrt{4\omega_0^2+3\omega_1^2}}{3} \approx -\frac{\omega_0}{3}\left(1+3\frac{\omega_1^2}{4\omega_0^2}\right)$$

corresponds to the counterclockwise rotating field, and, due to the fact that this field has very small magnitude, this resonance corresponds to a much weaker phenomenon.

It is important to note that the primary reason for this shift is that the orthogonal field modifies the primary field sufficiently to induce a non-negligible change of the Larmor frequency. Because the fields are orthogonal, the shift in the Larmor frequency is proportional to the square of the ratio of the field magnitudes. While this effect is usually negligible in HF NMR experiments, it could be (as we will see later) significant in the ULF NMR regime. Equivalently, this effect can be viewed as resulting in a non-negligible change in direction of the main static field.

Now, let us analyze this phenomenon quantitatively and proceed with solving the evolution equation. In the frame of reference associated with the rotating-wave approximation (see Eqn. 45) we have

(Eqn. 3.55)
$$\frac{d\mathbf{m}''}{dt}+\omega_1\cdot\mathbf{u}_1\cdot\mathbf{m}''=0,$$

where:

(Eqn. 3.56)
$$\mathbf{u}_1=-\boldsymbol{\alpha}_1+e^{\omega_1 t\boldsymbol{\alpha}_1}\cdot\left(e^{(\omega_0-\omega)t\boldsymbol{\alpha}_3}\cdot\boldsymbol{\alpha}_1\cdot e^{-(\omega_0-\omega)t\boldsymbol{\alpha}_3}+e^{-(\omega_0+\omega)t\boldsymbol{\alpha}_3}\cdot\boldsymbol{\alpha}_1\cdot e^{-(\omega_0+\omega)t\boldsymbol{\alpha}_3}\right)\cdot e^{-\omega_1 t\boldsymbol{\alpha}_1}.$$

We start with computing the terms $e^{(\omega_0\pm\omega)t\boldsymbol{\alpha}_3}\cdot\boldsymbol{\alpha}_1\cdot e^{-(\omega_0\pm\omega)t\boldsymbol{\alpha}_2}$. Recollecting that $e^{\psi\alpha_3}\cdot\hat{\mathbf{e}}_1$ is simply a vector $\hat{\mathbf{e}}_1$ rotated counterclockwise by angle ψ about the z-axis and using Eqn. 12f, this term can be easily calculated to be

$$e^{\omega' t\alpha_3}\cdot\boldsymbol{\alpha}_1\cdot e^{-\omega' t\alpha_3}=(e^{\omega' t\alpha_3}\cdot\hat{\mathbf{e}}_1)^{\times}=(\cos(\omega' t)\cdot\hat{\mathbf{e}}_1+\sin(\omega' t)\cdot\hat{\mathbf{e}}_2)^{\times}=\cos(\omega' t)\cdot\alpha_1+\sin(\omega' t)\cdot\alpha_2,$$

where $\omega'=\omega_0\pm\omega$.

Or, using exponential functions, we can rewrite this as

(Eqn. 3.57)
$$e^{\omega' t\alpha_3}\cdot\boldsymbol{\alpha}_1\cdot e^{-\omega' t\alpha_3}=e^{-i\omega' t}\cdot\boldsymbol{\sigma}_+^{(3)}+e^{i\omega' t}\cdot\boldsymbol{\sigma}_-^{(3)}.$$

Here the matrices $\boldsymbol{\sigma}_\pm^{(3)}$ are defined by

(Eqn. 3.58)
$$\boldsymbol{\sigma}_\pm^{(3)}=\frac{1}{2}\cdot(\boldsymbol{\alpha}_1\pm i\cdot\boldsymbol{\alpha}_2).$$

While this approach is workable, it is beneficial to use a more general approach that will provide a better insight into the mathematics involved and illuminate the similarities with the quantum mechanics.

It can be shown that for any square matrices **A** and **B**, a similarity transformation $e^{\psi\mathbf{A}}\cdot\mathbf{B}\cdot e^{-\psi\mathbf{A}}$, where ψ is an arbitrary scalar, can be expanded in a power-series:

(Eqn. 3.59)
$$e^{\psi\mathbf{A}}\cdot\mathbf{B}\cdot e^{-\psi\mathbf{A}}=\sum_{n=0}^{\infty}\frac{\psi^n}{n!}\mathbf{a}_n.$$

The expansion coefficients are computed using the following recurrent formula:

(Eqn. 3.60)
$$\mathbf{a}_{n+1}=\left[\mathbf{A},\mathbf{a}_n\right]\equiv\mathbf{A}\cdot\mathbf{a}_n-\mathbf{a}_n\cdot\mathbf{A},\ \mathbf{a}_0=\mathbf{B}$$

where the square brackets denote, as usual, a commutator of two matrices. Eqn. 3.60 is easily obtained by differentiating Eqn. 3.59. Thus the similarity transformation $e^{\psi\mathbf{A}}\cdot\mathbf{B}\cdot e^{-\psi\mathbf{A}}$ depends only on the commuting properties of the matrices **A** and **B**.

The easily verified commutation relationships for the matrices of basic rotations $\boldsymbol{\alpha}_1$, $\boldsymbol{\alpha}_2$, $\boldsymbol{\alpha}_3$ are

(Eqn. 3.61)
$$[\boldsymbol{\alpha}_k, \boldsymbol{\alpha}_l] = \sum_{m=1}^{3} \varepsilon_{k,l,m} \boldsymbol{\alpha}_m,$$

where the $\varepsilon_{k,l,m}$ are usual Levi-Civita symbols. $\varepsilon_{k,l,m}$ is defined as $\varepsilon_{k,l,m} = 1$ if (k, l, m) is an even permutation of $(1,2,3)$; $\varepsilon_{k,l,m} = -1$ if it is an odd permutation;[5] and $\varepsilon_{k,l,m} = 0$ if any index is repeated. Explicitly, Eqn. 3.61 states that

$$[\boldsymbol{\alpha}_1, \boldsymbol{\alpha}_2] = \boldsymbol{\alpha}_3, \; [\boldsymbol{\alpha}_1, \boldsymbol{\alpha}_3] = -\boldsymbol{\alpha}_2, [\boldsymbol{\alpha}_2, \boldsymbol{\alpha}_3] = \boldsymbol{\alpha}_1$$

Applying these relations to compute the term $e^{\omega' t \alpha_3} \cdot \boldsymbol{\alpha}_1 \cdot e^{-\omega' t \alpha_3}$ we will get

$$e^{\omega' t \alpha_3} \cdot \boldsymbol{\alpha}_1 \cdot e^{-\omega' t \alpha_3} = \boldsymbol{\alpha}_1 + \frac{\omega' t}{1} \boldsymbol{\alpha}_2 - \frac{(\omega' t)^2}{2!} \boldsymbol{\alpha}_1 - \frac{(\omega' t)^3}{3!} \boldsymbol{\alpha}_2 + \frac{(\omega' t)^4}{4!} \boldsymbol{\alpha}_1 + \ldots =$$
$$= \boldsymbol{\alpha}_1 \cdot \sum_{n=0}^{\infty} (-1)^n \frac{(\omega' t)^{2n}}{(2n)!} + \boldsymbol{\alpha}_2 \cdot \sum_{n=0}^{\infty} (-1)^n \frac{(\omega' t)^{2n+1}}{(2n+1)!} = \cos(\omega' t) \boldsymbol{\alpha}_1 + \sin(\omega' t) \boldsymbol{\alpha}_2 .$$

Using exponential functions, we can rewrite this as

(Eqn. 3.62)
$$e^{\omega' t \alpha_3} \cdot \boldsymbol{\alpha}_1 \cdot e^{-\omega' t \alpha_3} = e^{-i\omega' t} \boldsymbol{\sigma}_+^{(3)} + e^{i\omega' t} \boldsymbol{\sigma}_-^{(3)} .$$

Note that for these matrices we have the following similarity transformation:

(Eqn. 3.63)
$$e^{\psi \alpha_3} \cdot \boldsymbol{\sigma}_\pm^{(3)} \cdot e^{-\psi \alpha_3} = e^{\mp i \psi} \boldsymbol{\sigma}_\pm^{(3)} .$$

Similarly, for the other rotation axes are

(Eqn. 3.64)
$$e^{\psi \alpha} \cdot \boldsymbol{\sigma}_\perp^{(1)} \cdot e^{-\psi \alpha_1} = e^{\pm i \psi} \boldsymbol{\sigma}_\pm^{(1)} \boldsymbol{\sigma}_\pm^{(1)} = \frac{1}{2} (\boldsymbol{\alpha}_2 \perp i \boldsymbol{\alpha}_2)$$

$$e^{\psi \alpha_2} \cdot \boldsymbol{\sigma}_\pm^{(2)} \cdot e^{-\psi \alpha_2} = e^{\mp i \psi} \boldsymbol{\sigma}_\pm^{(2)}, \boldsymbol{\sigma}_\pm^{(2)} = \frac{1}{2} (\boldsymbol{\alpha}_3 \pm i \boldsymbol{\alpha}_1).$$

Or in general:

(Eqn. 3.65)
$$e^{\psi \alpha_k} \cdot \boldsymbol{\sigma}_\pm^{(k)} \cdot e^{-\psi \alpha_k} = e^{\mp i \psi} \boldsymbol{\sigma}_\pm^{(k)}, \boldsymbol{\sigma}_\pm^{(k)} = \frac{1}{2} (\boldsymbol{\alpha}_l \pm i \boldsymbol{\alpha}_m)$$

where (k, l, m) is an even permutation of $(1,2,3)$.

---

[5] Even permutations: (1,2,3), (2,3,1), and (3,1,2). Odd permutations: (1,3,2), (2,1,3), and (3,2,1)

Applying the same strategy to calculate similarity transformation $e^{\omega_1 t\alpha_1}\cdot\ldots\cdot e^{-\omega_1 t\alpha_1}$ we will get

(Eqn. 3.66)
$$\mathbf{u}_1=\{A_0(t)\cdot\boldsymbol{\alpha}_1+A_{+1}(t)\cdot\boldsymbol{\sigma}_+^{(1)}+A_{-1}\cdot\boldsymbol{\sigma}_-^{(1)}\}+c.c.$$

Here we use *c.c.* to denote the complex conjugate of the expression in the curly brackets, and time-dependent functions are

$$A_0(t)=\frac{1}{2}(e^{-i(\omega_0+\omega)t}+e^{-i(\omega_0-\omega)t}-1),\quad A_{\pm1}(t)=\frac{i}{2}(e^{-i(\omega_0+\omega\pm\omega_1)t}+e^{-i(\omega_0-\omega\pm\omega_1)t}).$$

Now we can solve Eqn. 3.55. In general the solution of this differential equation can be expressed through a time-dependent matrix:

(Eqn. 3.67)
$$\mathbf{m}''=\mathbf{R}(t)\cdot\mathbf{m}_0'',\quad \mathbf{m}_0''\equiv\mathbf{m}''(t=0),\quad \mathbf{R}(t=0)=\mathbf{I}$$

where the matrix $\mathbf{R}(t)$ satisfies the following differential equation:

(Eqn. 3.68)
$$\frac{\partial\mathbf{R}(t)}{\partial t}+\omega_1\cdot\mathbf{u}_1\cdot\mathbf{R}(t)=0,\quad \mathbf{R}(0)=\mathbf{I}.$$

Eqn. 3.68 can be rewritten in the integral form

(Eqn. 3.69)
$$\mathbf{R}(t)=\mathbf{I}-\omega_1\cdot\int_0^t\mathbf{u}_1\cdot\mathbf{R}(t')dt',$$

which can be solved by successive approximations:

(Eqn. 3.70)
$$(0)\quad \mathbf{R}^{(0)}(t)=\mathbf{I},$$
$$(1)\quad \mathbf{R}^{(1)}(t)=\mathbf{I}-\omega_1\cdot\int_0^t\mathbf{u}_1(t')\cdot\mathbf{R}^{(0)}(t')dt'=\mathbf{I}-\omega_1\cdot\int_0^t\mathbf{u}_1(t')dt',$$
$$(2)\quad \mathbf{R}^{(2)}(t)=\mathbf{I}-\omega_1\cdot\int_0^t\mathbf{u}_1(t')dt'+\omega_1^2\cdot\int_0^t\mathbf{u}_1(t')\cdot\int_0^{t'}\mathbf{u}_1(t'')dt''dt',$$
$$\ldots$$
$$(n)\quad \mathbf{R}^{(n)}(t)=\mathbf{I}-\omega_1\cdot\int_0^t\mathbf{u}_1(t')\cdot\mathbf{R}^{(n-1)}(t')dt',\ \text{etc.}$$

If we continue to assume that $\omega_1<\omega_0$, a few iterations should be enough. Note that this approach is equivalent to the well-known perturbative expansion of the evolution operator widely used in quantum mechanics. We see the time dependence is only in scalar functions, so we can implement integration in the successive approximation scheme (Eqn. 70):

$$\mathbf{R}^{(n)}(t)=\mathbf{I}-\omega_1\cdot\Delta\mathbf{R}^{(1)}+\omega_1^2\cdot\Delta\mathbf{R}^{(2)}-....=\sum_{k=0}^{n}\omega_1^k\cdot\Delta\mathbf{R}^{(k)}$$

(Eqn. 3.71)
$$\Delta\mathbf{R}^{(n)}=\int_0^t A_0(t')\boldsymbol{\alpha}_1\Delta\mathbf{R}^{(n-1)}(t')dt'+\int_0^t A_{+1}(t')\boldsymbol{\sigma}_+^{(1)}\Delta\mathbf{R}^{(n-1)}(t')dt'+\int_0^t A_{-1}(t')\boldsymbol{\sigma}_-^{(1)}\Delta\mathbf{R}^{(n-1)}(t')dt'+c.c.$$

Starting with $\Delta\mathbf{R}^{(0)}(t)=\mathbf{I}$, which is simply a rotating-wave approximation, we will compute the next step:

(Eqn. 3.72)
$$(1)\ \Delta\mathbf{R}^{(1)}(t)=\left\{C_0(t)\boldsymbol{\alpha}_1+C_{+1}(t)\cdot\boldsymbol{\sigma}_+^{(1)}+C_{-1}(t)\cdot\boldsymbol{\sigma}_-^{(1)}+c.c.\right\}$$

where:

$$C_0(t)\equiv\int_0^t A_0(t')dt'=\frac{i}{2}\left(\frac{e^{-i(\omega_0+\omega)t}-1}{\omega_0+\omega}+\frac{e^{-i(\omega_0-\omega)t}-1}{\omega_0-\omega}+it\right)$$
$$C_{\pm1}(t)\equiv\int_0^t A_\pm(t')dt'=-\frac{1}{2}\left(\frac{e^{-i(\omega_0+\omega\pm\omega_1)t}-1}{\omega_0+\omega\pm\omega_1}+\frac{e^{-i(\omega_0-\omega\pm\omega_1)t}-1}{\omega_0-\omega\pm\omega_1}\right).$$

As a first pass we only keep terms on the order of $\omega_1/\omega_0+\omega$ from the expansion in Eqn. 71. To do this we need to compute the second term, because integration of the $A_0\cdot C_\pm^*(t)$ and respective complex conjugates will result in terms proportional to $((\omega_0+\omega)\omega_1)^{-1}$ that need to be kept in the expansion. Multiplying and integrating many complex exponentials to compute the second iteration is too tedious, so we will simplify our formulas. First we assume that the frequency of the oscillating magnetic field is close to the Larmor frequency so that $|\omega_0-\omega|\ll 1$. In this case we have

$$A_0(t)\approx\frac{1}{2}e^{-i\omega' t},A_{\pm1}(t)\approx\frac{i}{2}e^{-i(\omega'\pm\omega_1)t},C_0(t)\approx\frac{i}{2}\frac{e^{-i\omega' t}-1}{\omega'},C_{\pm1}(t)\approx-\frac{1}{2}\frac{e^{-i(\omega'\pm\omega_1)t}-1}{\omega'\pm\omega_1},$$

where $\omega'=\omega_0+\omega$.

Using these functions in Eqn. 3.71 to compute $\Delta\mathbf{R}^{(2)}(t)$ and keeping only terms of order $1/\omega'\omega_1$ we will get

(Eqn. 3.73)
$$(2)\ \Delta\mathbf{R}^{(2)}(t)=-\frac{i}{2\omega'\omega_1}\left(e^{-i\omega_1 t}-1\right)\cdot[\boldsymbol{\alpha}_1,\boldsymbol{\sigma}_+^{(1)}]+c.c.$$

Combining everything together, and taking into account that $[\boldsymbol{\alpha}_1, \boldsymbol{\sigma}_+^{(1)}] = -i \cdot \boldsymbol{\sigma}_+^{(1)}$, we will get an approximation of the solution of Eqn. 3.55 to the first order in ω_1 / ω':

(Eqn. 3.74)
$$\mathbf{R}^{(1)}(t) = \mathbf{I} + \frac{\omega_1}{\omega'} \cdot \frac{1}{2} \{-i(e^{-i\omega' t} - 1) \cdot \boldsymbol{\alpha}_1 + (e^{-i(\omega'+\omega_1)t} - e^{-i\omega_1 t}) \cdot \boldsymbol{\sigma}_+^{(1)} + (e^{-i(\omega'-\omega_1)t} - 1) \cdot \boldsymbol{\sigma}_-^{(1)} + c.c.\}.$$

We recognize that the expression in the curly brackets in the last equation is a linear combination of basic rotations (i.e., matrices $\boldsymbol{\alpha}_1$, $\boldsymbol{\alpha}_2$, $\boldsymbol{\alpha}_3$), so for this last equation the result can be written as

(Eqn. 3.75)
$$\mathbf{R}^{(1)}(t) = \mathbf{I} + \frac{\omega_1}{\omega'} \cdot \mathbf{D}^{\times}(t), \text{ or}$$
$$\mathbf{R}^{(1)}(t) = \mathbf{I} + \frac{\omega_1}{\omega'} \cdot \{D_1(t)\alpha_1 + D_2(t)\alpha_2 + D_3(t)\alpha_3\}$$

where the rotation axis vector $\mathbf{D}(t)$ and, correspondingly, the rotation generator $\mathbf{D}^{\times}(t)$ are defined by

(Eqn. 3.76)
$$\mathbf{D}(t) = D_1(t)\hat{\mathbf{e}}_1 + D_2(t)\hat{\mathbf{e}}_2 + D_3(t)\hat{\mathbf{e}}_3$$
$$\mathbf{D}^{\times}(t) = D_1(t)\boldsymbol{\alpha}_1 + D_2(t)\boldsymbol{\alpha}_2 + D_3(t)\boldsymbol{\alpha}_3$$

and

$$D_1(t) = -\frac{i}{2}(e^{-i\omega' t} - 1) + c.c. = -\sin(\omega' t)$$
$$D_2(t) = \frac{1}{1}(e^{-i(\omega'+\omega_1)t} + e^{-i(\omega'-\omega_1)t} - e^{-i\omega_1 t} - 1) + c.c. = \cos(\omega' t) \cdot \cos(\omega_1 t) - \cos\left(\frac{\omega_1 t}{2}\right) \cdot \cos\left(\frac{\omega_1 t}{2}\right)$$
$$D_3(t) = \frac{i}{4}(e^{-i(\omega'+\omega_1)t} - e^{-i(\omega'-\omega_1)t} - e^{-i\omega_1 t} + 1) + c.c. = \cos(\omega' t) \cdot \sin(\omega_1 t) - \cos\left(\frac{\omega_1 t}{2}\right) \cdot \sin\left(\frac{\omega_1 t}{2}\right).$$

We remind the reader that the expression in the curly brackets in Eqn. 3.75 is simply a cross-product matrix for a time-dependent vector $\mathbf{D}(t) = (D_1(t), D_2(t), D_3(t))^T$: $\{\ldots\} \cdot \mathbf{v} = \mathbf{D}(t) \times \mathbf{v}$.

Here we need to point out that while the exact solution of Eqn. 3.68 is a rotation matrix and thus is an orthogonal matrix. However, the "rotation" matrix $\mathbf{R}^{(1)}(t)$, defined by Eqn. 75, is an approximate solution; it is not an orthogonal matrix and is not a truly rotation matrix. One way to "fix" this matrix is to use a Taylor series expansion for a matrix exponential:

(Eqn. 3.77)
$$e^{\mathbf{A}} = \mathbf{I} + \mathbf{A} + \frac{\mathbf{A}^2}{2} + \frac{\mathbf{A}^3}{6} + \ldots$$

Comparing Eqns. 3.75 and 3.77, we can define an approximate orthogonal solution of Eqn. 3.68 as

(Eqn. 3.78) $$\mathbf{R}^{(1)}(t)=e^{\frac{\omega_1}{\omega'}\mathbf{D}^{\times}(t)}.$$

Both Eqns. 3.75 and 3.78 give an approximate solution to Eqn. 3.68, and thus give an approximate solution to Eqn. 3.55, to the first order of ω_1/ω' in the rotating-wave approximation frame.[6]

It is instructive to ask: What is the behavior of this approximate solution? As a curiosity, we note that the trajectory of the magnetization vector is a 3D Lissajous curve, which is a graph of a complex harmonic motion. This is actually instructive because these curves are highly sensitive to the ratio ω'/ω_1, and if this ratio is rational (i.e., $\omega'/\omega_1=k/n$ where k and n are integers), then the function is periodic, with a period $T=2\pi n/\omega_1=2\pi k/\omega'$. The trajectory also depends on the direction of the initial vector $\mathbf{m}_0''$. To help understand these dependences, let us consider a few specific cases.

Initially we will assume the magnetization is aligned along the $\mathbf{B}_1(t=0)$ (i.e., along the x-axis). This is called a "spin-lock" mode. In this case, for the rotating-wave approximation, the magnetization simply follows the clockwise rotating component of the $\mathbf{B}_1(t)$. If the oscillation frequency is equal to the precession frequency, then the magnetization and the clockwise rotating component of the oscillating field are always parallel, meaning that the oscillating magnetic field has no effect on precession around $\mathbf{B}_0$. Assuming a unit magnetization, $\mathbf{m}_0''=\mathbf{e}_1$, we have the following formula for the magnetization evolution in the rotating approximation frame:

(Eqn. 3.79) $$\mathbf{m}''^{(1)}(t)=\underbrace{\hat{\mathbf{e}}_1+\frac{\omega_1}{2\omega'}\hat{\mathbf{e}}_3}_{\mathbf{a}}+\underbrace{\frac{\omega_1}{\omega'}\left(\cos(\omega' t)-\frac{1}{2}\right)\left(\sin(\omega_1 t)\hat{\mathbf{e}}_2-\cos(\omega_1 t)\hat{\mathbf{e}}_3\right)}_{\mathbf{b}}.$$

Here we used Eqn. 3.75 and thus neglected the normalization factor imposed by Eqn. 3.78. We see that the trajectory of the magnetization vector described by Eqn. 3.79 consists of a constant vector **a** and a vector **b** rotating counterclockwise about the x-axis with angular frequency ω_1. The amplitude of this rotating vector is modulated with angular frequency ω'. Let us now shift our perspective to the laboratory frame of reference where we have rotation about the x-axis with angular frequency ω_1, and rotation about the z-axis with angular frequency ω_0 superposed on top of the rotating frame perspective, given by $\mathbf{m}^{(1)}(t)=e^{-\omega_0 t\cdot\alpha_3}\cdot e^{-\omega_1 t\cdot\alpha_1}\cdot\mathbf{m}''^{(1)}(t)$.

Transforming Eqn. 3.79 into a laboratory frame, we will get

$$\mathbf{m}^{(1)}(t)=e^{-\omega_0 t\cdot\alpha_3}\cdot\left(\hat{\mathbf{e}}_1+\frac{\omega_1}{2\omega'}\cdot e^{-\omega_1 t\cdot\alpha_1}\cdot\hat{\mathbf{e}}_3\right)-\frac{\omega_1}{\omega'}\left(\cos(\omega' t)-\frac{1}{2}\right)\cdot\hat{\mathbf{e}}_3.$$

[6] Just a reminder: A rotating-wave approximation frame, defined by Eqn. 3.45, is the frame of reference following rotation of magnetization under rotation-wave approximation. Naturally, in this frame, the solution of Eqn. 3.68 using rotating-wave approximation is a constant vector.

The last expression can be rewritten as

$$\textbf{(Eqn. 3.80)}\qquad \mathbf{m}^{(1)}(t) = e^{-(\omega_0 t + \Delta\phi(t))\cdot\alpha_3}\cdot\hat{\mathbf{e}}_1 + m_{||}(t)\cdot\hat{\mathbf{e}}_3 + O\left(\left(\frac{\omega_1}{\omega'}\right)^2\right)$$

where

$$\Delta\phi(t) = -\arctan\left(\frac{\omega_1\sin(\omega_1 t)}{2\omega'}\right),\ \text{and}\ m_{||}(t) = \frac{\omega_1}{\omega'}\left(2\sin\left(\frac{\omega' t}{2}\right)^2 - \sin\left(\frac{\omega_1 t}{2}\right)^2\right).$$

Figure 3.5 illustrates an example of such a curve generated using typical ULF NMR parameters—$\omega/2\pi = \omega_0/2\pi = 4000\text{Hz}$ and $\omega_1/2\pi = 400\text{Hz}$. The red line shows the curve over one period of ω_0 and the blue dashed lines show successive periods. The first term of Eqn. 3.80 describes, apart from the additional phase shift $\Delta\phi(t)$, the trajectory typically observed in a spin-lock sequence at high fields, when the rotating-wave approximation holds. This is indicated by the black trace in Figure 3.5. However, because the rotating-wave approximation is not valid when the magnitude of the alternating field $\mathbf{B}_1(t)$ is not negligible compared to the magnitude of the static field $\mathbf{B}_0$ (as is often the case in the ULF NMR regime), we also have finite terms for $\Delta\phi(t)$ and $m_{||}(t)$. As was mentioned before, the term $\Delta\phi(t)$ produces an additional phase shift of the transverse component of magnetization, compared to the rotating wave approximation. This phase shift is a periodic function with a period in which $T = 2\pi/\omega_1$ and magnitude $\approx \omega_1/4\omega_0$. This phase shift translates into shift of the instantaneous angular frequency of magnetization rotation about the z-axis, ω_{inst}:

$$\omega_{\text{inst}} = \omega_0 + \frac{d\Delta\phi}{dt} \approx \omega_0\left(1 + \frac{\omega_1^2}{4\omega_0^2}\cos(\omega_1 t)\right).$$

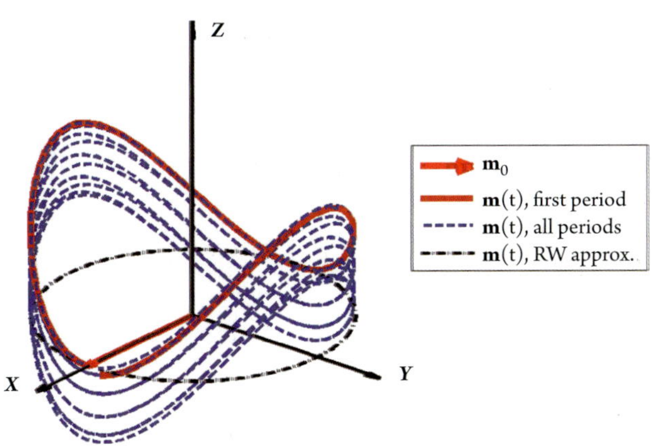

FIGURE 3.5 Effect of the counter-rotating field in a laboratory frame. Initially the magnetization is aligned with the x-axis.

It is easy to see that the magnitude of this frequency shift corresponds to the Bloch-Siegert frequency shift (compare with Eqn. 3.54). The frequency shift for the specific example considered in this section is shown in Figure 3.6.

The term $m_{\|}(t)$ produces a component of magnetization parallel to $\mathbf{B}_0$ that is a sum of two vectors oscillating with the frequencies ω_0 and $\omega_1/2$ with magnitudes $\approx \omega_1/\omega_0$ and $\approx \omega_1/2\omega_0$, resulting in the "saddle" shape in Figure 3.5.

We will give two short examples of how this effect would influence our observed results. In a spin-lock experiment, instead of measuring a constant-amplitude sine wave, the amplitude and phase of the obtained signal would vary. The next example concerns a CPMG sequence typically used to measure T_2 relaxation [18]. The method addresses imperfection of π-pulses (used to produce rephasing), preventing cumulative error by correcting the component of magnetization parallel to $\mathbf{B}_0$ after every even π-pulse. However, this sequence will not correct the term $m_{\|}(t)$, which could alter the measurement of T_2.

The second example sets the initial magnetization orthogonal to $\mathbf{B}_1(t=0)$ and aligned along $\mathbf{B}_0$ (i.e., along the z-axis). Assuming a unit magnetization, $\mathbf{m} = \hat{\mathbf{e}}_3$, we have the following formula for the magnetization evolution in the rotating-wave approximation frame:

$$\textbf{(Eqn. 3.81)}\quad \mathbf{m}''^{(1)}(t) = \hat{\mathbf{e}}_3 - \underbrace{\frac{\omega_1}{2\omega'}(1+\cos(\omega_1 t))\hat{\mathbf{e}}_1}_{a} + \underbrace{\frac{\omega_1}{\omega'}\cdot\{\cos(\omega_1 t)\cos(\omega' t)\hat{\mathbf{e}}_1 + \sin(\omega' t)\hat{\mathbf{e}}_2\}}_{b}.$$

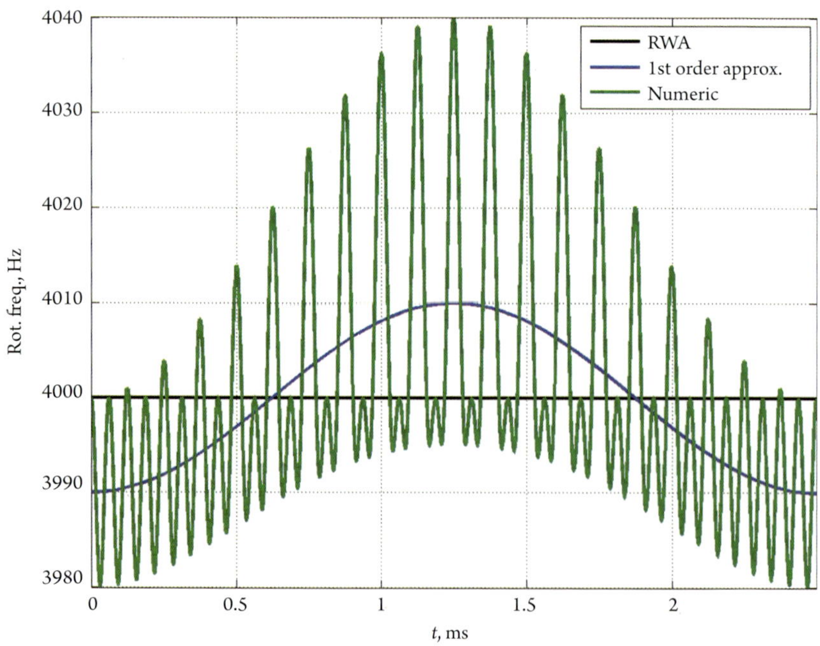

FIGURE 3.6 Instantaneous frequency of magnetization rotation about the z-axis.

The first term in this equation—vector $\hat{\mathbf{e}}_3$—is a constant vector that gives the rotating-wave approximation solution. The second term, vector **a**, is a vector counter-aligned with the x-axis; its magnitude oscillates between 0 and ω_1/ω' with angular frequency ω_1. The third term, vector **b**, describes a vector rotating, clockwise and counterclockwise, depending on the sign of $\cos(\omega_1 t)$, about the z-axis with angular frequency ω'. The end of the vector traces an ellipse with the major axis ω_1/ω' aligned with the y-axis and the minor axis aligned along the x-axis and modulated from 0 to ω_1/ω' with angular frequency ω_1. While the terms in Eqn. 3.81 are easy to interpret, it is it more beneficial to visualize the trajectory traced by the magnetization vector in the rotating frame (i.e., in the frame associated with precession about $\mathbf{B}_0$). Multiplying Eqn. 3.81 by $e^{-\omega_1 t\cdot\alpha_1}$ to impose clockwise rotation about the x-axis with angular frequency ω_1, we will get the formula for the magnetization in this frame:

$$\mathbf{m}'^{(1)}(t)=e^{-(\omega_1 t+\Delta\phi(t))\cdot\alpha_1}\cdot\hat{\mathbf{e}}_3+m_1(t)\cdot\hat{\mathbf{e}}_1+O\left(\left(\frac{\omega_1}{\omega'}\right)^2\right), \text{ where}$$

$$\Delta\phi(t)=\arctan\left(\frac{\omega_1\sin(\omega' t)}{\omega'}\right), \text{ and } m_1(t)=\frac{\omega_1}{\omega'}\left(\cos(\omega_1 t)\cos(\omega' t)-\frac{1}{2}(\cos(\omega_1 t)+1)\right).$$

The trace described by these equations for the resonance parameters used in the previous example (i.e., $\omega/2\pi = \omega_0/2\pi = 4000\text{Hz}$, $\omega_1/2\pi = 400\text{Hz}$) is shown in Figure 3.7, where the red line shows the trace over one period of ω_0, the blue dashed line shows subsequent periods, and the black dashed line corresponds to the RWA solution. One obvious observation from Figure 3.7 is that, in this example, the magnetization misses the point $-\hat{\mathbf{e}}_3$, indicated by the red dashed arrow. This means that applying a linear polarized field at the Larmor frequency associated with the static field $\omega_0 = \gamma\,|\mathbf{B}_0|$ does not completely invert the magnetization, and thus we do not achieve truly resonance conditions. Achieving the fully resonant condition is achieved by applying a circular polarized field with the same frequency. The minimal angle between the magnetization and the z-axis, which we denote α, in this case of a linear polarized field can be estimated as

$$\cos\alpha\approx-1+\frac{1}{2}\cdot\left(\frac{\omega_1}{2\omega_0}\right)^2.$$

It is interesting to compare this angle with the similar angle for the case of slightly off-resonance (i.e., $\omega = \omega_0 \pm \Delta\omega$) circular polarized field, which is defined by the following relation [5]:

$$\cos\alpha=1-2\frac{\omega_1^2}{\omega_1^2+\Delta\omega^2}\approx-1+2\left(\frac{\Delta\omega}{\omega_1}\right)^2.$$

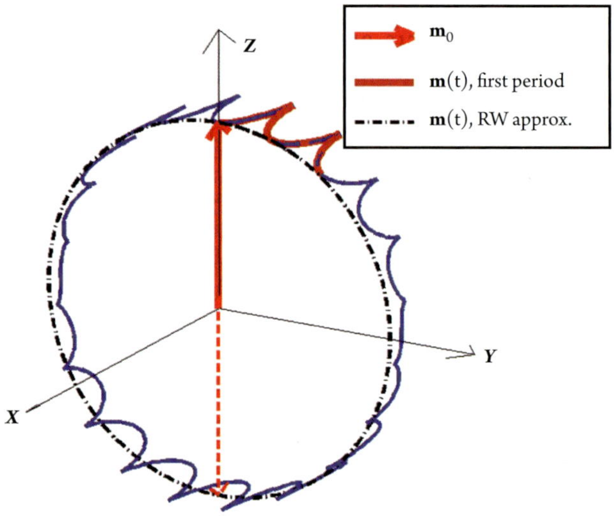

FIGURE 3.7 Effect of the counter-rotating field in a rotating frame. Initially magnetization is aligned with the *z*-axis.

Comparing these two last equations we can deduce that the minimal angle achieved in the linear polarized case corresponds to the following off-resonance frequency shift:

$$\Delta\omega = \omega_0 \cdot \left(\frac{\omega_1}{2\omega_0}\right)^2.$$

Comparing this last formula with Eqn. 3.54 we immediately see that this frequency shift again corresponds to the Bloch-Siegert frequency shift.

Finally let us consider this case in the laboratory frame. We now need to write the components of the magnetization vector explicitly:

(Eqn. 3.82)

$$\mathbf{m}^{(1)}(t) = \begin{bmatrix} \sin(\omega_1 t)\sin(\omega_0 t) - \frac{\omega_1}{2\omega'}\cdot(\cos(\omega_0 t)(1+\cos(\omega_1 t)) - 2\cos(\omega t)\cos(\omega_1 t)) \\ \sin(\omega_1 t)\cos(\omega_0 t) + \frac{\omega_1}{2\omega'}\cdot(\sin(\omega_0 t)(1+\cos(\omega_1 t)) + 2\sin(\omega t)\cos(\omega_1 t)) \\ \cos(\omega_1 t) - \frac{\omega_1}{\omega'}\cdot\sin(\omega_1 t)\sin(\omega' t) \end{bmatrix} + O\left(\left(\frac{\omega_1}{\omega'}\right)^2\right).$$

When the magnetization is in the *x*-*y* plane (i.e., when $\omega_1 t \approx \pi/2 + \pi k$, $k = 0,1,\ldots$), the angular frequency of precession about the *z*-axis is

$$\omega'' = \omega_0 + \frac{d\Delta\phi}{dt} \approx \omega_0\left(1 + \frac{\omega_1^2}{4\omega_0^2}\right)$$

which corresponds to the Bloch-Siegert frequency shift (see Eqn. 3.54).

3.2 QUANTUM MECHANICAL DESCRIPTION OF INTERACTION BETWEEN THE ELECTROMAGNETIC RADIATION AND THE NUCLEAR SPINS

While the classical approach allows us to predict very accurately what we can observe in the actual experiment, it is somewhat cumbersome and does not address the quantum nature of photon–spin interaction. Therefore, to illuminate the true nature of the interactions in NMR and MRI, we consider the problem using a quantum mechanical approach.

First let us review, without too many details and proofs, the underlying rules of quantum mechanics. After many years of research and debates in what Albert Einstein called "Real Black Magic Calculus," practitioners of the art agree on the following.

The state of a system is described by a unit vector in complex Hilbert space $\mathcal{H}$ (a generalization of a "wave function" conception). Using Dirac notation [25] these *state vectors* are denoted as $|a\rangle$, in which case they are called "ket," or as $\langle a|$, called "bra." The "ket" vectors belong to the $\mathcal{H}$ and the "bra" vectors belong to the "dual" Hilbert space denoted as $\mathcal{H}^*$. In this notation a denotes the collection of values of the physical quantities defining the state. These physical quantities can take continuous values, such as spatial coordinates of a particle, or discrete values, such as a spin projection on some axis. A pair of "bra" $\langle a|$ and "ket" $|b\rangle$ forms a scalar product denoted as $\langle a|b\rangle$. Note that $\langle a|b\rangle$ is simply a number. It is helpful to think of "ket" vectors as column vectors and "bra" vectors as row vectors. Then the correspondence between "bra" and "ket" for a given state a is given by Hermitian adjoint (complex-conjugate-transpose, denoted by † superscript): $\langle a|=|a\rangle^\dagger$. As state vectors are unit vectors, we have the following relation $\langle a|a\rangle = 1$, called the normalization condition. A simple but very important rule, called a *superposition principle*, states that if a system can be in states described by kets $|a\rangle$ and $|b\rangle$, then the system can also be in a "mixed" state described by a linear combination of those state vectors: $|\psi\rangle = \alpha\,|a\rangle + \beta|b\rangle$, where α and β are scalars. The physical meaning of state vectors and their scalar products will become clear shortly.

Observables (i.e., physical quantities measured in an experiment) are represented by linear operators on a Hilbert space $\mathcal{H}$. A linear operator **A** associates, according to a certain rule, to each vector $|a\rangle$ from Hilbert space $\mathcal{H}$ some vector $|b\rangle \equiv \mathbf{A}|a\rangle$ belonging to the same space $\mathcal{H}$. This association or mapping is linear; that is, the following relation holds for any two vectors $|a\rangle$ and $|b\rangle$, and two scalars α and β:

(Eqn. 3.83)
$$\mathbf{A}\big(\alpha|a\rangle+\beta|b\rangle\big)=\alpha\mathbf{A}|a\rangle+\beta\mathbf{A}|b\rangle.$$

If the state of a system is described by a state vector $|\psi\rangle$, then the expectation value $\langle A\rangle$ of an observable A is given by

(Eqn. 3.84)
$$\langle A\rangle=\langle\psi|\mathbf{A}|\psi\rangle.$$

Demanding that the expectation value of a physical observable is a real number means that the linear operator associated with the observable is a self-adjoint or Hermitian operator: $\mathbf{A}=\mathbf{A}^\dagger$. Given a linear operator, one recalls the concept of eigenvectors $|\gamma\rangle$ and eigenvalues γ, which are solutions of the equation

(Eqn. 3.85)
$$\mathbf{A}|\lambda\rangle=\lambda|\lambda\rangle.$$

Note that if a system is in the state described by an eigenvector $|\gamma\rangle$ of an operator **A** associated with some observable A, then the corresponding eigenvalue γ is the expectation value $\langle A\rangle$: $\langle A\rangle=\langle\gamma|\mathbf{A}|\gamma\rangle=\gamma\langle\gamma|\gamma\rangle=\gamma$. It could be proven (see, for, example [20]) that eigenvectors of a Hermitian operator form a complete orthonormal basis, meaning that any state vector can be represented as a superposition of those eigenvectors. Assuming that Hermitian operator A associated with some observable A has the eigenvectors $|a_i\rangle$ such as $\mathbf{A}|a_i\rangle = a_i\,|a_i\rangle$, then for any state vector $|\psi\rangle$ we have the following decomposition:

(Eqn. 3.86)
$$|\psi\rangle = \sum_i |a_i\rangle\langle a_i|\psi\rangle.$$

Using Eqns. 3.84 and 3.86, the expectation value of an observable A for a system in this state $|\psi\rangle$ can be computed as

(Eqn. 3.87)
$$\langle A\rangle = \sum_i a_i\,|\langle a_i|\psi\rangle|^2\,.$$

This last equation is simply interpreted; recalling that a_i is the expectation value $\langle A\rangle$ if the system is in the state $|a_i\rangle$, we can conclude that square modulus $|\langle a_i|\psi\rangle|^2$ is the probability to find the system in the state $|a_i\rangle$. Altogether this constitutes the third postulate of quantum mechanics, which can be formulated as follows: Values of any observable A measured in an experiment are drawn from the set of eigenvalues $\{a_i\}$ of the operator $\mathbf{A}$ associated with this observable. The probability to measure certain value a_i, $P(A = a_i)$, for a system in the state described by a vector $|\psi\rangle$, is defined by

(Eqn. 3.88)
$$P(A = a_i) = \sum_{j:a_j=a_i} \left|\langle a_j|\psi\rangle\right|^2$$

where the sum is over eigenvectors $|a_j\rangle$ such as $\mathbf{A}|a_j\rangle = a_i|a_j\rangle$.

The change of the system state with the time (i.e., the evolution of a system) is described by a continuous unitary[7] operator:

(Eqn. 3.89)
$$|\psi,t\rangle = \mathbf{U}(t,t_0)|\psi,t_0\rangle.$$

Here $\mathbf{U}(t,t_0)$ is a *time evolution operator*. Obviously this operator, being an operator defining the evolution of a system with time, should satisfy the following conditions: $\mathbf{U}(t,t_0) = \mathbf{U}(t,t')\mathbf{U}(t',t_0)$, and $\mathbf{U}^{-1}(t,t_0) = \mathbf{U}(t_0,t)$. A time evolution operator is determined by the Schrödinger equation:

(Eqn. 3.90)
$$i\hbar\frac{\partial}{\partial t}\mathbf{U}(t,t_0) = \mathbf{H}(t)\mathbf{U}(t,t_0)$$

where operator $\mathbf{H}(t)$ is called the Hamiltonian operator of the system and $\hbar \equiv h/2\pi$ is the reduced Planck's constant. If the Hamiltonian does not depend on time, it coincides with the energy operator. Multiplying this last equation by $|\psi,t_0\rangle$, we will get the traditional form of the Schrödinger equation:

(Eqn. 3.91)
$$i\hbar\frac{\partial}{\partial t}|\psi,t\rangle = \mathbf{H}(t)|\psi,t\rangle.$$

---

[7] An operator $\mathbf{A}$ is a unitary operator if $\mathbf{A}^{\dagger}\mathbf{A} = \mathbf{A}\mathbf{A}^{\dagger} = \mathbf{I}$, where $\mathbf{I}$ denotes a identity operator.

It is easy to check that if the Hamiltonian **H** does not depend on time, the evolution operator can be written as (compare with Eqn. 9)

(Eqn. 3.92)
$$\mathbf{U}(t,t_0)=e^{-\frac{i}{\hbar}(t-t_0)\mathbf{H}}.$$

As usual, the exponential of an operator is defined through its eigenvectors (compare with Eqn. 10):

(Eqn. 3.93)
$$e^{\mathbf{A}}=\sum_i e^{a_i}\,|a_i\rangle\langle a_i|.$$

The quantity $|a_i\rangle\langle a_i|$ is a projection operator on the state vector $|a_i\rangle$. In general, $|a\rangle\langle b|$ forms a linear operator called the "outer product" or "tensor product" operator.

Next, if the Hamiltonian **H** does depend on time, but in such a way that for any time moments t and t', we have $[\mathbf{H}(t), \mathbf{H}(t')] \equiv \mathbf{H}(t)\mathbf{H}(t') - \mathbf{H}(t')\mathbf{H}(t) = 0$, the evolution operator is

(Eqn. 3.94)
$$\mathbf{U}(t,t_0)=e^{-\frac{i}{\hbar}\int_{t_0}^{t}\mathbf{H}(t')dt'}.$$

Finally, in the general case, we can write an evolution operator using a "time-ordered exponential":

(Eqn. 3.95)
$$\mathbf{U}(t,t_0)= = T_D e^{-\frac{i}{\hbar}\int_{t_0}^{t}\mathbf{H}(t')dt'} \equiv \lim_{N\to\infty}\left\{\left(1-\frac{i}{\hbar}\mathbf{H}(t_N)\Delta t\right)\cdot\left(1-\frac{i}{\hbar}\mathbf{H}(t_{N-1})\Delta t\right)\right\}\cdots\left(1-\frac{i}{\hbar}\mathbf{H}(t_0)\Delta t\right)$$

where $\left(1-\frac{i}{\hbar}\mathbf{H}(t_j)\Delta t\right)$ is an evolution operator over infinitesimal interval time interval (t_j, t_{j-1}), the time moments $\{t_j\}_0^N$ are defined as $t_j = t_0 + j\Delta t$, $\Delta t = (t - t_0)/(N - 1)$, and T_D denotes the Dyson time-ordering operator.

So far we have considered evolution of a single particle; now let us consider a macroscopic sample consisting of a large number of identical particles. The state of each particle can be described by state vector $|\psi_i\rangle$, where index $i = (1,..,N)$ numerates particles. We can write these vectors as a linear combinations of some orthonormal basis state vectors $|\alpha_k\rangle$, $k = (1,..,M)$:

(Eqn. 3.96)
$$|\psi_i\rangle=\sum_{k=1}^{M}a_k^{(i)}\,|\alpha_k\rangle, i=(1,..,N).$$

The expectation value of any observable A for this macroscopic sample can be written as

(Eqn. 3.97)
$$\langle A\rangle\equiv\frac{1}{N}\sum_{i=1}^{N}\langle\psi_i|\mathbf{A}|\psi_i\rangle=\sum_{k,l=1}^{M}\rho_{l,k}\langle\alpha_k|\mathbf{A}|\alpha_l\rangle$$

where $\rho_{l,k} \equiv \frac{1}{N}\sum_{i=1}^{N} a_k^{(i)*} a_l^{(i)}$ are elements of a matrix called a density matrix and **A** is an operator associated with an observable A. It is now convenient to introduce a statistical operator defined by elements of the density matrix:

(Eqn. 3.98) $$\rho \equiv \frac{1}{N}\sum_{i=1}^{N} |\psi_i\rangle\langle\psi_i| = \sum_{k,l=1}^{M} \rho_{l,k} |\alpha_l\rangle\langle\alpha_k|.$$

A statistical operator defined according to Eqn. 3.98 is called a *density operator*. It is easy to show that for an expectation value we have

(Eqn. 3.99) $$\langle A\rangle = \sum_{k=1}^{M} \langle \alpha_k | \boldsymbol{\rho}\mathbf{A} | \alpha_k\rangle = trace\{\boldsymbol{\rho}\mathbf{A}\}.$$

Evolution of the density operator with time is described by

(Eqn. 3.100) $$i\hbar\frac{d}{dt}\rho = [\mathbf{H}, \rho]$$

where **H** is the Hamiltonian of an individual particle.

This concludes our brief overview of quantum mechanics conceptions. Now let's apply this formalism to describe a system of spin ½ particles (such as protons) with magnetic moment placed in an external magnetic field.

From the Stern-Gerlach experiment [28] we know that whenever we measure a projection of the spin vector of a spin ½ particle on some axis, we will get only $\hbar/2$ or $-\hbar/2$. Let's choose this axis to be the z-axis and denote the state vectors for those two states as $|s_z, \pm\rangle$. By definition those state vectors are eigenvectors of an operator corresponding to the measurement of the spin projection on the z-axis $\mathbf{S}_z : \mathbf{S}_z |s_z, \pm\rangle = \pm\frac{\hbar}{2}|s_z, \pm\rangle$. This allows us to write operator $\mathbf{S}_z$ using spectral decomposition as

(Eqn. 3.101) $$\mathbf{S}_z = \frac{\hbar}{2}\{|s_z,+\rangle\langle s_z,+| - |s_z,-\rangle\langle s_z,-|\}.$$

To complete the description, we introduce operators corresponding to the measurement of the spin projection on the x- and y-axis[8]: S_x, S_y. The isotropy of the space, meaning all directions in the space are equivalent, results in the following commutation relations for those operators (see, for example, [22] or [23]):

(Eqn. 3.102) $$[\mathbf{S}_x, \mathbf{S}_y] = i\hbar\mathbf{S}_z,\ [\mathbf{S}_y, \mathbf{S}_z] = i\hbar\mathbf{S}_x,\ [\mathbf{S}_z, \mathbf{S}_x] = i\hbar\,\mathbf{S}_y.$$

Note that the spin-projection operators obey the same commutation relations as basic rotation matrices, apart from the factor $i\hbar$—see Eqn. 3.61. This should not be surprising because the relationships in Eqn. 3.102 are derived requiring that a Hamiltonian of a closed system does not change due to rotation of the system as a whole at an infinitesimal angle

---

[8] *Nota bene*: Here and everywhere else in this chapter we use a right-handed Cartesian coordinate system.

about an arbitrary axis. Using the commutation relations in Eqn. 3.102 we can explicitly write operators S_x, S_y for a spin ½ system as[9]

(Eqn. 3.103)
$$\mathbf{S}_x = \frac{\hbar}{2}\{|s_z,+\rangle\langle s_z,-| + |s_z,-\rangle\langle s_z,+|\}$$
$$\mathbf{S}_y = i\frac{\hbar}{2}\{|s_z,-\rangle\langle s_z,+| - |s_z,+\rangle\langle s_z,-|\}.$$

Eigenvectors of the operators S_x, S_y could be also expressed through the eigenvectors of the operator S_z:

(Eqn. 3.104)
$$|s_x,\pm\rangle = \frac{1}{\sqrt{2}}\{|s_z,+\rangle \pm |s_z,-\rangle\}$$
$$|s_y,\pm\rangle = \frac{1}{\sqrt{2}}\{|s_z,+\rangle \pm i|s_z,-\rangle\}.$$

Let us now use a simple example to illustrate how to use these relations to compute a quantity measurable in an experiment. Assuming a system is in the state with spin projection on the z-axis equal to $\hbar/2$, described by the state vector $|s_z, \pm\rangle$. The expectation value $\langle S_z\rangle \equiv \langle s_z, +|\mathbf{S}_z|s_z, +\rangle = \hbar/2$, and the probability to measure spin projection on the z-axis equal to $\hbar/2$ is $P(S_z = \hbar/2) = |\langle s_z,+|s_z,+\rangle|^2 = 1$, and the probability to measure $-\hbar/2$ is $P(S_z = -\hbar/2) = |\langle s_z,-|s_z,+\rangle|^2 = 0$. Then we can compute the expected value of the spin projections on the x-axis:

(Eqn. 3.105)
$$\langle S_x\rangle \equiv \langle s_z,+|\mathbf{S}_x|s_z,+\rangle = \left\langle s_z,+\left|\frac{\hbar}{2}\{|s_z,+\rangle\langle s_z,-| + |s_z,-\rangle\langle s_z,+1|\}\right|s_z,+\right\rangle =$$
$$= \frac{\hbar}{2}\left\{\langle s_z,+|s_z,+\rangle\langle s_z,-|s_z,+\rangle + \langle s_z,+|s_z,-\rangle\langle s_z,+|s_z,+\rangle\right\} = 0.$$

The probability to measure spin projection on the x-axis equal to $\hbar/2$ is $P(S_x = \hbar/2) = |\langle s_z,+|s_x,+\rangle|^2 = |1/\sqrt{2}\{\langle s_z,+|s_z,+\rangle + \langle s_z,+|s_z,-\rangle\}|\rangle^2 = 1/2$, and, similarly, the probability to measure $-\hbar/2$ is $P(S_x = -\hbar/2) = 1/2$. The same is true for the projection of the spin vector on the y-axis $\langle S_y\rangle = 0$, $P(S_y = \pm\hbar/2) = 1/2$. These results are consistent with the physical experiment: if we prepare a system with defined spin projection of some axis, as in the Stern-Gerlach experiment, then a projection on an orthogonal axis is undefined.

---

[9] The idea is to write $\mathbf{S}_x$ and $\mathbf{S}_y$ as sums of all combinations $|s_z, \pm\rangle\langle s_z, \pm|$ and find the decomposition coefficients using the commutation relationships in Eqn. 3.97, keeping in mind that $\mathbf{S}_x$ and $\mathbf{S}_y$ are self-adjoint operators.

The scalar operators $\mathbf{S}_x$, $\mathbf{S}_y$, and $\mathbf{S}_z$ represent measurements of the particle spin vector on corresponding axes (i.e., scalar value) and can be combined into a vector operator, **S**:

(Eqn. 3.106)
$$\mathbf{S} \equiv \mathbf{S}_x \hat{\mathbf{e}}_1 + \mathbf{S}_y \hat{\mathbf{e}}_2 + \mathbf{S}_z \hat{\mathbf{e}}_3$$

where $\hat{\mathbf{e}}_1$, $\hat{\mathbf{e}}_2$, and $\hat{\mathbf{e}}_3$ are unit vectors corresponding to the *x*-, *y*-, and *z*-axes. We also introduce an operator corresponding to the square modulus of the spin vector: $\mathbf{S}^2 \equiv \mathbf{SS} = \mathbf{S}_x^2 + \mathbf{S}_y^2 + \mathbf{S}_z^2$. If, for example, the system is in the $|s_z, +\rangle$ state, then for the expectation values of these operators in the case of spin ½ particle we have $\langle \mathbf{S} \rangle = \hbar / 2\hat{e}_3$, and $\langle \mathbf{S}^2 \rangle = 3\hbar^2/4 \equiv \hbar^2 1/2(1/2+1)$.

If a particle has an intrinsic magnetic moment, this magnetic moment is parallel to the spin vector, and we can write an operator corresponding to this magnetic moment:

(Eqn. 3.107)
$$\boldsymbol{\mu} = \gamma \mathbf{S}$$

where the scalar γ denotes, of course, the magnetogyric ratio.

Now if we apply a magnetic field to such a particle, the interaction energy of its magnetic moment with the field will be $-\boldsymbol{\mu} \cdot \mathbf{B}$, and the Hamiltonian operator is

(Eqn. 3.108)
$$\mathbf{H} = -\gamma \mathbf{S} \cdot \mathbf{B} \equiv -\gamma(\mathbf{S}_x B_x + \mathbf{S}_y B_y + \mathbf{S}_z B_z).$$

To illustrate the link between the quantum mechanics formalism described above and an experiment, let us consider a couple of special cases. First let us assume that the magnetic field is constant and aligned with the *z*-axis (i.e., $\mathbf{B} = B_0\hat{\mathbf{e}}_3$). In this case we can write a solution of the Schrödinger equation as

(Eqn. 3.109)
$$|\psi, t\rangle = e^{\frac{i}{\hbar}(t-t_0)\gamma B_0 S_z} |\psi, t_0\rangle.$$

The system is initially in the state with spin projection on the *z*-axis equal to $\hbar/2$: $|\psi, t_0\rangle = |S_z, +\rangle$ (i.e., low energy state). The expected magnetic moment, the quantity we measure in an experiment, in this state is $\langle \boldsymbol{\mu}(t_0) \rangle \equiv \gamma \langle s_z, + | \mathbf{S} | s_z, + \rangle = \gamma(\hbar/2)\hat{\mathbf{e}}_3$. Then, using the definition of an exponential operator (see Eqn. 3.93), the state of the system during the following time is described by the vector $|\psi, t\rangle = e^{it\omega_0/2} |s_z, +\rangle$, where we choose $t_0 = 0$ to shorten the notation, and denote $\omega_0 \equiv \gamma B_0$. We see that state vector $|\psi, t\rangle$ at any time *t* differs from the initial state vector $|\psi, t_0\rangle$ only by a scalar complex multiplier $e^{it\omega/2}$, meaning that the state of the system is the same for all the consequent time moments and all physical observables are constant. In particular, the probability to find the system in the state with spin projection on the *z*-axis equal to $-\hbar/2$ (i.e., the high energy state) is nonexistent: $P_-(t) \equiv |\langle s_z, - | \psi, t \rangle|^2 = |e^{it\omega_0/2} \langle s_z, - | s_z, + \rangle|^2 = 0$. Similarly, if the system was initially in the high energy state, the probability to find the system in the low energy state in the presence of a static magnetic field is zero.[10] The expected value of the magnetic moment at time *t* is $\langle \boldsymbol{\mu}(t) \rangle \equiv \gamma \langle s_z, + | e^{-it\omega_0/2} \mathbf{S} e^{it\omega_0/2} | s_z, + \rangle = \gamma \langle s_z, + | \mathbf{S} | s_z, + \rangle = \gamma(\hbar/2)\hat{\mathbf{e}}_3$.

Second, initially the system is in the state with spin projection on the x-axis equal to $\hbar/2$: $|\psi, t_0\rangle = |s_x, +\rangle$. As was shown before, this state can be written as a combination of eigenvectors of the $\mathbf{S}_z$; see Eqn. 3.104. The evolution of the system in this case is described by the following time-dependent state vector: $|\psi,t\rangle = 1/\sqrt{2}\{e^{it\omega_0/2}|s_z,+\rangle + e^{-it\omega_0/2}|s_z,-\rangle\}$. The expected value of magnetic moment at time t is easy to calculate (hint: Use Eqn. 3.103 to get $S_x|s_z,\pm\rangle = \hbar/2|s_z,\mp\rangle$ and $S_y|s_z,\pm\rangle = \pm i\hbar/2|s_z,\mp\rangle$):

(Eqn. 3.110)

$$\langle \boldsymbol{\mu}(t)\rangle \equiv \langle \psi,t|\mathbf{S}|\psi,t\rangle = \gamma\frac{\hbar}{2}\left\{\frac{e^{it\omega_0}+e^{-it\omega_0}}{2}\hat{\boldsymbol{e}}_1 + i\frac{e^{it\omega_0}-e^{-it\omega_0}}{2}\hat{\boldsymbol{e}}_2\right\} = \\ = \gamma\frac{\hbar}{2}\{\cos(t\omega_0)\hat{\boldsymbol{e}}_1 - \sin(t\omega_0)\hat{\boldsymbol{e}}_2\}.$$

This last equation is easy to interpret: if the average magnetization was initially orthogonal to the magnetic field, then the average magnetization subsequently rotates clockwise (assuming γ is positive) about the magnetic field with angular frequency $\omega_0 \equiv \gamma B_0$—which, of course, is the Larmor frequency.

In general, using the fact that the spin operator does not explicitly depend on time, we can obtain the equation describing the evolution of the expected magnetic moment. First let's compute the derivative of this quantity:

(Eqn. 3.111)

$$\frac{d}{dt}\langle\boldsymbol{\mu}(t)\rangle \equiv \gamma\frac{d}{dt}\langle\psi|\mathbf{S}|\psi\rangle = \gamma\langle\psi|\mathbf{S}|\dot{\psi}\rangle + \langle\dot{\psi}|\mathbf{S}|\psi\rangle$$

where the dot denotes differentiation with respect to time: $|\dot{\psi}\rangle \equiv \frac{d}{dt}|\psi\rangle$. According to the Schrödinger equation (Eqn. 3.91), we have $|\dot{\psi}\rangle = -\frac{i}{\hbar}\mathbf{H}(t)|\psi\rangle$, and $\langle\dot{\psi}| = \frac{i}{\hbar}\langle\psi|\mathbf{H}(t)$. Substituting these formulas into Eqn. 3.111, we get

(Eqn. 3.112)

$$\frac{d}{dt}\langle\boldsymbol{\mu}(t)\rangle = \gamma\frac{i}{\hbar}\langle\psi|[\mathbf{H}(t),\mathbf{S}]|\psi\rangle.$$

Using the commutation relationships (Eqn. 3.102), we can explicitly compute the operator $[\mathbf{H}(t),\mathbf{S}]$:

$$[\mathbf{H}(t),\mathbf{S}] = -\gamma i\hbar\{(B_z\mathbf{S}_y - B_y\mathbf{S}_z)\hat{e}_1 + (B_x\mathbf{S}_z - B_z\mathbf{S}_x)\hat{e}_2 + (B_y\mathbf{S}_x - B_x\mathbf{S}_y)\hat{e}_3\} = \gamma i\hbar\mathbf{B}\times\mathbf{S}.$$

---

[10] Here we neglected the possibility of a spontaneous emission, which is actually very low. To account for this effect we need to introduce a Hamiltonian for electromagnetic field, describing the radiation of a magnetic dipole. In this model the probability of spontaneous emission per unit time can be calculated as $W = (2/3)\gamma^2 h/(\lambda/2\pi)^2$, where $\lambda = c/2\pi\omega$ is the wavelength of the emitted photon. Assuming a 1T field, we have a probability of spontaneous emission for a proton $W \sim 10^{-25}$ 1/s, which is quite negligible.

Finally, we obtain the equation that describes the expected magnetic moment evolution:

(Eqn. 3.113)
$$\frac{d}{dt}\langle \boldsymbol{\mu}(t)\rangle = \gamma \langle \boldsymbol{\mu}(t)\rangle \times \mathbf{B}.$$

In this equation, we finally see the quantum and classical approaches converge, since this last equation is exactly Eqn. 3.4 describing the magnetic moment evolution.

Next let us complicate the experiment and assume that the magnetic field consists of a constant aligned with z-axis field $\mathbf{B}_0$, and the field $\mathbf{B}_1(t)$ orthogonal to the z-axis and rotating clockwise about it with angular frequency ω—that is, $\mathbf{B}_1(t) = B_1\cos(\omega t)\hat{\mathbf{e}}_1 - B_1\sin(\omega t)\hat{\mathbf{e}}_2 + B_0\hat{\mathbf{e}}_3$. It is convenient to introduce operators $\mathbf{S}_{\pm} \equiv \mathbf{S}_x \pm i\mathbf{S}_y$ to write the Hamiltonian as

(Eqn. 3.114)
$$\mathbf{H}(t) = -\left\{\omega_0 \mathbf{S}_z + \frac{\omega_1}{2}(e^{+i\omega t}\mathbf{S}_+ + e^{-i\omega t}\mathbf{S}_-)\right\}.$$

Similar to the classical approach, we seek a solution of the Schrödinger equation in the rotating frame. We transform to the rotating frame by substituting $|\psi',t\rangle = e^{-(i/\hbar)\omega_0 t S_z}|\psi,t\rangle$, where the prime denotes that the state vector belongs to the rotating frame (compare with Eqn. 3.35). The Schrödinger equation in this rotating frame is

(Eqn. 3.115)
$$i\hbar\frac{\partial}{\partial t}|\psi',t\rangle = \left\{e^{-\frac{i}{\hbar}\omega_0 t \mathbf{S}_z}\mathbf{H}(t)e^{\frac{i}{\hbar}\omega_0 t \mathbf{S}_z} + \omega_0\mathbf{S}_z\right\}|\psi',t\rangle.$$

The term $e^{-\frac{i}{\hbar}\omega_0 t \mathbf{S}_z}\mathbf{H}(t)e^{\frac{i}{\hbar}\omega_0 t \mathbf{S}_z}$ is easy to compute using the commutation relationships in Eqn. 3.102 and taking into account that Eqn. 3.59 for a similarity transformation $e^{\psi \mathbf{A}}\mathbf{B}e^{-\psi \mathbf{A}}$ involving square matrices **A** and **B** can be generalized for linear operators.[11] We obtain the Schrödinger equation in this rotating frame:

(Eqn. 3.116)
$$i\hbar\frac{\partial}{\partial t}|\psi',t\rangle = -\frac{\omega_1}{2}(e^{+i\Delta\omega t}\mathbf{S}_+ + e^{-i\Delta\omega t}\mathbf{S}_-)|\psi',t\rangle$$

where $\Delta\omega \equiv \omega - \omega_0$. We look for the solution of Eqn. 3.116 in the form:

(Eqn. 3.117)
$$|\psi',t\rangle = u_+|s_z,+\rangle + u_-|s_z,-\rangle.$$

The square modulus of the time-dependent coefficients $p_\pm$ represents the probability to find the system in the state $|s_z,+\rangle$ at the time t. Using relations $\mathbf{S}_\pm|s_z,\pm\rangle = \hbar\,|s_z,\pm\rangle$ and $\mathbf{S}_\pm|s_z,\pm\rangle = 0$ it is easy to get equations for the coefficients $u_\pm$:

(Eqn. 3.118)
$$\begin{cases}\dfrac{\partial}{\partial t}u_+ = i\dfrac{\omega_1}{2}e^{+i\Delta\omega t}u_- \\ \dfrac{\partial}{\partial t}u_- = i\dfrac{\omega_1}{2}e^{-i\Delta\omega t}u_+\end{cases}.$$

---

[11] Explicitly we have $e^{-\frac{i}{\hbar}\omega t s_z}\mathbf{S}_z e^{\frac{i}{\hbar}\omega t s_z} = \mathbf{S}_z$, and $[\mathbf{S}_z, \mathbf{S}_\pm] = \pm\hbar\mathbf{S}_\pm$ resulting in $e^{-\frac{i}{\hbar}\omega t \mathbf{S}_z}\mathbf{S}_\pm e^{\frac{i}{\hbar}\omega t \mathbf{S}_z} = e^{\pm i\omega t}\mathbf{S}_\pm$. Compare this with Eqn. 3.63.

The solution of the system of the differential equations in Eqn. 3.118 is given by

(Eqn. 3.119)

$$\begin{cases} u_+ = -\dfrac{2\omega'_-}{\omega_1} C_- e^{+i\omega'_+ t} - \dfrac{2\omega'_+}{\omega_1} C_+ e^{+i\omega'_- t} \\ u_- = C_+ e^{-i\omega'_+ t} + C_- e^{-i\omega'_- t} \end{cases}$$

where $\omega'_\pm \equiv \frac{1}{2}\left(\Delta\omega \pm \sqrt{\Delta\omega^2 + \omega_1^2}\right)$ and the constants $C_\pm$ are defined by the initial state of the system:

(Eqn. 3.120)

$$\begin{cases} -\dfrac{2\omega'_-}{\omega_1} C_- - \dfrac{2\omega'+}{\omega_1} C_+ = \langle s_z, + | \psi, t_0 \rangle \\ C_+ + C_- = \langle s_z, - | \psi, t_0 \rangle \end{cases}.$$

Assuming that the system was initially in the state with minimal energy (i.e., $|\psi, 0\rangle = |s_z, +\rangle$), we get

(Eqn. 3.121)

$$C_- = -C_+ = \frac{\omega_1}{2\sqrt{\Delta\omega^2 + \omega_1^2}}.$$

Using this last equation to compute probabilities $P_\pm(t)$ to find the system at the time t in the state $|s_z, \pm\rangle$ correspondently, we will get the Rabi's formula [35] for a two-level system:

(Eqn. 3.122)

$$\begin{cases} P_+(t) \equiv |u_+|^2 = 1 - \dfrac{\omega_1^2}{\alpha^2} \sin^2\left(\dfrac{\alpha t}{2}\right) \\ P_-(t) \equiv |u_-|^2 = \dfrac{\omega_1^2}{\alpha^2} \sin^2\left(\dfrac{\alpha t}{2}\right) \end{cases}$$

where $\alpha = \sqrt{\Delta\omega^2 + \omega_1^2}$.

From Eqn. 3.122 we see that the probability to find the system in the high energy state oscillates between 0 and $\omega_1^2/(\Delta\omega^2 + \omega_1^2)$ with the angular frequency $\sqrt{\Delta\omega^2 + \omega_1^2}$, known as Rabi frequency. Unless we tune the frequency of the rotating field $\mathbf{B}_1(t)$ close to the Larmor frequency, this probability is rather small. Once we tune the rotating-field frequency close enough to the Larmor frequency, the maximum value of $P_-(t)$ becomes noticeable, reaching 1 at $\omega = \omega_0$, making it a resonance phenomenon. We note that "close enough" means that the difference between the Larmor frequency and the frequency of the $\mathbf{B}_1(t)$ rotation is comparable to the Rabi frequency: $\Delta\omega \equiv \omega - \omega_0 \sim \omega_1$. The width of this resonance is described by the Lorentzian $1/(1+(\varepsilon\omega_0/\omega_1)^2)$, where $\varepsilon = \Delta\omega/\omega_0$ is relative detuning. The lower the ratio ω_0 / ω_1 is, the broader, in relative sense, is the resonance width. Thus in ULF regime, where often $\omega_0 \sim \omega_1$, we have very broad resonance.

In practice, one deals more often with oscillating rather than rotating fields. In this case, assuming $\mathbf{B}_1(t) = B_1 \cos(\omega t)\hat{\mathbf{e}}_1 + B_0\hat{\mathbf{e}}_3$, we can write the Hamiltonian of the system as

(Eqn. 3.123) $$\mathbf{H}(t) = -\left\{\omega_0 \mathbf{S}_z + \frac{\omega_1}{4}(e^{+i\omega t}\mathbf{S}_+ + e^{-i\omega t}\mathbf{S}_-) + \frac{\omega_1}{4}(e^{-i\omega t}\mathbf{S}_+ + e^{+i\omega t}\mathbf{S}_-)\right\}.$$

Naturally in this last formula the term $(e^{+i\omega t}\mathrm{S}_+ + e^{-i\omega t}\mathrm{S}_-)$ represents the clockwise rotating field and the term $(e^{-i\omega t}\mathrm{S}_+ + e^{+i\omega t}\mathrm{S}_-)$ represents the counterclockwise rotating field. Using the same approach as before we will get the following equations for the coefficients $u_\pm$:

(Eqn. 3.124) $$\begin{cases} \dfrac{\partial}{\partial t}u_+ = i\dfrac{\omega_1}{2}(e^{+i\Delta\omega t} + e^{-i\omega' t})u_- \\ \dfrac{\partial}{\partial t}u_- = i\dfrac{\omega_1}{2}(e^{-i\Delta\omega t} + e^{+i\omega' t})u_+ \end{cases}$$

where $\omega' \equiv \omega + \omega_0$. The solution of the system of the differential equations in Eqn. 3.124 cannot be given in terms of elementary functions, and we need to resort to a successive approximation scheme similar to that in Eqn. 3.70.

3.3 NMR RELAXATION

We conclude this chapter by moving from the realm of simplistic interactions between single spins and electromagnetic fields to the more realistic case of ensembles of spins in a complex "soup" of electromagnetic fields. In the previous section we considered equations of motion for isolated and ensemble spins in an external magnetic field. This simple model of nuclear magnetization evolution allows description of some aspects of the nuclear magnetism, such as precession of free spins, and resonant interaction of free spins with rotating or oscillating magnetic field. However, it completely ignores the interaction of the spins with their surroundings (beyond that of a homogenous uniform external magnetic field). Spins in the real world do not exist in such a uniform field. For example, spins are surrounded by magnetic moments, both electron and nuclear, of neighboring atoms, which generate local magnetic fields. The magnitude of these local fields varies from $\sim 10^{-2}\mu$T in liquids to $\sim 10^{2}\mu$T in solids. These local magnetic fields, which vary in space and time, lead to a phenomenon called relaxation. In NMR the term *relaxation* describes a variety of processes by which a spin system (or an ensemble of spins) returns to the thermal equilibrium (i.e., the most probable state). The following simple observations illustrate the main aspects of such a phenomenon.

If we place a macroscopic sample in an external magnetic field $\mathbf{B}_0$ and we observe the sample, we find that the sample acquires a magnetic moment aligned with this magnetic field over some time period that is characteristic of the sample. This magnetic moment is due to the imbalance between the number of spins being in the state with minimal energy (i.e., spin projection on the magnetic field direction is positive) and the number of spins being in the state with maximal energy (in a two-state system)—that is, with the opposite projection. At the thermal equilibrium, we find that the distribution of spins among energy states follows the Boltzmann distribution. This distribution is described by

(Eqn. 3.125)
$$\frac{N_m}{N} = \frac{e^{\frac{\gamma \hbar m B_0}{k_B T}}}{Z}$$

where N_m is the number of particles with projection of spin moment on magnetic field direction equal m; for a particle with a spin moment I, this projection takes the values $m = -I, I-1, \ldots, I$; $N = \sum_{m=-1}^{I} N_m$ is the total number of particles; γ is the magnetogyric ratio, $\hbar \equiv h/2\pi$ is the reduced Planck's constant; k_B is the Boltzmann constant; T is the temperature of the system; and $Z = \sum_{m=-I}^{I} e^{(\gamma \hbar m B_0/k_B T)}$ is the normalization factor.

Using Eqn. 3.125 we can compute the expected magnetic moment $\langle M \rangle$ of this macroscopic sample at the thermal equilibrium:

(Eqn. 3.126)
$$\langle M \rangle = \gamma \hbar N \frac{\sum_{m=-I}^{I} m e^{\frac{\gamma \hbar m B_0}{k_B T}}}{Z} \approx N \frac{\gamma^2 \hbar^2 I(I+1)}{3 k_B T} = \chi_0 B_0$$

where the constant $\chi_0 = N\gamma^2(\hbar^2 I(I+1)/3k_B T)$ is called a *static nuclear susceptibility*.[12]

This example shows that the spins in the sample are initially distributed equally between the $2I + 1$ energy levels, resulting in zero magnetic moment. After some time the spins are redistributed on the energy levels according to the Boltzmann distribution, giving magnetic moment according to Eqn. 3.126. This process of spin redistribution is called the *longitudinal* or *spin-lattice relaxation*. It is important to note the following two properties of this process. First, as shown in our discussion of Eqn. 3.109, the projection of a spin moment along some axis cannot be changed in the absence of a magnetic field (or some component thereof) orthogonal to this axis. Stated in another way, for the longitudinal relaxation to take place, the magnetic field experienced by the spin must contain components orthogonal to B_0. Secondly, the change of the population of energy levels results in change of the energy of the spin system. In the case of the longitudinal relaxation, the energy flows between the spin system and some other system to which the spins are coupled, usually referred to as a reservoir or lattice, that will accept this energy. This coupling is mediated by magnetic fields orthogonal to B_0. The interactions mediated by these "orthogonal" local fields are called *spin-lattice interactions*. The process of longitudinal relaxation in time is described by an exponential:

(Eqn. 3.127)
$$\langle M_{\|}(t) \rangle = \chi_0 B_0 \left(1 - e^{-\frac{t}{T_1}} \right).$$

[12] Note that in SI units, the static nuclear susceptibility defined here has dimensions of $A \cdot m^{-1} \cdot T^{-1}$. Sometimes it is convenient to define dimensionless static nuclear susceptibility: $\chi_0 = N(\gamma^2 \hbar^2 I(I+1)/3k_B T)\mu_0$, where $\mu_0 \equiv 4\pi \times 10^{-7}\ T^2 J^{-1} m^3$ is the vacuum permeability constant.

Here $\langle M_{\|}(t)\rangle$ is longitudinal magnetization (i.e., the component of the magnetization vector parallel to B_0), and the constant T_1, called the longitudinal (or spin-lattice) relaxation time, characterizes the rate at which the longitudinal magnetization recovers. If we revisit our statement earlier in this paragraph where we said that the Boltzmann distribution is attained "after some time," that time would be $t \gg T_1$.

Now consider the following example: after we polarize a sample (i.e., established magnetic moment [see Eqn. 3.127]) by applying magnetic field B_0 for the time much longer than the longitudinal relaxation time T_1 of the sample, we somehow change the direction of this static magnetic moment with respect to the applied magnetic field (various methods for changing or "tipping" the moment are discussed elsewhere in the text), so that the magnetic moment of the sample becomes orthogonal to the magnetic field. We assume that the projection of magnetic moment of the sample on the direction of the applied magnetic field (i.e., longitudinal magnetization) is zero, meaning that the spins in the sample are again equally distributed on the $2I+1$ energy levels. However, the induced magnetic moment did not disappear, so we have non-zero projection of this moment on some axis orthogonal to the magnetic field (i.e., transverse magnetization). The system described is not in the thermal equilibrium state; the relaxation process described above will start redistributing spins on the energy levels towards Boltzmann distribution, thereby increasing the longitudinal magnetization with time. At the same time a transition between energy levels changes the phase of the corresponding state vector, resulting in decay of the transverse magnetization. The longitudinal magnetization increases while the transverse magnetization decays as a consequence of transitions between energy levels that progresses exponentially with the time constant T_1. In addition to this, the local fields parallel to B_0, while not changing energy level population, induce different precession frequency for different spins. The interactions mediated by these "parallel" local fields, called spin-spin interactions, result in additional dephasing of the transverse magnetization. The process by which the transversal magnetization decays is called transversal relaxation and described by an exponential:

(Eqn. 3.128)

$$\langle M_{\perp}(t)\rangle = \langle M_{\perp}(t=0)\rangle e^{-\frac{t}{T_2}}$$

where $\langle M_{\perp}(t)\rangle$ is transversal magnetization (i.e., the component of the magnetization vector orthogonal to B_0) and the constant T_2, called the transversal relaxation time, characterizes the rate at which the transversal magnetization decays.

It is important to note that, as we described above, spin-lattice interactions contribute both to the recovery of longitudinal magnetization and to the decay of transversal magnetization, but spin-spin interactions contribute only to the dephasing (i.e., decay) of the transversal magnetization. That is why longitudinal relaxation time is always longer than or equal to the transversal relaxation time: $T_1 \geq T_2$.

REFERENCES

1. Bene GJ, Denis PM, Extermann CR (1950). Upper Limit of Spin-Spin Interaction Factor. *Phys Rev* 77(2): 288.
2. Bene GJ, Denis PM, Extermann RC (1950). Caractéristiques des noyaux stables. *J Phys Radium* *11*(10): S1–S7.
3. Brown RM (1950). Nuclear Magnetic Resonance in Weak Fields. *Phys Rev* 78(5): 530–532.
4. Abragam A (2002). Principles of Nuclear Magnetism, Oxford University Press, 1961. (reprinted 2002, p. 97).

5. Kimmich R, Anoardo E (2004). Field-cycling NMR relaxometry. *Progress in Nuclear Magnetic Resonance Spectroscopy* 44: 257–320.
6. Slichter CP (1990). *Principles of Magnetic Resonance.* Springer-Verlag.
7. Noak F (1986). NMR field cycling spectroscopy: principles and applications. *Progress in NMR Spectroscopy* 18: 171–276.
8. Jaynes ET (1955). Matrix treatment of nuclear induction. *Phys Rev* 98(4): 1099–1105.
9. Korn GA, Korn TM (2000). *Mathematical Handbook for Scientists and Engineers,* 2nd ed. New York: Dover Publications, Inc.
10. Liu S, Trenkler G (2008). Hadamard, Khatri-Rao, Kronecker and other matrix products. *International Journal of Information and System Sciences* 4(1): 160–177.
11. Kahan W (2008). "Notes for Math H110, Computing Cross-Products and Rotations in 2- and 3-Dimensional Euclidean Spaces." Available online at: http://www.cs.berkeley.edu/~wkahan/MathH110/Cross.pdf
12. Gelfand IM, et al. (1963). *Representations of the Rotation and Lorentz Groups and Their Applications.* Pergamon Press.
13. Sternberg S (1994). *Group Theory and Physics.* Cambridge University Press.
14. Gantmacher FR (2000). *The Theory of Matrices.* AMS Chelsea Publishing.
15. Suter D, Chingas GC, Harris RA, Pines A. (1987). Berry's phase in magnetic resonance. *Molecular Physics* 61(6): 1327–1340.
16. Berry MV (1984). Quantal phase factors accompanying adiabatic changes. *Proc R Soc Lond A 392,* 45–57.
17. Bloch F, Siegert A (1940). Magnetic resonance for nonrotating fields. *Physical Review* 57: 522–527.
18. Meiboom S, Gill D (1958). Modified spin-echo method for measuring nuclear relaxation times. *Review of Scientific Instruments* 29(8).
19. Dirac PA (1947). *Quantum Mechanics.* Oxford University Press.
20. Akhiezer NI, Glazman IM (1981). Theory of Linear Operators in Hilbert Space, Pitman.
21. Gerlach W, Stern O (1922). Das magnetische Moment des Silberatoms. *Zeitschrift für Physik A Hadrons and Nuclei* 9(1): 353–355.
22. Landau LD, Lifshitz EM (1977). *Quantum Mechanics: Non-Relativistic Theory.* Pergamon Press.
23. Bohm A (2001). *Quantum Mechanics: Foundation and Applications.* New York: Springer-Verlag.
24. Rabi II (1936). On the Process of Space Quantization. *Physical review* 49: 324–328.

CHAPTER 4

IMAGING TECHNIQUES AT ULF

4.1 INTRODUCTION

One of the most powerful applications of NMR is MRI. At the heart of the MRI is the NMR signal. However, in MRI, magnetic field gradients are also applied to spatially encode the frequency and phase of the NMR signal. While an image based purely on the signal intensity represents primarily the spin density, images also contain other material specific (chemical environment) information about transverse (T_2) and longitudinal (T_1) relaxation, spin-spin effects, flow, diffusion etc., which can be extracted with appropriate sequences of magnetic field pulses. This image information content, or contrast, is what allows MRI to encode such a wealth of information. Since its first demonstration in the 1970s [1], the use of MRI as a powerful diagnostic tool has expanded significantly. It is now perhaps best known as a medical imaging tool, as it is uniquely suited to noninvasively measure and distinguish soft-tissue anatomy without the use of ionizing radiation. Such images are usually based on some combination of proton density and relaxation (T_1/T_2) contrast. This information complements information available from x-ray imaging, which differentiates density and atomic species but typically has poor contrast for soft tissues. As noted earlier, MRI is also used as a noninvasive method of monitoring physiological function via associated changes in blood flow, perfusion (see for example reference [2]), or oxygenation[3].This approach, known as fMRI, is widely used as a tool to map the functional architecture of the brain.

As with all NMR approaches, the MRI signal scales proportionally with the applied magnetic field, and the magnetization of a voxel is directly proportional to the polarization field (Eqn. 1.8). Thus, the trend in NMR and MRI has been toward higher and higher magnetic fields for improved signal and spatial resolution (Fig. 1.2), most commonly provided by either permanent magnets or superconducting magnets. However, despite this overwhelming trend toward higher field strengths, there remain compelling reasons and interest for undertaking imaging at low (mT) and even ultra-low (μT) magnetic fields, as outlined in Chapter 1. In this chapter, we will discuss the primary motivations for ULF in MRI: (1) the MRI contrast can be measured at varied field strengths because the magnetic fields are easier to manipulate, (2) the information obtained at these lower field strengths is different than at high field strengths, and (3) in the absence of large magnetic fields, certain applications are enabled (e.g., imaging in combination with MEG or in the presence of metal, the potential for portable systems for rural or emergency settings, etc.).

At the time of this writing, a handful of groups have demonstrated anatomical imaging at ULF [4–8]. Because the signal scales with the polarization magnetic field strength, the obvious challenge for ULF MRI as compared with traditional HF MRI, is signal. There are many variables (coil configuration, pulse sequence, subject variability, etc.) between different imaging systems and methodologies that make direct comparison between images difficult. But here, to provide the general flavor of how things scale with field, we compare brain images at 1.5T with those at 46μT (which used a 30mT pre-polarization) in Figure 4.1 (data are from reference [7]). It is immediately obvious from this figure that the overall quality of the 1.5T image seems better. This is not surprising given the 50-fold increase in polarization field (1.5T vs. 30mT).

Table 4.1 lists some of the parameters for the two images, including voxel SNR, voxel size, the readout and phase-encoding steps, and the acquisition time. We will discuss each of these in great detail in Section 4.2. According to Table 4.1 we see that the voxel SNR of our ULF brain images shown in Figure 4.1 is about 10 (for a single scan), in a 3 × 3 × 6mm³ voxel. For the 1.5T image it is about 30, in a 1 × 1 × 6mm³ voxel. Let's look a little closer at what this means. While it is generally challenging to rigorously compare images (for example, factors such as T_1, T_2, k-space filtering, slice definition, etc., must be taken into account), even a very simple comparison immediately brings up several interesting points about ULF MRI. As we will discuss further in Section 4.2, the acquired signals and

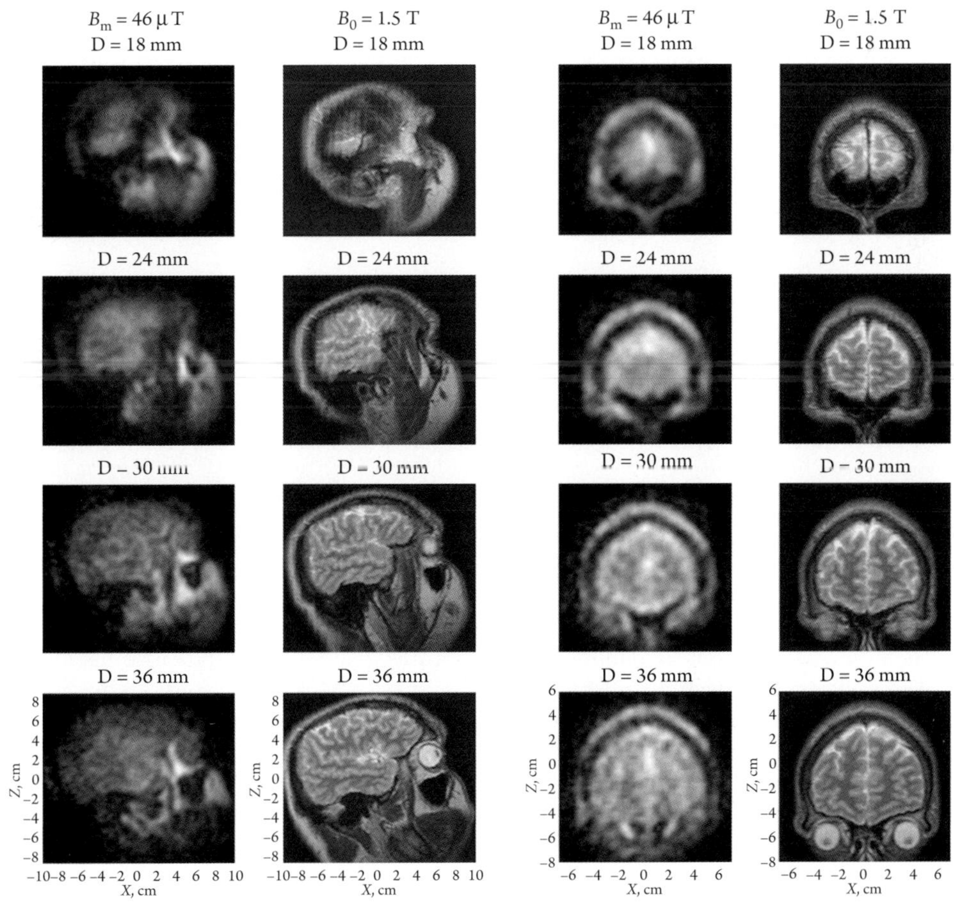

FIGURE 4.1 Comparison of images of the human brain at 46mT and 1.5T. Data are from reference [7].

TABLE 4.1 Image Parameters from Figure 4.1

Field strength	1.5T	30mT (46μT)
Voxel size (mm^3)	1 × 1 × 6	3 × 3 × 6
N_x (readout steps)	128	90
$N_{y,z}$ (phase steps)	128 × 128	61 × 11
t_a (ms)	10	50
SNR (voxel)	30	10

reconstructed image are linked by a discrete Fourier transform from which it follows that (for a single voxel)

(Eqn. 4.1)
$$\left(\frac{I_0}{\sigma_i}\right) = SNR_{\text{voxel}} = \sqrt{N_x N_y N_z}\left(\frac{S_0}{\sigma_s}\right)$$

where I_0/σ_i is the SNR for the image voxel and $N_{x,y,z}$ is the number of pixels (readout and phase-encode steps), S_0 is the signal in the time domain (for example, a sinewave from precessing magnetization, neglecting relaxation). S_0 is proportional to the voxel volume, dV, and the magnetic field,

(Eqn. 4.2)
$$S_0 \approx dV \cdot \chi_0 .$$

The noise in the acquisition bandwidth, σ_s, can also be expressed

(Eqn. 4.3)
$$\sigma_s = \sqrt{\sigma_n^2 \cdot \frac{N_x}{t_a}}$$

where σ_n is system noise, N_x is the number of readout steps, and t_a is the acquisition time. The relation N_x/t_a is the acquisition bandwidth.

Putting Eqns. 4.1, 4.2, and 4.3 together we find that we can describe the SNR of a device as

(Eqn. 4.4)
$$\left(\frac{\chi_0}{\sqrt{\sigma_n^2}}\right) = SNR_{\text{voxel}} \Big/ dV \cdot \sqrt{N_y N_z t_a} .$$

We can compare what this value is between the ULF and HF images, and we see it is about 12. A couple observations then follow. We might think that the ULF image is somehow not as bad as we expect, given the 50-fold difference in signal due to polarization. But several other things about this image are different. We took fewer steps at ULF, largely driven by the fact that the acquisition time was five times longer and it would have taken a really long time. Why must our acquisition time be so much longer? Because (as we shall also hear about again in Section 4.2) we are bandwidth limited compared to HF MRI. What does this mean? Imagine for a moment that we have a ball of water that we want to image. To produce a 1D image we will apply a gradient in our MRI machine and get an image in the frequency domain similar to that shown in Figure 4.2. In a HF scanner, 1.5T, our gradients are typically 10^{-2}T/m (10^{-4}T/cm). Using the fact that there the gyromagnetic ratio is 42.6MHz/T for protons, this gradient is about 4.2kHz/cm, so if our ball is 10cm in diameter we have $\Delta\omega$

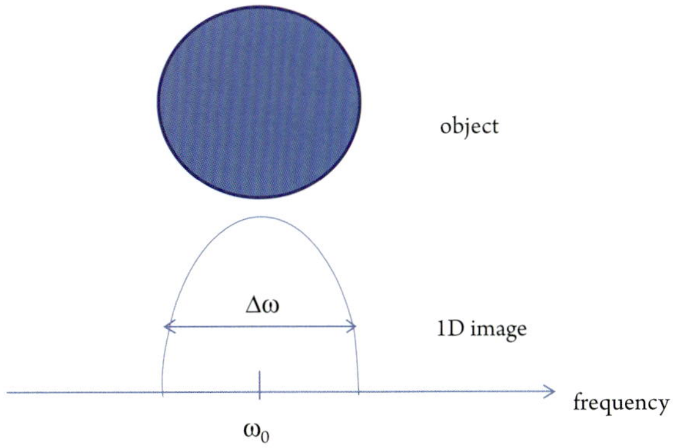

FIGURE 4.2 Example of a 1D NMR image in the frequency domain.

or about 42kHz. From the Nyquist theorem we know that to sample this we will need to sample at

(Eqn. 4.5)
$$t_a = \frac{1}{2\Delta\omega}.$$

Thus, to take 100 steps we will have $\Delta\omega = 420\text{Hz}$ and t_a needs to be 1.2 ms. On the other hand, in ULF MRI our gradients are much smaller (usually ~100 times smaller), and thus we have to sample for 120ms to take the same steps across the sample. This analysis, while by no means rigorous, gives the general flavor of the issue of scaling with magnetic field: there is less signal, less bandwidth, and image comparison can be a subtle business.

Imaging techniques used in ULF MRI are generally similar to those used for traditional HF MRI. One key difference, however, is that the ULF NMR/MRI methods typically utilize different magnetic fields for polarization, spin evolution, and measurement. In this regard it bears some resemblance to and maintains many of the advantages for novel contrast of field-cycling NMR/MRI. A description of fast field-cycling MRI relying on more traditional permanent and superconducting magnet technologies can be found in reference [9]. However, acquiring a "useful" image with ULF can be more challenging due to lower signal amplitude and less bandwidth with which to acquire it, as we saw in the simple example of Figure 4.1. And of course, dealing with SQUID sensors in the presence of relatively large and time-varying magnetic fields is always an added challenge. The definition of "useful" will be discussed shortly (Section 4.3.1.1), but ULF MRI will likely always be at a disadvantage in terms of spatial resolution and SNR simply because of these challenges.

The areas where ULF MRI may provide an advantage over HF MRI can roughly be broken into two categories: hardware and contrast mechanisms. ULF MRI offers a distinct advantage with imaging specifically enabled by lower magnetic fields (e.g., in the presence of metal, combined with other modalities such as MEG or EEG, or in an operating room), and with flexible field generation, such as the ability to reorient or even remove the magnetic field in real time. Contrast refers to differences between tissue types for both changes in T_1 and T_2. At ULF, one has the unique ability to explore contrast associated with changing magnetic field as given by traditional MRI theory, and also (unique to ULF) phenomena enabled by overlapping the Larmor frequency with processes of interest such as fluctuations in the neural magnetic field. These differences in hardware and contrast may be interrelated, and indeed they are also the very things that pose significant challenges for ULF

MRI. The key decision criteria for pursuing imaging at ULF are whether the benefits(e.g., contrast) outweigh the drawbacks (e.g., reduced SNR).

In Section 4.2 we will cover the basics of MRI in the context of a typical ULF MRI pulse sequence. In Section 4.3 we will discuss some the significant challenges, such as low signal, low bandwidth, and the fact that the magnetic fields used are comparable in strength to other unwanted but unavoidable magnetic fields (e.g., concomitant gradients and ghost artifacts). Section 4.4 will focus on imaging techniques to make the most of the signal, and Section 4.5 will elaborate on the unique advantages of ULF MRI. We will discuss proven and potential applications to brain imaging (and others) enabled by ULF MRI in Chapter 5.

4.2 GENERAL IMAGING CONCEPTS (HOW TO DO MRI)

In general. the principles used for ULF MRI are largely similar to those used for traditional MRI. The primary differences with ULF include (1) less signal and lower bandwidth, (2) simpler and more diverse manipulation of magnetic fields (novel pulse sequences), (3) differences in detector technology, and (4) differences in T_1 contrast.

The general concepts for NMR/MRI (and ULF MRI) were discussed in Chapters 1 (physics) and 2 (hardware). Here we review the general physical principles of MRI, highlighting the differences between traditional HF and ULF approaches. An excellent and far more complete description of conventional MRI can be found in reference [12].

The principal aim of all MRI is to spatially encode the NMR signal. The spatial variation in NMR properties (e.g. T_1, T_2, or density) is what underlies the information available in the MRI images. While the ULF MRI images we presented in Chapter 1 were primarily based on density contrast, as we have since seen, T_1 and T_2 can be used to provide information on the chemical environment (Chapter 3).

MRI is fundamentally based on the fact that the Larmor frequency over the sample depends on the spatial profile of the applied magnetic field over the sample, $\omega = \gamma B$, and thus provides a mechanism for such encoding.

Recall that, neglecting relaxation effects, the NMR signal $S(t)$ in a single voxel (dV) will be

(Eqn. 4.6) $$dS(t) \propto \rho(\mathbf{r}) e^{i\int_0^t \omega(\mathbf{r},t')dt'} dV$$

where $\rho(\mathbf{r})$ is the spin density and $\omega(\mathbf{r}, t')$ is the Larmor frequency over the sample during the measurement. For most pure NMR applications, without imaging, the Larmor frequency does not vary appreciably in space or time over the sample during the experiment such that $\omega(\mathbf{r}, t') = \omega_0$ and the NMR signal is

(Eqn. 4.7) $$S(t) \propto \iiint \rho(\mathbf{r}) e^{i\omega_0 t} \, dV.$$

If we wish to spatially encode the NMR signal, we intentionally apply a magnetic field gradient $\mathbf{G}(t)$ (assumed to be a linear gradient for these discussions) that causes the local Larmor frequency (magnetic field) to vary in a known way, such that

(Eqn. 4.8) $$\omega(\mathbf{r},t) = \omega_0 + \gamma \mathbf{G}(t) \cdot \mathbf{r}.$$

In Eqn. 4.8 we assume that the primary Larmor frequency established by B_m does not vary with time or position *during* the signal measurement time. However, the ability to manipulate the measurement field in strength and orientation *between* measurements to extract different information from the image is a key feature of the ULF MRI approach that typically differs from HF approaches.

The signal from the sample becomes

(Eqn. 4.9)
$$S(t)=\iiint C(\mathbf{r})\rho(\mathbf{r})e^{i\int_0^t[\omega_0 t'+\gamma\mathbf{G}(t')\cdot\mathbf{r}]dt'}dV,$$

(Eqn. 4.10)
$$S(t)=e^{i\varphi(t)}\iiint q(\mathbf{r})e^{i\int_0^t\gamma\mathbf{G}(t')\cdot\mathbf{r}dt'}dV.$$

In Eqn. 4.10 we have used the contrasted spin density $q(\mathbf{r}) = C(\mathbf{r})\,\rho(\mathbf{r})$. $q(\mathbf{r})$ is primarily proportional to the local spin density $\rho(\mathbf{r})$ of the observed nuclides. When a suitable preparatory sequence is used, $q(\mathbf{r})$ can also be made to depend on the relaxation times $T_1(\mathbf{r})$ and $T_2(\mathbf{r})$ and on the diffusion coefficient $D(\mathbf{r})$, all local properties at point $\mathbf{r}$. For simplicity, $C(\mathbf{r})$ contains all of these aspects of contrast information. In general $C(\mathbf{r})$ could also vary with time, but we will neglect this for now. We have also assumed that the integral over the main Larmor frequency can be expressed as a time-varying phase $\int_0^t \omega_0(t')dt' = \varphi(t)$.

It should be mentioned that in the approach detailed in Eqn. 4.7 we are assuming that the signal is obtained from the entire sample. Another way to extract information is through the excitation of a sub-space of the sample, for example by slice selection, as described in Chapter 1. In this approach a "slice select" gradient is applied in conjunction with a specific RF pulse to excite only a slab of the sample. In this case the information from Eqn. 4.10 would simply involve a 2D integration over the slab.

We next introduce the concept of the reciprocal space vector [10,11]:

(Eqn. 4.11)
$$\mathbf{k}\equiv(2\pi)^{-1}\,\gamma\int_0^t\mathbf{G}(t')dt'$$

and following the outline in Callaghan (and references therein) [12] we rewrite Eqn. 4.10 as

(Eqn. 4.12)
$$S(\mathbf{k})=e^{i\varphi(t)}\iiint q(\mathbf{r})e^{i2\pi\mathbf{k}\cdot\mathbf{r}}dV, \text{ where}$$

(Eqn. 4.13)
$$q(\mathbf{r})=e^{i\varphi(t)}\iiint S(\mathbf{k})e^{-i2\pi\mathbf{k}\cdot\mathbf{r}}\,d^3k.$$

Eqns. 4.12 and 4.13 are a Fourier transform pair showing that the signal and spin density are mutually conjugate, which is a fundamental formulation underlying MRI. In MRI the pulse sequence is typically thought of as the trajectory covering this *k*-space, from which the MRI image is derived. Just as we can describe the trajectory of a particle as $\mathbf{r}(t)=\int_0^t\mathbf{v}(t')dt'$ where $\mathbf{v}(t)$ is the velocity, we can think of $\mathbf{k}(t)$ as a trajectory through the image, where the gradient is like the velocity term. How we apply the gradients will determine the course [13].

An example of the 3D Fourier Imaging pulse sequence used to produce many of our ULF MRI images (including those shown in Fig. 4.1 and Chapter 1, Fig. 1.1) is shown in Figure 4.3. The magnetic field coil hardware used to implement this pulse sequence is shown schematically in Figure 4.4. B_p denotes the magnetic field coils to generate the sample

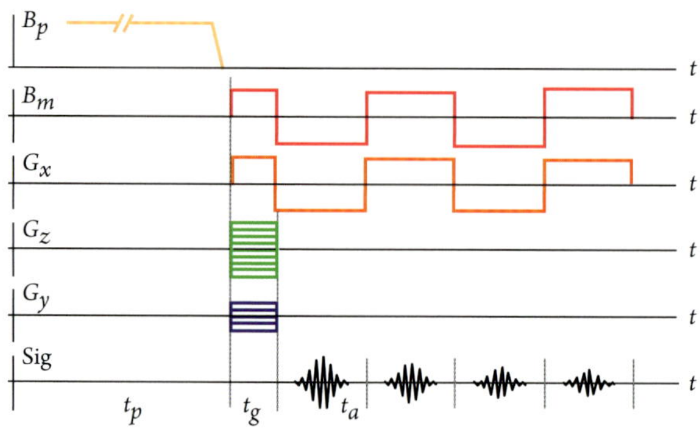

FIGURE 4.3 Fourier imaging sequence for ULF MRI.

magnetization, in this example along the x-axis. B_m denotes the measurement magnetic field coils, along the z-axis. The additional $G_{x,y,z}$ coils are for gradient encoding in the $B_z/dx,y,z$ directions, respectively. In HF MRI there is a single fixed field providing both B_p and B_m, typically provided by a large superconducting magnet. In ULF MRI the field generation is typically produced by simple electromagnets and allows for different field orientations and strengths provided by separate B_p and B_m coils. The pulse sequence shown in Figure 4.3 produces the trajectory in k-space, shown in Figure 4.5 with only the x and z dimensions for simplicity. Let us now go through the ULF MRI pulse sequence in more detail to further highlight the similarities and differences between traditional and ULF MRI.

4.2.1 Pre-polarization

In the first time period, t_p, a pre-polarization field is applied to recruit spins. To develop equilibrium magnetization, the pre-polarization time t_p must be long compared to T_1. (We

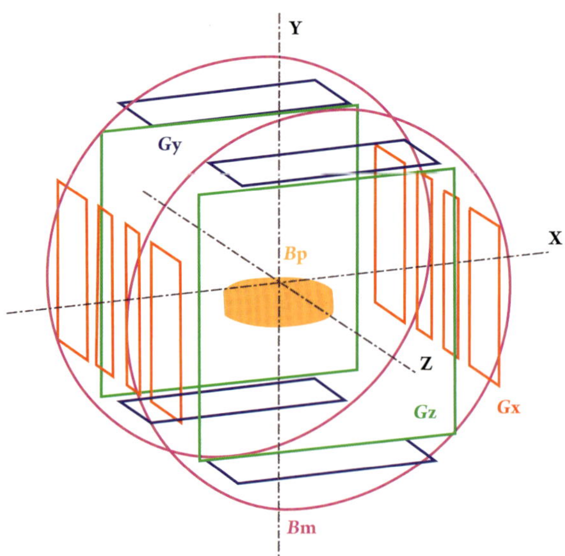

FIGURE 4.4 Schematic of ULF MRI field generation hardware for the pulse sequence in Figure 4.3.

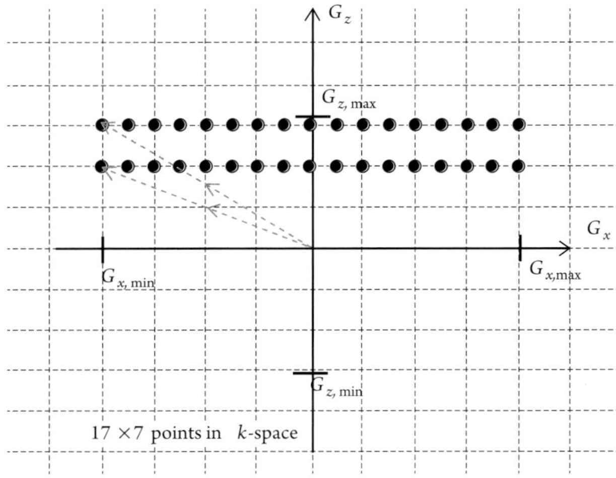

FIGURE 4.5 Trajectory in k_x-k_z-space corresponding to the pulse sequence shown in Figure 4.3.

use the term "develop" to denote the change of a given physical parameter with time.) The first step to any NMR/MRI application, regardless of magnetic field strength, is recruitment of the spin population to produce a measurable magnetization (Chapter 1, Eqns. 1.6–1.8). This is the "preparation" time before we begin our travels through *k*-space and image acquisition. With ULF MRI, as with many field-cycling methods, sample preparation is done by application of a pre-polarization field, a method by which we can apply a larger (typically 10–100mT) field, B_p, for some time t_p, to recruit more spins. Readout is then at lower Larmor frequencies (magnetic fields) chosen to derive certain benefits (contrast, compatibility, penetration through metal, etc.).

To briefly review, when placed in an external magnetization field B_p, magnetization of the *N* spins in a voxel will result.

We remind the reader that the equilibrium magnetization is given by

(Eqn. 4.14)
$$M_{eq} = \frac{N\hbar^2 \gamma^2 I(I+1) B_p}{3k_B T}.$$

For the case where we start with no initial magnetization and apply this field along some axis (in Fig. 4.4 it is the *x*-axis).the magnetization develops as

(Eqn. 4.15)
$$M_x(t) = M_{x,eq}\left(1 - e^{-t/T_1}\right)$$

where $k_B = 1.381 \times 10^{-23}$ J/K and $\hbar = 1.055 \times 10^{-34}$J-sec, and γ is in the Rad/T-sec form (267.513 for the spin $I = ½$ protons), and T is the temperature. We note that in HF MRI polarization and measurement are usually performed by the same field. A discussion of how one might produce the pulsed pre-polarization field can be found in Chapter 2.

Relating back to our imaging Eqns. 4.12 and 4.13, the contrasted spin density develops during this stage as $q(\mathbf{r})\rho(\mathbf{r})(1-\exp(-t_p/T_1(\mathbf{r})))$.

As Eqn. 4.15 shows, the magnetization asymptotically approaches equilibrium inverse–exponentially. Hence a common rule of thumb is to polarize for several T_1 times to attain the maximum signal (at least $3 \times T_1$ is common). While the most obvious implication of ULF MRI is lower SNR due to small polarizing fields, T_1 (and hence contrast) also changes with field, typically decreasing with reduced fields. Therefore, an advantage at ULF is that shorter T_1 leads to shorter required polarization times and the potential for a higher duty cycle. For example, in brain tissue at 1.5T, T_1 is ~1s [14], whereas at ULF is it ~100ms [15]. Another advantage of the ULF approach is that the T_1 contrast in the image can be selected by the user to correspond to that of either the polarization field or the measurement field, depending on the pulse sequence. This can provide additional information about tissue based on how T_1 changes with field strength (T_1 dispersion). The topic of T_1 in the context of image contrast, and the advantages and disadvantages that it confers at ULF, will be discussed more completely in Section 4.5.

It is also worth noting that the B_p used to recruit spin in the pre-polarization method can be relatively inhomogeneous with almost no ill effects on the image, as the field that affects image quality is the measurement field in which the sample magnetization is recorded. This field is typically 1,000 times smaller than B_p at ULF (100μT measurement vs. 100mT pre-polarization). In traditional MRI the polarization field and the measurement field are the same, and thus there is a requirement for B_p to be not only large but highly uniform (better than 1ppm uniformity). At ULF this is not necessarily the case; for a fixed relative homogeneity, the NMR line width scales linearly with the strength of the magnetic field [16]. This will be discussed more completely in Section 4.2.2. Typically it is much easier to generate the large B_p field when the requirement for homogeneity is removed.

After B_p is removed, spin evolution and/or readout begins. B_p can be removed either adiabatically or non-adiabatically. This was described in detail in Chapter 3 but one simple way to visualize this is that if the rotation of the field orientation during B_p removal (e.g., transitioning from B_p to B_m) is much faster than the Larmor frequency, it is non-adiabatic ($dB_p/dt \gg \gamma B_m^2$). In this case, the magnetization cannot follow the field direction change. In the pulse sequence example shown in Figure 4.3, adiabatic removal leaves the spins aligned with the much weaker measurement field (the z-axis shown in Fig. 4.4). In the case of non-adiabatic removal, the spins are left in their original orientation (e.g., the x-axis shown in Fig. 4.4) and precession about the z-axis would begin immediately.

The approach taken to remove B_p is a key part of how precession is started in ULF MRI. Since B_p is typically 10 to 100mT and is removed within 10 to 100ms (depending on the approach), the field changes dB/dt may range from 0.1 to 10 T/s. It is worth noting that the FDA initially limited dB/dt to 20T/s [17], but now these guidelines have been relaxed and dB/dt should avoid discomfort, pain, or nerve stimulation [18]. In our experience B_p removal is generally too slow to produce unwanted physiological effects (none that we have observed). However, a rapid change in B_p can induce eddy currents and transient magnetic fields in nearby conductors and/or affect the sensors, each of which may impose a "dead time" for these effects to settle after B_p is switched off. A discussion on correction for artifacts associated with these transients will be presented in Section 4.3. Section 4.4 will discuss the merits of adiabatic versus non-adiabatic B_p in terms of phase stability and loss of signal (in the presence of the shorter T_1 times of ULF).

4.2.2 Begin Precession (Spin Reorientation)

Upon completion of the polarization, the MRI pulse sequence begins. As we described in Chapter 1, the measurable signal is derived from the precession of the magnetization when spins are tipped such that there is a component of magnetization transverse to the applied magnetic field. This process is described by the Bloch equations:

(Eqn. 4.16)
$$\frac{d\mathbf{M}}{dt}=\gamma\mathbf{M}\times\mathbf{B}-\left[\frac{1}{T_1}(M_z-\chi_0 B_z)\hat{\mathbf{z}}+\frac{1}{T_2}(M_x\hat{\mathbf{x}}+M_y\hat{\mathbf{y}})\right]$$

where B_z is the measurement field (here defined to be along the z-axis), and T_1 is the value in the measurement field.

The first term describes the precession about any transverse magnetization and the second the effects of spin relaxation. We need to begin this spin precession to produce our signal and start our trajectory through k-space.

In the implementation of the pulse sequence shown in Figure 4.3 we begin precession by removing B_p (along the x-axis) non-adiabatically leaving the magnetization along this direction, and applying B_m orthogonally to B_p (along the z-axis). This immediately begins the precession of the magnetization about the z-axis of the measurement field at the start of the encoding period, t_g. By repeating the subsequent pulse sequence for different values of t_p, and using the initial amplitude of the precession signal, one can determine T_1 at the value of the polarization field.

Alternately, if the B_p ramp-down had been adiabatic, spins would end up aligned with the z-axis and a spin-reorientation (also known as "spin tipping" or "spin-flip") would be required at the transition between t_p and t_g in Figure 4.3. Spin-flip is also routine in HF MRI, where B_p and B_m are the same field. The ultimate goal of spin-reorientation is to result in some component of the magnetization orthogonal to the measurement field. Typically the spin flip is 90 degrees (or $\pi/2$) for maximum signal, but it can be any value. Any component of the magnetization vector tipped away from the measurement field axis will begin to precess and provide a measurable signal. In HF MRI the first spin-flip is typically a 90-degree($\pi/2$) pulse, and in the case of spin-echo imaging that pulse is followed by a series of refocusing 180-degree(π) RF pulses. To initiate the spin-flip, the coils are oriented orthogonal to the axis of the polarization field. Although not shown, in the ULF MRI configuration a spin-flip coil would be oriented along the y-axis orthogonal to both B_p (x-axis) and B_m (z-axis).

The spin reorientation can be provided by either resonant or nonresonant methods. In the resonant case, a magnetic field time varying at the Larmor (resonant) frequency is applied in a fixed orientation orthogonal to the measurement field. In the nonresonant case, a field that varies slowly in time and orientation, and does not contain Larmor frequency content, is applied. It is worth emphasizing that the second (nonresonant) approach to spin-reorientation is totally unique to the ULF approach. Both approaches are described below.

1. **Resonant spin-tipping:** This approach is similar to traditional MRI, as described in Chapter 1. After the removal of B_p a time-varying field B_1 (or B_{RF}) is applied orthogonally to B_m at the Larmor frequency for a desired period of time to reorient the magnetization. The measurement field of the system may be reduced such that the Larmor frequency is low enough that both the applied magnetic field and the resulting NMR signal can penetrate through conductive containers (such as a soda can or foil-lined packaging), or are not appreciably distorted by the presence of conducting materials [19,20].

2. **Nonresonant spin-tipping:** The nonresonant spin-reorientation can be implemented several ways. Here we present two examples. (1) The original orientation of the measurement field B_m is changed to some new direction adiabatically (the field changes slowly enough that the magnetization can follow). The orientation of B_m is then non-adiabatically restored to its original orientation, leaving the magnetization "tipped." (2) B_p and B_m are orthogonal, as shown in Figure 4.4, and the non-adiabatic switch-off of B_p is followed by application of orthogonal B_m. Spins remain at 90 degrees and simply begin precession.

Regardless of how precession is induced, it is useful to reiterate that pre-polarization, spin-reorientation, and the subsequent evolution can all be at different field strengths, which in turn determines the field-dependent contrast for the material. This is a very powerful experimental "knob," as the contrast might vary strongly with magnetic field (as described in Chapter 3).

Before we move on to the rest of the pulse sequence, let us briefly revisit the issue of the field homogeneity requirement of B_m, in the context of imaging. As we mentioned in Chapter 1, the inherent line width is proportional to the inverse of the measured relaxation time, $1/T_2^*$,

(Eqn. 4.17)
$$\Delta\omega_l \approx \frac{2}{T_2^*}.$$

For simplicity we can consider the 1D imaging case, where we have two objects separated by Δx, and we apply a gradient G_x. If one then looks at a Fourier transform of the signal, there will be two peaks separated by $\gamma G_x \Delta x$, from Eqn. 4.8. The minimum ability to resolve them spatially will be

(Eqn. 4.18)
$$\gamma G_x \Delta x = \Delta\omega_l .$$

Thus the spatial resolution can be expressed as

(Eqn. 4.19)
$$\Delta x = \frac{\Delta\omega_l}{\gamma G_x} = \frac{2}{\gamma G_x T_2^*}.$$

If T_2^* is dominated by T_2, the resolution can be improved only by raising the applied gradient. But if field inhomogeneities across the sample, ΔB, are the primary cause of dephasing, then making B_m more homogeneous will improve resolution. The field inhomogeneity of B_m can be written as $B_m(\Delta B/B_m)$, where $\Delta B/B_m$ is the relative homogeneity. Thus

(Eqn. 4.20)
$$\Delta\omega_l = \gamma\Delta B = B_m\left(\frac{\Delta B}{B_m}\right)$$

and

(Eqn. 4.21)
$$\Delta x = \frac{B_m}{G_x}\left(\frac{\Delta B}{B_m}\right).$$

Because magnet design determines the relative homogeneity, the resolution can be improved either by improving the homogeneity of the magnet or by reducing the field strength B_m. Even when T_2 limits the resolution, an LF MRI system will be able to employ less homogeneous magnets to obtain the same resolution as an HF system. In this case, because B_m is very low (microtesla), inhomogeneous fields can be employed and excellent line widths obtained.

4.2.3 Encoding and Acquisition

To realize the information in the image, or to traverse *k*-space, one must apply and vary the gradients along multiple axes that spatially encode the NMR signal, and collect the data before the signal has dephased (limited by T_2). These periods are shown as t_g (time during application of gradient fields) and t_a (acquisition time) respectively, in Figure 4.3. Finally, a 2D or 3D Fourier transform must be performed on the data to extract the image. Echo pulses are also routinely employed to help remove the effects of field inhomogeneity.

To begin the discussion, let us revisit the various types of echoes. In HF MRI two types of echoes are routinely used. (1) The spin echo, as described in Chapter 1, uses a 180-degree spin-tip to produce refocusing. This is shown schematically in Figure 4.6a. The spins are shown precessing in the *x-y* plane about a magnetic field oriented into the page. The spins have dephased due to gradients. After the 180-degree reorientation (imagine flipping the paper over), the faster spins are behind the slower, and will catch up, producing the echo. This sort of echo is also referred to as a "pancake" echo because it can also be visualized as flipping the orientation of the spins, like flipping a pancake. (2) The gradient echo, Figure 4.6b, is also routinely used in HF MRI where we assume we have a large homogeneous field and then a smaller gradient. The reversal of the gradient can change the precession speed, thus causing the echo.

A third type of echo, Figure 4.6c, is unique to ULF MRI and is known as the "field echo." This echo is possible if one can reverse the orientation of the measurement field as well. In this case the precession direction is changed. An analogy is to runners on a racetrack who suddenly reverse direction in the middle of the race (with faster ones now being behind and the echo happening when they catch up). For this reason the field echo is also referred to as the "racetrack" echo.

In HF MRI the field echo is not an option due to the inability to reorient the main magnetic field, but a field echo can be quite valuable. For example, a gradient echo alone cannot remove inhomogeneity associated with the main magnetic field, but a field echo can.

In the sequence shown in Figure 4.3, the NMR signal is spatially encoded by application of the magnetic gradient fields during the time t_g. The period t_g, indicated in Figure 4.5 by a dashed line, represents moving to a starting place in *k*-space. The G_z (and G_y) phase-encoding gradient moments provide the intercept along the k_z and k_y axis, respectively. The G_x dephasing gradient moment sets our starting place for the acquisition of the line in *k*-space along k_x. Upon completion of phase encoding, t_g, the phase-encoding gradients (G_z and G_y) are removed and B_m and G_x are inverted to produce a field echo. During the acquisition time, t_a, we acquire a single line along k_x. The dephasing gradient moment is half the readout gradient moment (by using t_g that is half the length of t_a). This ensures that the echo signal refocuses in the center of the readout gradient, as we cross $k_x = 0$. The signals from multiple echoes can be acquired and averaged to improve the SNR, as shown in Figure 4.3, where the subsequent field echoes are trips back and forth along the same line in *k*-space, or multiple lines in *k*-space can be encoded in a single acquisition to accelerate encoding. Acquisition of multiple echoes is efficacious only for as long as sufficient signal remains from the decaying

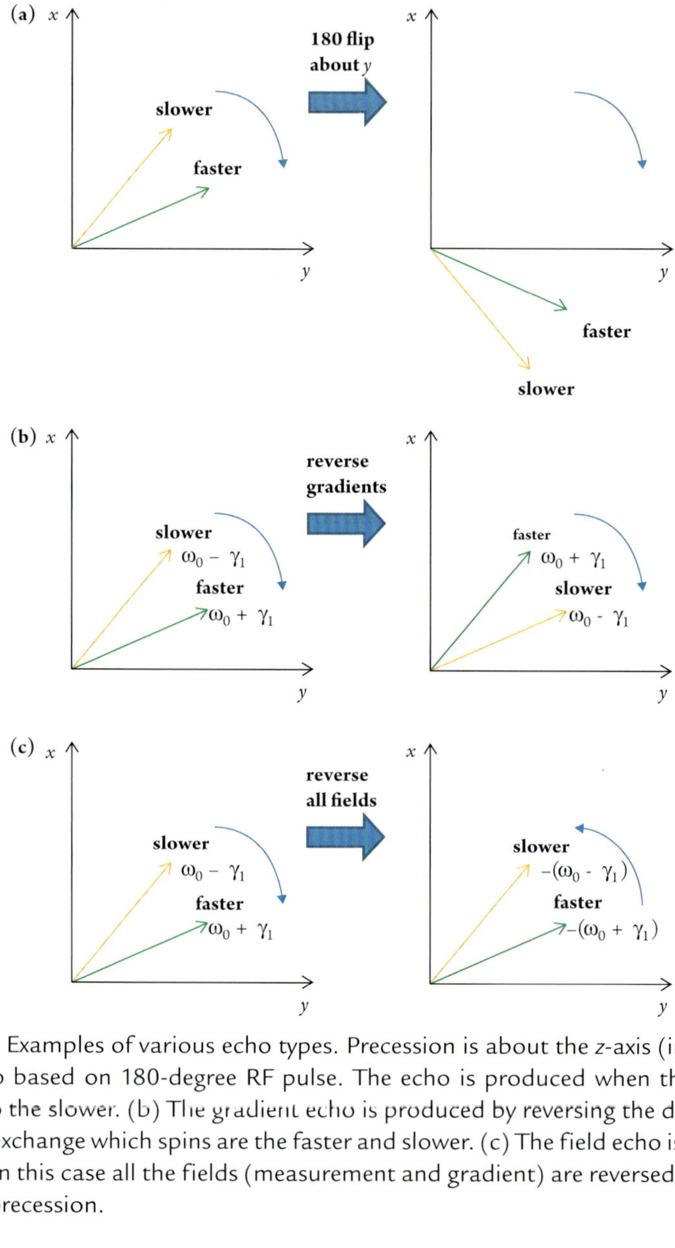

FIGURE 4.6 Examples of various echo types. Precession is about the *z*-axis (into the page). (a) Spin-echo based on 180-degree RF pulse. The echo is produced when the faster spins "catch up" to the slower. (b) The gradient echo is produced by reversing the direction of the gradients to exchange which spins are the faster and slower. (c) The field echo is possible only in ULF MRI. In this case all the fields (measurement and gradient) are reversed, changing the direction of precession.

magnetization. Acquisition of multiple echoes can also be used for more precise estimation of T_2. The echoes produced by reversing both G_x and B_m are noteworthy because while the gradient echo is routinely used in HF MRI, the field echo is unique to ULF. Acquiring data for the full MRI image requires that we step through the above sequence for all required values of G_y to fully populate *k*-space (unless multiple lines are encoded in a single excitation).

In terms of encoding and acquisition, ULF MRI can use methods very similar to traditional HF MRI. Typically one uses both the frequency and phase of the voxel to encode an image, as shown in Figure 4.3. However, one could also use projection reconstruction encoding by rotating the encoding gradients between excitations to produce the trajectory through *k*-space shown in Figure 4.7. Alternatively one could also rotate the sample, but

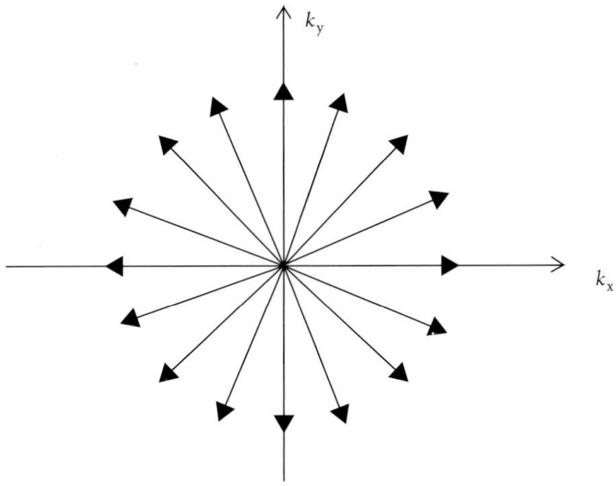

FIGURE 4.7 Sketch of projection imaging *k*-space trajectory (for FID acquisition). http://www.urmc.rochester.edu/smd/rad/mriweb

that is not practical for most applications. Another technique that is uniquely enabled by the low field strengths used in ULF MRI is the possibility of rotating the main magnetic field (instead of the sample or gradients). This could be useful if there were multiple sensors in a variety of orientations around the sample and one were trying to optimize signal in all of them. In projection reconstruction encoding the *k*-space vector begins at the origin after the start of precession, travels along the diagonal line determined by the gradients, and is then inverted through the origin by the 180-degree pulse. Data is acquired as the *k*-space vector passes through the origin again and then retraces the same line.

4.2.4 Image Reconstruction in ULF MRI: Spatial Resolution and Field of View

To illustrate some simple examples of image reconstruction techniques at ULF, let us first consider the simple 1D imaging case where a linear gradient is applied to encode spatial position by frequency variation. Frequency encoding occurs during the readout of the signal and produces a single line in *k*-space. If we wish to acquire in more than a single dimension, we have numerous choices about how to proceed. For example, as we show in Figure 4.7, we can use three orthogonal gradients to produce the frequency encode (readout) gradient in any orientation (projection imaging) to get different lines in *k*-space. Or we can implement more complicated patterns to travel through *k*-space. We can, in principle, leverage any pulse sequence from HF MRI if we have the hardware and signal time available. On the other hand, maybe we can invent new approaches, such as reorienting B_m.

Regardless of our choice of pulse sequence, there are few key imaging parameters that are intimately interrelated and must be considered to understand the type of image we will end up with. These are field-of-view (FOV) and spatial resolution. To illustrate them, we chose the familiar Fourier imaging approach, as shown in Figure 4.5, for the remaining discussion. In this case we apply short phase-encoding gradients before readout encoding. This approach results in different voxels having different phase shifts, which provides the spatial information orthogonal to readout encoding. Phase-encoding gradients can be applied before or during the signal readout in the case of multiple echo encoding (used to accelerate overall image encoding). During an acquisition time, we are then recording the free induction decay (FID) encoded with position information via frequency and/or phase.

If the direction of the measurement field B_m is along the z-axis, these gradients are typically longitudinal to the main field, dB_z/dx, dB_z/dy, and dB_z/dz, and are typically referred to as G_x, G_y, and G_z, respectively. The gradient used for encoding the lines in k-space is typically known as the "read" gradient and by our convention is along the x-axis (or readout axis), G_x.

From Eqn. 4.13 we can write that the contrasted spin density is

(Eqn. 4.22)
$$q(\mathbf{r})=e^{i\varphi(t)}\int_{-\infty}^{\infty}\int_{-\infty}^{\infty}S(k_x,k_z)e^{-i2\pi(k_x x+k_z z)}dk_x\,dk_z$$

In this example we perform 2D imaging using a simple Cartesian raster of k-space. The G_z is used to encode phase. G_x describes a line through k-space and G_z will set the intercept of that line on the coordinate system. We then remind the reader of Eqns. 4.12 and 4.13, which define the relationship between the spatial and frequency domain by a Fourier transform pair. From the Nyquist theorem it then follows that for any real signal (using the x-direction as an example)

(Eqn. 4.23)
$$\Delta x=\frac{1}{2W_x}=\frac{1}{2(k_{x,\max}-k_{x,\min})}$$

and

(Eqn. 4.24)
$$\Delta k_x=\frac{1}{2L_x}=\frac{1}{2(x_{\max}-x_{\min})}$$

where W_x is the extent of the image in the k-space domain and L_x is the extent of the image in the spatial domain. What Eqns. 4.23 and 4.24 illustrate is that the extent of the image in the spatial domain (FOV) is related to the resolution in the k-space domain. And conversely, the spatial resolution is related to the extent of the image in the k-space domain. This is illustrated schematically in Figure 4.8.

Recall from Eqn. 4.11, assuming that the gradient does not change over the acquisition time, that

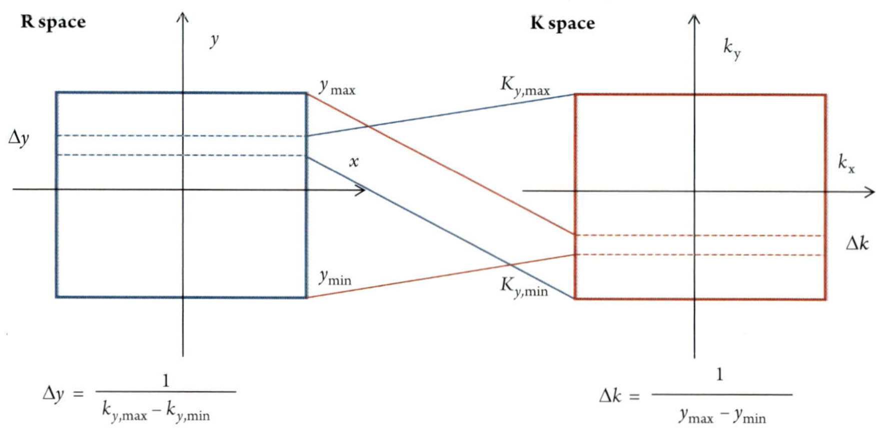

FIGURE 4.8 Schematic diagram showing relationship between R-space and k-space.

(Eqn. 4.25)

$$k_{x,z}(t) \equiv (2\pi)^{-1}\gamma G_{x,z} t_{x,z}$$

where $t_{x,z}$ describes the time during which the gradient is switched on. Specifically, in the readout (x) direction, this leads to

(Eqn. 4.26)

$$k_{x,\max} - k_{x,\min} = \frac{\gamma}{2\pi} G_x t_a .$$

Thus we can describe the spatial resolution, Eqn. 4.23, in the readout direction as

(Eqn. 4.27)

$$\Delta x = \frac{2\pi}{2(\gamma G_x t_a)} .$$

We remind the reader that G_x is the value of the readout gradient and t_a is the acquisition time.

The resolution in the phase-encoding direction(s) is arrived at similarly.

(Eqn. 4.28)

$$\Delta z = \frac{1}{2(k_{z,\max} - k_{z,\min})}$$

where

(Eqn. 4.29)

$$k_{z,\max} - k_{z,\min} = \frac{\gamma}{2\pi}(G_{z,\max} - G_{z,\min})\, t_g = \frac{\gamma}{2\pi}(2G_{z,\max})t_g .$$

One difference between readout and phase encoding is that the phase gradient values are incremented between some maximum and minimum values, and typically $G_{z,\min} = -G_{z,\max}$.

(Eqn. 4.30)

$$\Delta z = \frac{2\pi}{2(2G_{z,\max} t_g)} .$$

We note that usually, but not always, $t_a = 2t_g$.

Now let us return to the discussion of FOV. From Eqn. 4.24 we can write

(Eqn. 4.31)

$$L_x = \frac{1}{2\Delta k_x} .$$

In the readout direction we can write, using Eqn. 4.25,

(Eqn. 4.32)

$$\Delta k_x = \frac{\gamma}{2\pi} G_x \Delta t$$

where

(Eqn. 4.33)

$$\Delta t = \frac{1}{F_s} = \frac{t_a}{(N_x - 1)} .$$

F_s is the sampling frequency and N_x is the number of data points.

Combining Eqns. 4.31, 4.32, and 4.33 we can write the FOV in the readout direction as

(Eqn. 4.34)
$$L_x = \frac{2\pi}{2(\gamma G_x t_a)}(N_x - 1).$$

In the phase-encoding direction(s) we can write

(Eqn. 4.35)
$$\Delta k_z = \frac{\gamma}{2\pi}\Delta G_z t_g$$

where

(Eqn. 4.36)
$$\Delta G_z = \frac{\left(G_{z,\max} - G_{z,\min}\right)}{\left(N_z - 1\right)} = \frac{2G_{z,\max}}{\left(N_z - 1\right)}$$

and N_z is the number of encoding steps.

Combining Eqns. 4.35 and 4.36 we can write the FOV in the phase-encoding direction as

(Eqn. 4.37)
$$L_z = \frac{2\pi}{2(\gamma 2G_{z,\max} t_g)}(N_z - 1).$$

The key point here is that FOV, L, is defined by the distance between lines in k-space, Δk. The spatial resolution Δr, conversely, is defined by the entire span in k-space, and the two are related as

(Eqn. 4.38)
$$L = (N - 1)\Delta r.$$

Now let's look at a practical example, the ULF MRI pulse sequence (shown in Fig. 4.3) for protons used to produce the images in Figure 4.1. In these examples we had $G_x \sim 100\mu T/m$ and $t_a \sim 0.1s$, for spatial resolution $\Delta x \sim 2.4mm$.

At HF we can apply large gradients (for $B_0 \approx 3T$, typical values of these gradients are $dB/dz \approx 10^{-2}T/m$; i.e., 40mT/m is typical). At ULF these gradients are typically much smaller ($B_m \sim 10^{-4}T$, $dB/dz \approx 10^{-4}T/m$). Thus, to obtain the same spatial resolution as at HF one needs a proportionally longer time for phase encoding or acquisition. Practically speaking in ULF MRI this represents ~10 to 100ms. In general one cannot just "turn up" the gradients because of distortions caused by concomitant gradients and bandwidth limitations. These will be further discussed in Section 4.3. The key point we wish to make here is that for many materials, waiting the encode time can cause appreciable signal decay due to T_2^* effects, as described in Chapter 1. Thus, our signal is disappearing just as we are requiring longer times to measure. We also note that the Fourier imaging approach shown in Figure 4.3 has the disadvantage that one must wait the phase-encode time before reading out the signal, as well as being time-consuming for requiring repeated excitations.

Now that we have gone through some of the basic steps required to obtain an image, let's move on to further discuss some of the unique challenges to imaging at ULF.

4.3 ULF MRI

4.3.1 What's So Hard?

We have already shown that the fields at which ULF MRI endeavors to acquire imagines not only buck the current trend of very high field strengths that has dominated MRI since its discovery, but seem contradictory to the notion that more signal is better. While the greatest challenge facing wide application of ULF MRI is the issue of decreasing signal with decreasing magnetic field, there are factors that drive the further exploration and development of MRI at ULF. We have already mentioned some of the unique benefits inherent in ULF MRI; however, while SNR is likely the greatest hurdle for successful ULF MRI, there are a variety of additional challenges. Before delving into the details of what we believe to be the compelling motivations for ULF MRI, we believe a discussion of the challenges is warranted. We will explore some of the greatest challenges and hurdles facing ULF MRI in this section. You, the reader, can then examine some of the benefits of ULF MRI, presented in Section 4.5, with your "eyes wide open."

Let's examine an expression for SNR in a single voxel, adapted from reference [21], assuming a single sensor:

(Eqn. 4.39)
$$SNR_{\text{voxel}} \sim \frac{g \cdot M \cdot V_{\text{voxel}} \sqrt{N_{\text{av}} N_x N_y t_{\text{a}} / 2}}{S_B^{1/2}}.$$

In this expression g is a sensor geometry factor, M is the magnetization, V_{voxel} is the voxel volume, N_{av} is the number of averages, N_x and N_y are the number of lines in k-space, t_{a} is the acquisition time, and S_B is the spectral noise density.

4.3.1.1 The SNR Is Really Lower

Let us first think about signal and where the challenges presented in acquiring the maximal signal in ULF MRI originate. The magnetization, M, will be inherently lower because it depends linearly on polarization. One can also see in Eqn. 4.39 that SNR is sacrificed to speed up imaging (shorter t_{a}) or improve spatial resolution (smaller voxel volumes). Ultimately, without enough SNR you are doomed to poor resolution and/or long imaging times. We repeatedly dwell on this message because low SNR is the major confound for ULF MRI.

Let's look again at some published brain images from 96μT [22], 0.15T [23], 1.5T[23], and 3.0T[22], shown in Figure 4.9. The FOVs, subjects, and exact protocols vary—but a key point is well illustrated. At 96μT (with 30mT pre-polarization) the voxel size is $3 \times 3 \times 6$ mm^3 and the SNR inside a voxel is only ~11 (using seven sensors). The image, while a milestone, doesn't look very good in comparison to the higher-field MRI images to the right. At 3T (second from left) the voxel is $1.5 \times 1.5 \times 3$ mm^3 (just two times smaller in each dimension) and the SNR is ~30. Needless to say, the 3T (and even 1.5T) images obviously appear far better. But even by 0.15T (far right) the qualitative impression of the image is greatly improved over ULF.

While obviously interrelated, the relationship between SNR and spatial resolution is complex, as one might infer from Figure 4.9. Nonetheless, one relationship is clear from Eqn. 4.39 and in practice: with sufficient SNR you can "buy" spatial resolution. This begs the question: How much SNR is "enough" for a good MRI? Additionally we must ask: Can ULF MRI provide sufficient SNR, or is there a different relative measure of image quality at ULF?

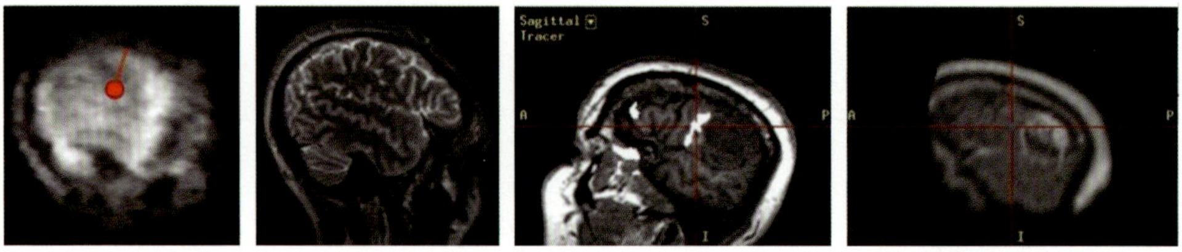

FIGURE 4.9 MRI images from left to right: 96μT ULF MRI with MEG co-registration (red dot) [22]; same brain with 3T[22]; images of a brain glioma at 1.5T [23]; images of the same brain with glioma at 0.15T[23].

Before we further contemplate that issue, let's briefly remind ourselves how we determine SNR in an image. The NEMA standard defines it several ways [24,25]. For surface coils (such as the SQUIDs in ULF MRI) the first proposed method is to take the same image of an object twice and calculate the average pixel signal (S) from one image and the average pixel standard deviation (SD) between the images:

(Eqn. 4.40)
$$SNR = \frac{S\sqrt{2}}{SD}.$$

However, because this method involves the subtraction of two images it can be subject to instabilities and systematic errors. An alternate approach is to use a single image. S is calculated as before, but the noise SD is calculated from a background region of the image. In this method,

(Eqn. 4.41)
$$SNR = \frac{0.66S}{SD}.$$

There are issues with the latter approach; for example, not all noise is independent of the signal amplitude. Furthermore, one should be aware that the selection of the "background" region can be the subject of significant debate.

Now let's consider the difference between SNR and spatial resolution. In Figure 4.10 we start in the upper left with an image from a 3T HF MRI system. This image has a voxel SNR of ~37 and size (resolution) of 1 × 1 mm^2. In the columns moving from left to right we add noise to decrease the SNR. Each row shows the same image filtered to reduce the voxel size as noted. The image gives some indication of the impact of SNR versus resolution. For example, all of the images in the left column (SNR 37) provide some reasonable anatomical detail (for example, about the cerebellum or corpus callosum) even when the spatial resolution is degrading. One might also argue that the images in the top row with good spatial resolution but decreasing SNR are still acceptable in terms of distinguishing anatomical features, but it is pretty clear that by the lower right (poor SNR and low spatial resolution) the images are not useful. How has ULF MRI compared so far? The images of the human brain shown in Figure 4.1 are sadly more like those in the lower right (SNR ~5 and spatial resolution ~4 × 4 mm^2), whereas the minimal requirement for a "useful" image might look more like SNR of 20 and 2 × 2 × 2 mm^3, and requires at least 30 times more SNR (~3 × for the voxel SNR and another order of magnitude to shrink the voxel size). Admittedly we have a way to go.

Based on these discussions, let us somewhat arbitrarily assign an SNR of more than 20 and a spatial resolution of ~2 × 2 × 3 mm^3 to be those that would result in a "good"

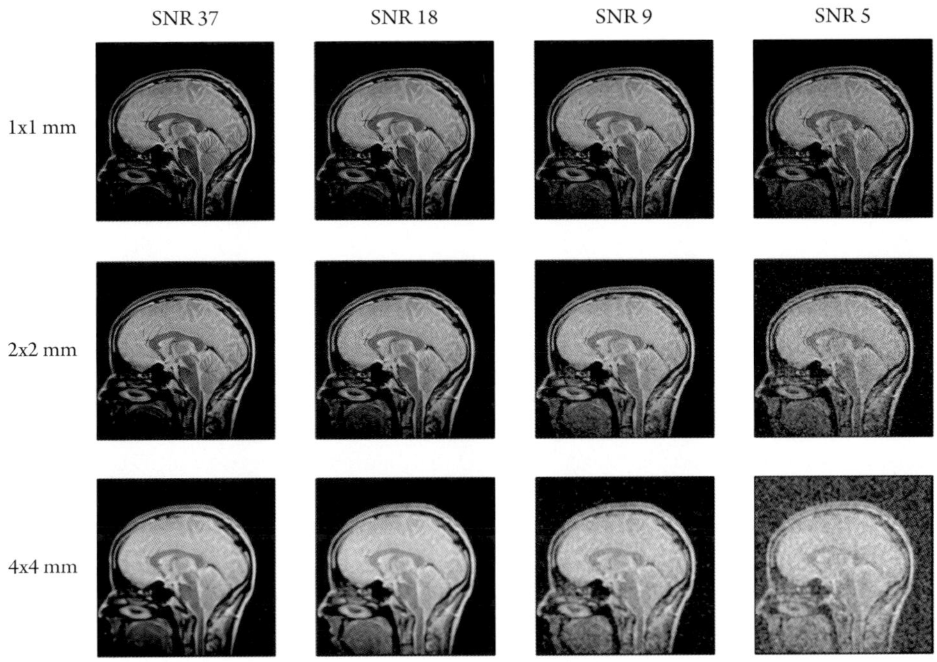

FIGURE 4.10 SNR (columns) versus spatial resolution (rows).

MRI, where "good" is loosely defined as able to provide reasonable anatomical detail of key brain structures. In Figure 4.10 this keeps us to approximately the upper left images. Given this target, how do we get there? Examining Eqn. 4.39 again, we can ask: What parameters do we have access to that will improve SNR and hence the image? For this discussion we set aside any discussion on improving the sensor. With respect to the images we have published thus far, we could potentially increase the magnetization by greater pre-polarization, implement a faster acquisition sequence to access more signal, consider additional averaging, and possibly reduce noise. We consider each of these in turn.

We can increase M by increasing the pre-polarization, but we must take care that we don't increase the noise in the process! This can probably be realistically accomplished by increasing B_p to the 100mT to 200mT level. To date the practical limits are magnet switching, cooling, and dB/dt (and associated physiological and noise induction effects), among others. Increasing B_p to this level would increase our magnetization by a factor of 3 to 6 over existing images acquired with $B_p \sim 30$mT. The images we presented in Figure 4.1 used a signal that was acquired after an encoding time. This delay of ~30ms sacrificed ~50% of our signal given the short (~50–100ms) T_2 of tissue at ULF. It is possible to implement a projection imaging sequence that does not require the initial encoding time, which could potentially recover more of the signal. The drawback of this approach is the need to keep the current sources to power all three gradients on, which may increase the noise. Assuming we could implement projection imaging without significantly increasing the noise during the signal acquisition, we would increase our SNR by another factor of 2.

Eqn. 4.39 also leads us to conclude that by increasing t_a, the acquisition time, we would also improve our SNR by simply acquiring the signal for a longer time. In practice this is not feasible. As we describe in the next section, signal acquisition at ULF is bandwidth-limited, requiring t_a of at least ~100ms. This is already on the order of T_2 for tissue. In simplistic terms, this means the signal is dying out while we are acquiring it, and increasing the acquisition time further does not significantly improve the signal measurement. Alternatively, we can average by repeating the entire pulse sequence multiple times; however, this has the undesirable effect of increasing the scan time. Ultimately, this tradeoff appears to be a no-win situation, and we'll take that off the table.

The last "knob" we have available to us is the noise, which appears an easy approach to increasing SNR. In principle, the SQUID sensors typically used in ULF MRI are capable of sub-femtotesla sensitivity. The problem is that noise originates from multiple sources: the sample itself, the sensor, and the environment (including the ULF MRI system itself). While we have some measure of control over the sensor and system noise, we have no practical control over sample noise (as noted in Chapter 1). Myers et al. [26] published a thorough analysis of sensor versus source noise (Fig. 4.11). The noise presented in the brain image in Figure 4.1 was ~2 to 3fT/√Hz, depending on sensor position, at our measuring frequencies of a few kHz. Based on this discussion, it would seem we have room to substantially improve on this noise level. However, our group has observed some practical limitations to reaching the SQUID noise floor. For example, to shield the SQUIDs from ambient noise, an RF shield is required. However, this introduces noise (primarily Johnson noise) inherent in the shield. As discussed in Chapter 2 we routinely wrap our cryostat with Mylar coated with 90nm of gold to shield the SQUIDs from RF interference. The Johnson

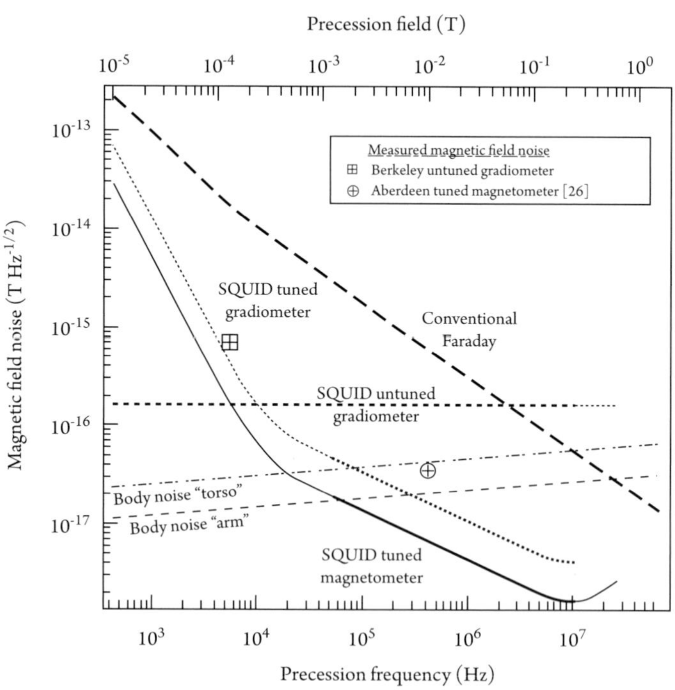

FIGURE 4.11 Calculated magnetic field noise of tuned and untuned SQUID detectors and conventional Faraday detector compared to modeled sample noise. From Myers W, et al. 2007 reference [26] used with permission from Elsevier.

noise originating in the gold-coated Mylar increased the noise from 0.5fT to 3fT at the outer SQUIDs around the edge of the cryostat (closest to the Mylar). In addition to the RF shield, all the field generation coils contribute to the total ambient noise. This is not considered at all in the curve above. While there are innumerable sources of ambient magnetic field noise, there may still be significant room for improvement based on the noise reported by Clarke's group [26] of 0.5fT. Ultimately, our experience is that any practical system that doesn't require an exotic MSR or other heroic measures to reduce ambient noise will likely attain a practical noise limit of 0.5 to 1fT. Attaining this noise performance might win us an additional improvement of a factor of 2 to 3 in our hunt for high SNR.

Now that we have examined all the practical knobs, let us consider Eqn. 4.39 again. If we assume that we can realize 100mT pre-polarization field, we gain an improvement of a factor of 3 over the pre-polarization presented in Figure 4.1. Let us also assume that the noise level can be reduced by a factor of 2 relative to that same figure. Further, let us assume that we can acquire the image using projection imaging to achieve another factor of 2 in signal. These relatively simple system improvements can provide ~12 times more SNR. However, as we discussed previously, we also need a total improvement of ~30 times in the SNR to achieve both ~20 voxel SNR *and* a smaller ($2 \times 2 \times 2\ mm^3$) voxel. Thus, even at this point, we are left with a relatively mediocre (at best) image or a very long (impractical) imaging time to attain a "good" image.

In Section 4.4 we will explore additional approaches to making the most of the available signal, including the use of more sensors to try to further improve the SNR without increasing scan time. The obvious win for SQUID-based systems is to use an array of sensors (typical for MEG systems, for example). Arrays of sensors can virtually increase N without increasing the scan time—or alternatively one can use the array to speed up imaging or increase the FOV (while keeping the SNR approximately the same). Parallel imaging will be discussed in Section 4.4.3.

4.3.1.2 Bandwidth Issues

To start the discussion of bandwidth, let us first consider the issue of FOV:

(Eqn. 4.42)
$$FOV_{imaging} = \frac{F_s}{\gamma G_x}$$

where F_s is the sampling frequency and G_x is the readout gradient strength. At ULF, because the Larmor frequencies during readout are typically low (e.g., ~2kHz for Earth's field), it is not necessary to heterodyne to read out the signal; rather, standard data acquisition systems (DAQs) and methods can be used. At HF MRI the signals of interest are typically many tens of MHz and typically too high frequency for standard data acquisition (analog-to-digital converters [ADCs]). In heterodyning approaches the high-frequency signals are converted to lower frequencies by mixing with a reference. In ULF MRI, however, sampling at 20kHz with off-the-shelf DAQ systems is adequate. Thus, the FOV described by Eqn. 4.42 is significantly larger than our actual region of interest. For example, with 20kHz sampling and 100μT/m gradients, we find the FOV for protons is ~4.7m, which typically is much larger than the sample(usually only 10–20cm).

The imaging bandwidth can be expressed, similarly to Eqn. 4.42, as:

(Eqn. 4.43)
$$\Delta L = \frac{\mathrm{BW}}{\mathrm{G}} \quad \text{or} \quad \mathrm{BW} = \Delta L \cdot \mathrm{G}.$$

The actual bandwidth (BW) over a typical 10cm sample size, and assuming 10^{-4}T/m gradients, is really only ~425Hz. This tells us that we are getting a lot more information in *k*-space (when we compare FOV from sampling to that from imaging) than we actually use. A plus side to working well below these limits and using direct signal acquisition is that many higher-frequency noise sources (associated with ambient fields or transients) are prevented from being aliased into the signal.

In HF MRI the gradients are typically 100 times larger than those used in ULF MRI. These larger gradients result in two related effects: the BW is 100 times smaller at ULF, and as per Eqn. 4.27 the spatial resolution attainable for the same readout time, t_a, at HF is inherently 100 times better than ULF MRI. To mitigate this effect at ULF, one can and does increase t_a. Typically $t_a \sim$ 10ms in HF MRI is commonly used, and this is increased to $t_a \sim$ 100ms in ULF. However, the T_2 of the material being imaged often provides a fundamental limit to how much one can increase t_a at ULF. For example, because the T_2 time for most biological tissue is on the order of 100ms, and the signal will die out, there is no point for t_a extending beyond the point that measurable signal exists. One might consider increasing G_x (and hence sample bandwidth). The low Larmor frequency of ULF MRI, however, limits the extent to which one can increase G_x strength. For example, if the gradients are comparable or larger than the measurement field, concomitant gradients cause severe image distortions (discussed in the next section) and the sample BW leads to frequencies that approach zero. While it is possible to measure signal at or near zero frequencies, the noise is dramatically higher at lower frequencies and consequently reduces the available SNR.

4.3.1.3 *Limitations from Relaxation Times*

We have already pointed out that it is not productive to increase t_a beyond the point at which there is measurable signal. While the changing of T_1 (getting shorter) at ULF can be the source of new contrast, T_1 and T_2 can also pose limitations on imaging that aren't as significant at high fields. As fields approach the ULF regime, T_1 approaches T_2, and they get shorter. Ultimately, this provides less time during which to acquire measurable signal. At HF, we have already shown that $t_a \sim$ 10ms provides reasonable SNR. At ULF, we need to acquire signal for $t_a \sim$ 100ms (or longer) for reasonable SNR. The need for longer t_a and decreasing relaxation times at ULF work against our need for better SNR.

The "silver lining" to the generally shorter T_1 at ULF is that the spin population is polarized faster; hence one can cycle through the polarization and acquisition pulse sequence faster. As with most HF and ULF differences, another challenge presented by the short relaxation times is manifest during flow-based experiments. For example, during a flow-based experiment in which a spin population is polarized, then allowed flow, and finally readout, one is more limited in how long the flow-based evolution is allowed to progress.

4.3.2 Stray Fields that Are Negligible in HF MRI Become Significant at ULF

Due to the low strength of the measurement field, acquisition of MRI at ULF is more susceptible to ambient fields. There are several sources of the ambient fields, both static and dynamic. The next two issues associated with ULF MRI are related to the fact that the magnetic fields used to acquire the MRI are comparable to unwanted magnetic fields. These magnetic fields are (1) a consequence of the environment (ambient) or (2) an inevitable consequence of producing gradients (the "concomitant" gradient issue) or (3) transients created by the pulsed B_p. In any case, these unwanted stray fields may produce artifacts and distortions in the image that must be understood and corrected.

The most widely used technique to measure NMR signal at low fields consists of polarizing the sample in a large field B_p, then switching off B_p in a time short compared to T_1 and observing the FID from the sample at an LF B_m. The use of a relatively strong polarization field will induce pseudo-static fields in the permeable materials in the vicinity of the polarizing coils. Additionally, rapidly switching off B_p inevitably results in the transient fields that arise from the currents proportional to dB/dt induced in any conductive materials (e.g., other components of the experimental apparatus and surrounding equipment). To date we have typically conducted our ULF NMR experiments inside an MSR or enclosure, which consists of several layers of μ-metal and/or aluminum. The residual magnetization of the high-permeability layers results in pseudo-static residual field, while eddy currents in the high-conductivity layers induced by the polarization field ramp-down result in transient fields.

In addition to the ambient and transient magnetic fields, there are also stray magnetic fields that arise as the inevitable result of applying imaging gradients (concomitant gradients).

There is a significant difference in approaches to evaluate the effects of the stray fields in HF and ULF MRI. In HF MRI the primary field (B_0) dominates all the stray fields so that only components parallel to the primary field typically cause any measurable effect on spin evolution. These fields are corrected for by simply accounting for the variation in the Larmor frequency caused by these parallel components. In ULF MRI the stray fields may be comparable in magnitude to the measurement field, B_m, so one must take into account not only parallel components of these fields but also the components orthogonal to B_m.

4.3.2.1 Concomitant Gradients

At ULF one must account not only for the "useful" encoding gradients applied in directions we desire, but also the additional gradients that occur as an inevitable consequence of their application. These are the so-called "concomitant" gradients transverse to the applied encoding gradients (see for example [28–30]) discussed briefly in Chapter 1.

For every set of (assumed linear) gradients that we apply to image (dB_z/dx, dB_z/dy, or dB_z/dz), Maxwell's equations predict that any coil system generating gradients will always generate gradients of transverse components (dB_x/dx, dB_x/dy, etc.) that have the same field strength as B_z gradients. As we discussed in Chapter 1, these effects may be neglected at HF, but at ULF these effects can become 10% of the signal and result in significant distortions in the image.

There has been previous work on concomitant gradient effects and corrections [27,28] for the case of LF MRI. These assumed that the direction of the measurement field is unperturbed by the gradient, focusing instead on the effect that the amplitude change has on encoding phase, or used parabolic approximations. A paper specific to the effects at ULF [28] approached the problem from the impact that "deflection" of the magnetic field has on the precession, and we follow that approach here as well.

The problem of concomitant gradients was introduced to the MRI community by Norris and Hutchison in 1990. The general MRI technique relies on applying magnetic field gradients to spatially encode the precession frequency. Maxwell's equations predict that any coil system generating gradients of one component of magnetic field, say dB_z/dx, dB_z/dy, or dB_z/dz, will always generate gradients of transverse components, such as dB_x/dx, dB_x/dy, etc. This can be illustrated by considering the fields generated by two common gradient coils: Maxwell coil and Golay coil (Figs. 4.12 and 4.13).

These and similar systems are widely used in MRI to produce gradient fields that are axi-symmetrical, with an origin placed in the plane of symmetry. Since the volume is free from electrical currents, the Maxwell equations must hold: $\nabla \times \mathbf{B}(\mathbf{r}) = 0$ and $\nabla \cdot \mathbf{B}(\mathbf{r}) = 0$. For this to be true, the components of the gradient tensor $\mathbf{G}$ are defined by

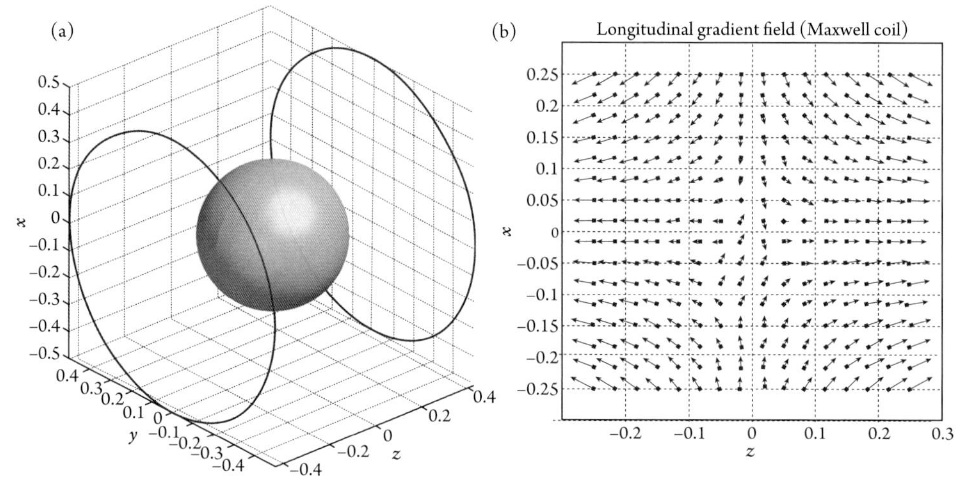

FIGURE 4.12 Diagram of a Maxwell coil (a) and the longitudinal gradient field produced by such a coil set (b). The field varies linearly (gradient) along the direction of the primary field (longitudinal gradient dB_z/dz).

(Eqn. 4.44)
$$\mathbf{G} \equiv \frac{\partial \mathbf{B}}{\partial \mathbf{r}} \equiv \begin{bmatrix} dB_x/dx & dB_x/dy & dB_x/dz \\ dB_y/dx & dB_y/dy & dB_y/dz \\ dB_z/dx & dB_z/dy & dB_z/dz \end{bmatrix}$$

and should satisfy the following conditions:

(Eqn. 4.45)
$$\frac{dB_x}{dx} + \frac{dB_y}{dy} + \frac{dB_z}{dz} = 0, \quad \frac{dB_x}{dy} - \frac{dB_y}{dx} = 0, \quad \frac{dB_x}{dz} - \frac{dB_z}{dx} = 0, \quad \frac{dB_y}{dz} - \frac{dB_z}{dy} = 0.$$

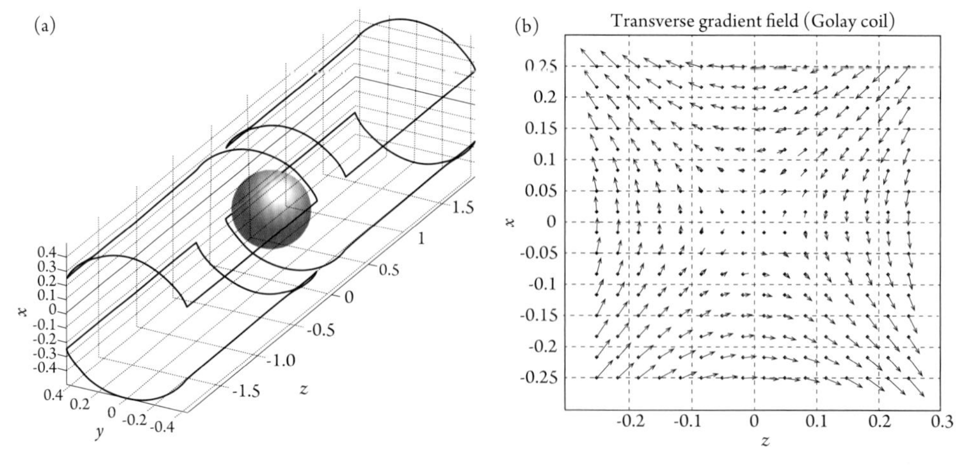

FIGURE 4.13 Diagram of a Golay coil (a) and the transverse gradient field produced by such a coil set (b). The field varies linearly (gradient) along the direction orthogonal to the field (transverse gradient dB_z/dx).

These conditions mean that the gradient tensor is symmetrical and traceless: $\mathbf{G} = \mathbf{G}^T$ and $Tr\{\mathbf{G}\} = 0$.

In the case of a cylindrical geometry [27,28] aligned with the z-axis, the gradient tensor can be written as

(Eqn. 4.46)
$$\mathbf{G} = \begin{bmatrix} -g_z/2 & 0 & g_x \\ 0 & -g_z/2 & g_y \\ g_x & g_y & g_z \end{bmatrix}.$$

Neglecting the higher orders of spatial dependence, we can write the total magnetic field as

(Eqn. 4.47)
$$\mathbf{B}(\mathbf{r}) = \mathbf{B}_0 + \mathbf{G}\cdot\mathbf{r}.$$

In this section, for consistency with our previously published work, we use the field notation (common to HF MRI) where $\mathbf{B}_0$ is the magnetic field applied during the acquisition of the signal. Separating the desirable gradient from concomitant gradients yields the equivalent form

(Eqn. 4.48)
$$\mathbf{B}(\mathbf{r}) = \mathbf{B}_0 + \mathbf{P}_{||}\mathbf{G}\mathbf{r} + \mathbf{P}_{\perp}\mathbf{G}\mathbf{r}$$

where $\mathbf{P}_{||} \equiv \hat{\mathbf{b}}_0 \hat{\mathbf{b}}_0^T$ is the projection operator on magnetic field direction, $\mathbf{P}_{\perp} \equiv \mathbf{I} - \hat{\mathbf{b}}_0 \hat{\mathbf{b}}_0^T$ is the projection operator on a plane orthogonal to magnetic field vector, $\hat{\mathbf{b}}_0 \equiv \mathbf{B}_0 / |\mathbf{B}_0|$ is the unit vector in along the static measurement field, and $\mathbf{I}$ is the identity matrix.

The resulting Larmor frequency for spins in the volume is given by

(Eqn. 4.49)
$$\omega(\mathbf{r}) = \gamma\sqrt{(B_0 + \Delta B_{||})^2 + \Delta B_{\perp}^2}.$$

Here $\Delta B_{||}$ is the component of the gradient field parallel to the primary field, and $\Delta B_{\perp}$ is the orthogonal component of the gradient field. The parallel component can be written as

(Eqn. 4.50)
$$\Delta B_{||} |\mathbf{P}_{||}\mathbf{G}\mathbf{r}| = \mathbf{g}^T\mathbf{r}.$$

where $\mathbf{g} \equiv (\nabla(\hat{\mathbf{b}}_0^T\mathbf{B}))^T = \mathbf{G}^T\hat{\mathbf{b}}_0$ is the gradient of the component of the total magnetic field parallel to the static measurement field $\mathbf{B}_0$ (i.e., desirable gradient).

The orthogonal component (i.e., concomitant gradient) is equal to

(Eqn. 4.51)
$$\Delta B_{\perp} = |\mathbf{P}_{\perp}\mathbf{G}\mathbf{r}|.$$

We can approximate the frequency variation (that affects the spatial encoding) as

(Eqn. 4.52)
$$\Delta\omega \equiv \omega(\mathbf{r}) - \omega_0 = \gamma\Delta B_{||} + \frac{\gamma}{2B_0}\Delta B_{\perp}^2 + O\left(\frac{\Delta B_{\perp}^2}{B_0^3}\right) \approx \Delta\omega_{||} + \Delta\omega_{\perp}$$

where $\omega_0 \equiv \gamma B_0$ is the Larmor frequency associated with the primary field, which is supposed to be uniform over the volume of interest.

This is true regardless of MRI magnetic field regime. For MR imaging in high fields ($B_0 \approx 1$T), typical values of these gradients are $dB/dz \approx 2 \cdot 10^{-2}$T/m, and a region of interest (ROI) of size D $\approx$ 0.5m. For such a typical HF case, the $\Delta B_{||}/B_0 \ll 1$, $\Delta B_{\perp}/B_0 \ll 1$, and

$\omega_{||}/\omega_{\perp}$ and the frequency variation is approximately only $\Delta\omega_{||}$. This is a key assumption in HF MRI and the reason why most often the concomitant gradients are negligible, as we noted above.

However, in ULF MRI, $B_0 \sim 10^{-4}$T, $dB/dz \approx 10^{-4}$T/m, and the ROI is slightly smaller, $D \approx$ 0.2m. Thus $\Delta\omega_{||} \approx 851$Hz, whereas $\Delta\omega_{\perp} \approx 84$Hz. This example illustrates that the effect from concomitant gradients can be 10% of the total frequency shift due to the primary gradient; thus, concomitant gradients in ULF MRI can result in significant distortions of the frequency and phase encoding, with correspondingly large displacement and distortion artifacts.

The magnitude of the distortions associated with the concomitant gradients can be characterized by the parameter $\varepsilon = LG_m/B_0$, where L is the size of the FOV and G_m max$|\mathbf{g}|$ is the maximum applied imaging gradient.

In general, the phase of the spins during the readout can be written as

(Eqn. 4.53) $$\phi(\mathbf{r},t)=-\omega_e(\mathbf{r})T_e+\omega_r(\mathbf{r})t=-\gamma\left|\mathbf{B}_0+\mathbf{G}_e\mathbf{r}-\mathbf{G}_r\mathbf{r}\right|T_e+\gamma\left|\mathbf{B}_0+\mathbf{G}_r\mathbf{r}\right|t$$

where $\mathbf{G}_e$ and $\mathbf{G}_r$ are correspondingly magnetic field gradient tensors associated with the phase-encoding and readout gradients and T_e is the duration of the phase-encoding interval.

Expanding this expression into Tailor series and retaining only terms up to the second order of the parameter ε, we get

(Eqn. 4.54)

$$\phi(\mathbf{r},t)=-\gamma B_0T_e-\gamma\hat{\mathbf{b}}_0^T\mathbf{G}_e\mathbf{r}T_e-\gamma\hat{\mathbf{b}}_0^T\mathbf{G}_r\mathbf{r}T_e-\gamma\frac{\mathbf{r}^T\mathbf{G}_r^T\mathbf{P}_\perp\mathbf{G}_r\mathbf{r}}{2B_0}T_e-\gamma\frac{\mathbf{r}^T\mathbf{G}_e^T\mathbf{P}_\perp\mathbf{G}_e\mathbf{r}}{2B_0}T_e$$
$$-\gamma\frac{\mathbf{r}^T\mathbf{G}_e^T\mathbf{P}_\perp\mathbf{G}_r\mathbf{r}}{2B_0}T_e-\gamma\frac{\mathbf{r}^T\mathbf{G}_r^T\mathbf{P}_\perp\mathbf{G}_e\mathbf{r}}{2B_0}T_e+\gamma B_0t+\gamma\hat{\mathbf{b}}_0^T\mathbf{G}_r\mathbf{r}t+\gamma\frac{\mathbf{r}^T\mathbf{G}_r^T\mathbf{P}_\perp\mathbf{G}_r\mathbf{r}}{2B_0}t.$$

Next we split phase-encoding gradients into two orthogonal gradients $\mathbf{G}_e = \mathbf{G}_{ph1} + \mathbf{G}_{ph2}$, and introduce the reciprocal k-space vector $\mathbf{k}$ as

(Eqn. 4.55) $$\mathbf{k}=k_r\hat{\mathbf{e}}_r+k_{ph1}\hat{\mathbf{e}}_{ph1}+k_{ph2}\hat{\mathbf{e}}_{ph2}$$

where the unit vectors in the direction of the readout and phase-encoding gradients $\{\hat{\mathbf{e}}_r, \hat{\mathbf{e}}_{ph1}, \hat{\mathbf{e}}_{ph2}\}$ are defined as

(Eqn. 4.56) $$\hat{\mathbf{e}}_\cdot=\mathbf{G}_\cdot^T\hat{\mathbf{b}}_0\Big/\left|\mathbf{G}_\cdot^T\hat{\mathbf{b}}_0\right|=\mathbf{g}_\cdot\Big/\left|\mathbf{g}_\cdot\right|$$

and $k_r = \gamma|\mathbf{g}_r|(t - T_e)$, $k_{ph1} = \gamma|\mathbf{g}_{ph1}|T_e$, $k_{ph2} = \gamma|\mathbf{g}_{ph2}|T_e$ are components of the k-space vector in the $\{\hat{\mathbf{e}}_r, \hat{\mathbf{e}}_{ph1}, \hat{\mathbf{e}}_{ph2}\}$ basis.

It is now convenient to introduce a unit gradient tensor $\hat{\mathbf{G}}\equiv\mathbf{G}/\left|\mathbf{G}^T\hat{\mathbf{b}}_0\right|$. It should be noted that for a given gradient this quantity depends only on coil geometry; thus it is constant during the MRI experiment.

Using this definition of a k-space vector and assuming that the readout and phase-encoding dimensions are orthogonal, Eqn. 4.54 can be rewritten as

(Eqn. 4.57) $$\varphi(\mathbf{K},\mathbf{r})=\mathbf{K}^T\{\mathbf{r}+\mathbf{r}_0+\mathbf{u}(\mathbf{r})+\mathbf{V}(\mathbf{K},\mathbf{r})\}$$

where

(Eqn. 4.58)
$$\mathbf{r}_0 = \frac{B_0}{|\mathbf{g}_r|} \cdot \hat{\mathbf{e}}_r$$

(Eqn. 4.59)
$$\mathbf{U}(\mathbf{r}) = \frac{|\mathbf{g}_r|}{2B_0}\left[\left(\mathbf{r}^T \hat{\mathbf{G}}_r^T \mathbf{P}_\perp \hat{\mathbf{G}}_r \mathbf{r}\right) \times \hat{\mathbf{e}}_r + 2\left(\mathbf{r}^T \hat{\mathbf{G}}_{\mathrm{ph}1}^T \mathbf{P}_\perp \hat{\mathbf{G}}_r \mathbf{r}\right) \times \hat{\mathbf{e}}_{\mathrm{ph}1} + 2\left(\mathbf{r}^T \hat{\mathbf{G}}_{\mathrm{ph}2}^T \mathbf{P}_\perp \hat{\mathbf{G}}_r \mathbf{r}\right) \times \hat{\mathbf{e}}_{\mathrm{ph}2}\right]$$

and

(Eqn. 4.60)
$$\mathbf{v}(\mathbf{k},\mathbf{r}) = \frac{|\mathbf{g}_{\mathrm{ph}1} + \mathbf{g}_{\mathrm{ph}2}|}{2B_0}\left[\mathbf{r}^T\left(\hat{\mathbf{G}}_{\mathrm{ph}1}^T \mathbf{P}_\perp \hat{\mathbf{G}}_{\mathrm{ph}1} + 2\hat{\mathbf{G}}_{\mathrm{ph}1}^T \mathbf{P}_\perp \hat{\mathbf{G}}_{\mathrm{ph}2} + \hat{\mathbf{G}}_{\mathrm{ph}2}^T \mathbf{P}_\perp \hat{\mathbf{G}}_{\mathrm{ph}2}\right)\mathbf{r}\right] \cdot \left(k_{\mathrm{ph}1}\hat{\mathbf{e}}_{\mathrm{ph}1} + k_{\mathrm{ph}2}\hat{\mathbf{e}}_{\mathrm{ph}2}\right).$$

We can analyze the effects of the terms inside the curly brackets in Eqns. 4.59 and 4.60 considering that the measured signal $S(\mathbf{k})$ and the contrasted spin density $q(\mathbf{r})$ (i.e., MR image) are linked by the Fourier transform:

(Eqn. 4.61)
$$\mathbf{S}(\mathbf{k}) \propto \int_V q(\mathbf{r}) e^{i\varphi(\mathbf{k},\mathbf{r})} d^3 r = \int_{\mathbf{V}} q(\mathbf{r}) e^{2\mathbf{k}^\Gamma\{\Gamma + \Gamma_0 + \mathbf{u}(\mathbf{r}) + \mathbf{v}(\mathbf{k},\mathbf{r})\}} d^3 r.$$

The constant $\mathbf{r}_0$ (Eqn. 4.58) represents a shift of the origin of the coordinate system of the reconstructed image and is typically removed by demodulation of the MRI signal. We note that while in HF MRI such demodulation happens at the hardware level (before recording the signal), in ULF MRI this hardware demodulation is not required (due to the lower acquisition frequencies). However, we do demodulate the recorded signals in software during reconstruction of the image.

The term $\mathbf{u}(\mathbf{r})$ (Eqn. 4.59) is proportional to the strength of the readout gradient and does not depend on vector $\mathbf{k}$. By changing the integration variable and neglecting the term $\mathbf{v}(\mathbf{k},\mathbf{r})$ (Eqn. 4.60) in the integral (Eqn. 4.61), it is easy to show that concomitant gradients associated with the readout gradient do not introduce blurring of the image and are limited to the *reversible* geometric $q(\mathbf{r}) \Rightarrow q(\mathbf{r} + \Delta\mathbf{r}(\mathbf{r}))$ and multiplicative $q(\mathbf{r}) \Rightarrow J(\mathbf{r})q(\mathbf{r})$ distortions:

(Eqn. 4.62)
$$\tilde{q}(\mathbf{r}) = \frac{1}{(2\pi)^3}\int_K S(\mathbf{k}) e^{-i\mathbf{k}^T\mathbf{r}} d^3k = \frac{1}{(2\pi)^3}\int_K\int_V q(\mathbf{r}') e^{i\mathbf{k}^T\{\mathbf{r}' + \mathbf{u}(\mathbf{r}') - \mathbf{r}\}} d^3k\, d^3r = \int_V q(\mathbf{r}')\delta(\mathbf{r}' + \mathbf{u}(\mathbf{r}') - \mathbf{r}) d^3r' =$$
$$/\mathbf{r}'' = \mathbf{r}' + \mathbf{u}(\mathbf{r}') \Leftrightarrow \mathbf{r}' = \mathbf{r}'' - \tilde{\mathbf{u}}(\mathbf{r}'')/ = \int_V q(\mathbf{r}'' - \Delta\tilde{\mathbf{u}}(\mathbf{r}''))J(\mathbf{r}'')\,\delta(\mathbf{r} - \mathbf{r}'')d^3r''$$
$$= q(\mathbf{r} - \tilde{\mathbf{u}}(\mathbf{r}))J(\mathbf{r})$$

where the Jacobian J is defined by

$$\text{(Eqn. 4.63)}\quad J(\mathbf{r}) \equiv \det\left(\frac{\partial \mathbf{r}'}{\partial \mathbf{r}''}\right)\Bigg|_{\mathbf{r}''=\mathbf{r}} \equiv \det\left(\begin{bmatrix} \partial x'/\partial x'' & \partial x'/\partial y'' & \partial x'/\partial z'' \\ \partial y'/\partial x'' & \partial y'/\partial y'' & \partial y'/\partial z'' \\ \partial z'/\partial x'' & \partial z'/\partial y'' & \partial z'/\partial z'' \end{bmatrix}\right)\Bigg|_{\mathbf{r}''=\mathbf{r}}$$

and $\delta(\mathbf{r})$ is Dirac's delta-function.

Taking into account that $\det(\delta\,\mathbf{r}'/\delta\,\mathbf{r}'') = [\det(\delta\,\mathbf{r}'/\delta\,\mathbf{r}'')]^{-1}$ and

$\frac{\delta}{\delta\,\mathbf{r}}\left((\mathbf{r}^T\mathbf{A}\mathbf{r})\cdot\mathbf{a}+\mathbf{b}\right) = \mathbf{a}\cdot\mathbf{r}^T\cdot(\mathbf{A}+\mathbf{A}^T)$, it is easy to calculate amplitude distortion:

(Eqn. 4.64)

$$J(\mathbf{r}) = \left[\det\left(\mathbf{I}+\frac{\partial u}{\partial \mathbf{r}}\right)\right]^{-1} = \left[\det\left(\mathbf{I}+\frac{|\mathbf{g}_r|}{B_0}\left[\hat{\mathbf{e}}_r\mathbf{r}^T\left(\widehat{\mathbf{G}}_r\mathbf{P}_\perp\widehat{\mathbf{G}}_r^T\right)+\hat{\mathbf{e}}_{ph1}\mathbf{r}^T\left(\widehat{\mathbf{G}}_r\mathrm{P}_\perp\widehat{\mathbf{G}}_{ph1}^t+\widehat{\mathbf{G}}_{ph1}\mathbf{P}_\perp\widehat{\mathbf{G}}_r^T\right)\right.\right.\right.$$
$$\left.\left.\left.+\hat{\mathbf{e}}_{ph2}\mathbf{r}^T\left(\widehat{\mathbf{G}}_r\mathbf{P}_\perp\widehat{\mathbf{G}}_{ph2}^T+\widehat{\mathbf{G}}_{ph2}\mathbf{P}_\perp\widehat{\mathbf{G}}_r^T\right)\right]\right)\right]^{-1}.$$

Let us illustrate these results using a practical example. We consider the seven-channel ULF MRI system used for concurrent detection of the MEG signals [7,22]. In this system the measurement field is along the z-axis: $\hat{\mathbf{b}}_0 = (0,0,1)^T$, the readout gradient is along the x-axis: $\hat{\mathbf{e}}_r = (1,0,0)^T$, and the phase-encoding gradients are along the z- and y-axes: $\hat{\mathbf{e}}_{ph1} = (0,0,1)^T$ and $\hat{\mathbf{e}}_{ph2} = (0,1,0)^T$. In this case the unit gradient tensors are

$$\text{(Eqn. 4.65)}\quad \widehat{\mathbf{G}}_r = \begin{bmatrix} 0 & 0 & 1 \\ 0 & 0 & 0 \\ 1 & 0 & 0 \end{bmatrix},\quad \widehat{\mathbf{G}}_{ph1} = \begin{bmatrix} -1/2 & 0 & 0 \\ 0 & -1/2 & 0 \\ 0 & 0 & 1 \end{bmatrix},\quad \widehat{\mathbf{G}}_{ph2} = \begin{bmatrix} 0 & 0 & 0 \\ 0 & 0 & 1 \\ 0 & 1 & 0 \end{bmatrix}.$$

Using these values we obtain the geometric distortion factor:

$$\text{(Eqn. 4.66)}\quad \mathbf{u}(\mathbf{r}) = \frac{|\mathbf{g}_r|}{2B_0}\left(z^2, 0, -xz\right)^T$$

and the multiplicative factor:

$$\text{(Eqn. 4.67)}\quad J(\mathbf{r}) = \left[1-\frac{|\mathbf{g}_r|x}{2B_0}-2\left(\frac{|\mathbf{g}_r|z}{2B_0}\right)^2\right]^{-1}.$$

Thus, pixels in the x-z plane, farther away from the x-y plane, appear shifted along the direction of the readout gradient, resulting in quadratic distortion of the $x = const$

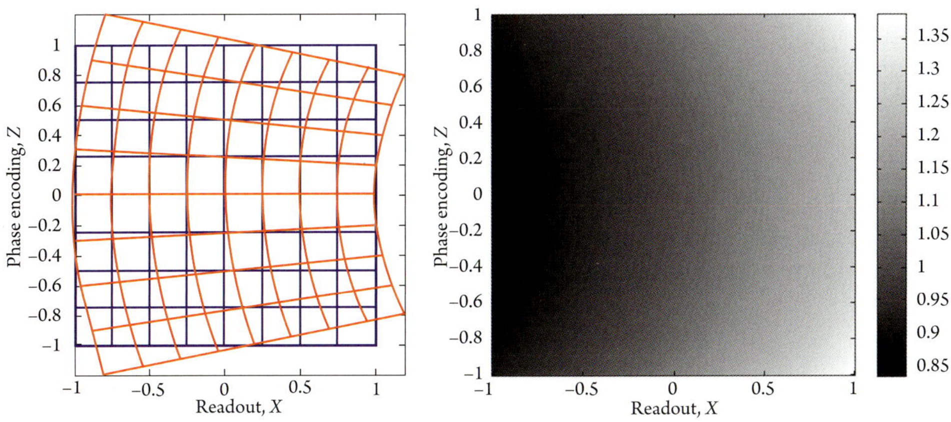

FIGURE 4.14 Distortions due to readout concomitant gradients: geometric (left) and multiplicative (right).

lines. In addition, the pixels farther along the readout dimension and farther away from the x-y plane appear shifted toward the x-y plane, resulting in the tilt of the $z = const$ lines [29]. The amplitude scaling of the reconstructed image determined by the Jacobian (Eqn. 4.63) reflects changes of the voxel volume over FOV. These effects are illustrated in Figure 4.14.

Thus the distortions caused by the readout concomitant gradients can be easily corrected in a post processing step after the reconstruction of the image. This is illustrated in Figure 4.15, showing reconstruction of a uniform phantom and a human hand before and

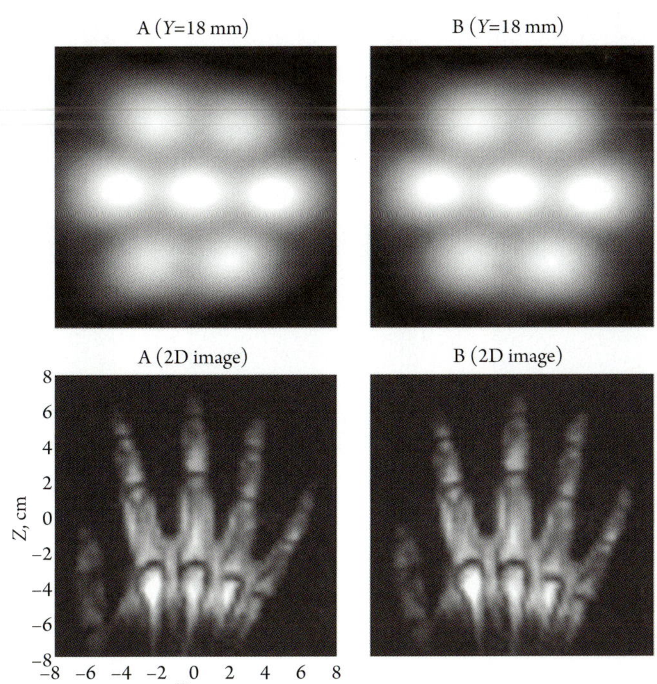

FIGURE 4.15 Images before and after correction of concomitant gradients [41].

after correction of geometric distortions associated with concomitant gradients during the readout. The phantom data were obtained at a 46μT measurement field with the following imaging gradients: readout gradient $G_x = 23.5\mu T/m$ (10 Hz/cm), readout time $t_a = 500ms$, phase-encoding gradient $\max|G_z| = 23.5\mu T/m$, number of phase-encoding steps $N_z = 73$, and phase-encoding time $t_e = 250ms$. This 2D imaging sequence provided $2 \times 2mm^2$ resolution in the *X-Z* plane. The hand images were obtained with a 94μT/m (40Hz/cm) readout gradient (readout time $t_a = 84ms$), and 94μT/m (40Hz/cm) and 47μT/m (20Hz/cm) phase-encoding gradients (encoding time $t_e = 42ms$). These imaging parameters provided $3 \times 3 \times 6mm^3$ resolution [41].

Finally, let us analyze the effects of the concomitant gradients associated with the phase-encoding gradients. Because the phase encoding employs a different gradient for each encoding step, the shift of the pixels—that is, the term $\mathbf{v}(\mathbf{k},\mathbf{r})$ (Eqn. 4.60)—is different for each step, resulting in blurring of the image [29]. This effect is illustrated in Figure 4.16 [28]. Here the top row simulates the typical HF MRI and bottom row is a typical ULF MRI case.

In contrast to distortions caused by readout concomitant gradients, which can be corrected after image reconstruction, the blurring caused by phase-encoding concomitant gradients is much more challenging to correct for. The reason for this difference is that readout distortion does not change the resolution of the image and correction does not involve solving an inverse problem; thus it is fast and accurate. Distortions caused by the phase-encoding gradients do decrease resolution of the image, and to correct those we

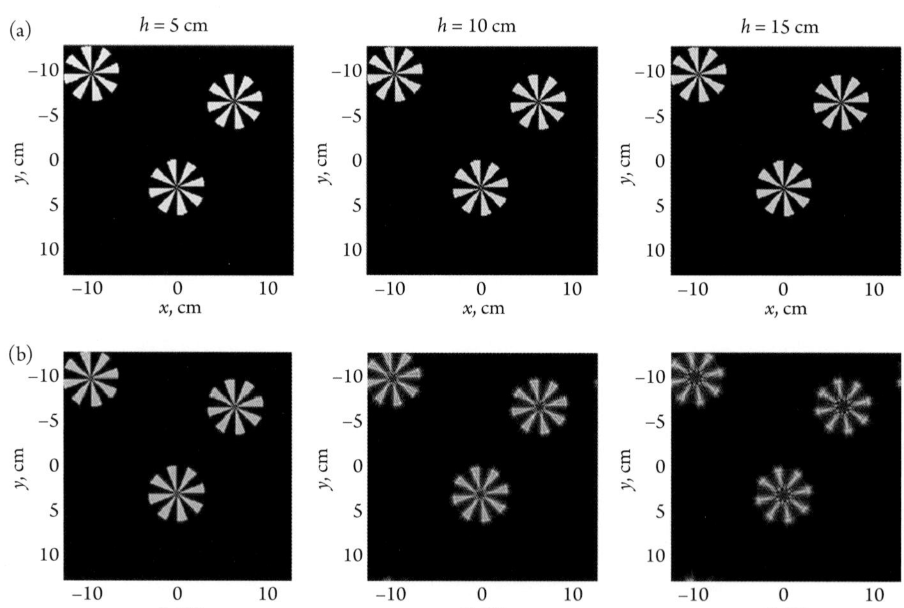

FIGURE 4.16 Comparison of computed distortions due to frequency shift caused by concomitant gradients in the phase-encoding step of a gradient-echo image for three different distances from the origin along the frequency-encoding axis (figure columns). The figure rows represent typical HF and ULF MRI examples, respectively: (row A) B_0 = 1T, $\max|G|$ = $2{\cdot}10^{-2}$T/m; (row B) B_0 = 100μT, $\max|G|$ = 50μT/m.

need to solve an inverse problem, which is computationally expensive and results in noise amplification.

We have developed one approach to correct these distortions by employing the general algebraic reconstruction method; it produces good results even when the artifacts caused by concomitant gradients are severe [30]. In general the solution of the Bloch equations (i.e., the evolution of the nuclear magnetization $\mathbf{m}(t)$ with time) can be written as

(Eqn. 4.68)
$$\mathbf{m}(t)=\mathrm{U}(t,t_0)\cdot\mathbf{m}_0+\chi_0\int_0^t\alpha_1(t')\mathbf{U}(t,t')\mathbf{B}(t')dt'$$

where $\mathbf{m}_0$ is the magnetization at time $t = t_0$.

$a_1(t)\equiv T_1(|\mathbf{B}(t)|)^{-1}$ is the longitudinal relaxation rate, and χ_0 is static magnetic susceptibility.

The evolution matrix $\mathbf{U}(t^{(2)}, t^{(1)})$ can be defined as a time-ordered exponential:

(Eqn. 4.69)
$$\mathbf{U}\left(t^{(2)},t^{(1)}\right)=T_D\exp\left(\int_{t(1)}^{t(2)}\mathbf{A}(t')dt'\right)\equiv \lim_{N\to\infty}\left\{\left(1+\mathbf{A}(t_N)\Delta t\right)\cdot\left(1+\mathbf{A}(t_{N-1})\Delta t\right)\ldots\left(1+\mathbf{A}(t_0)\Delta t\right)\right\}$$

where $1 + \mathbf{A}(t_j)\Delta t$ is the evolution matrix over an infinitesimal time interval $[t_j, t_{j+1}]$, the time moments $\{t_0, t_1, ..t_N\}$ are defined as $t_j = t^{(1)} + j\Delta t$, Δt, $=(t^{(2)} - t^{(1)})/(N - 1)$, and T_D denotes the Dyson time-ordering operator.

The evolution matrix generator (i.e., the matrix $\mathbf{A}(t)$), is defined as

(Eqn. 4.70)
$$A(t)=\Omega^{x}(t)-\frac{1}{\mathrm{T}_1}\mathbf{P}_{\|}(t)-\frac{1}{\mathrm{T}_2}\mathbf{P}_{\perp}(t),\text{ where}$$

(Eqn. 4.71)
$$\boldsymbol{\Omega}^{\times}(t)\equiv\gamma\begin{bmatrix}0 & -B_z(t) & B_y(t)\\ B_z(t) & 0 & -B_x(t)\\ -B_y(t) & B_x(t) & 0\end{bmatrix}.$$

We note that if the direction of the magnetic field is constant—that is, the unit vector $\hat{\mathbf{b}}\equiv\mathbf{B}(t)/|\mathbf{B}(t)|$ in the direction of the magnetic field, is constant—the evolution matrix $\mathbf{U}(t^{(2)}, t^{(1)})$ can be expressed as

(Eqn. 4.72)
$$\mathbf{U}\left(t^{(2)},t^{(1)}\right)=\exp\left(\hat{\mathbf{b}}^{\times}\phi\right)\cdot\exp\left(-\mathbf{P}_{\|}(\mathbf{r})\mu_1\right)\cdot\exp\left(-\mathbf{P}_{\perp}(\mathbf{r})\mu_2\right)$$

where $\phi = \int_{t^{(1)}}^{t^{(2)}} \omega(t')dt'$ is the phase integral, $\omega(t) = \gamma|\mathbf{B}(t)|, \hat{\mathbf{b}}^{\times} \equiv \frac{\mathbf{\Omega}^{\times}(t)}{\omega(t)}$; $\mu_1 = \int_{t^{(1)}}^{t^{(2)}} \alpha_1(t')dt'$ and $\mu_2 = \int_{t^{(1)}}^{t^{(2)}} \alpha_2(t')dt'$ are longitudinal and transversal relaxation integrals, and $\alpha_2(t) \equiv \frac{1}{T_2(|\mathbf{B}(t)|)}$ is the transversal relaxation rate.

Taking into account that matrices $\hat{\mathbf{b}}^{\times}, \mathbf{P}_{\|} = \hat{\mathbf{b}}\hat{\mathbf{b}}^{T}$, and $\mathbf{P}_{\perp} \equiv \mathbf{I} - \hat{\mathbf{b}}\hat{\mathbf{b}}^{T}$ share the same eigenvectors $\{\mathbf{v}_k\}_{-1}^{1}$:

(Eqn. 4.73) $$\hat{\mathbf{b}}^{\times} \cdot \mathbf{v}_k = \lambda_k \mathbf{v}_k,\ (k = -1,0,1),\ \lambda_k = (-i,0,i)$$

(Eqn. 4.74) $$\mathbf{P}_{\|} . \mathbf{v}_k = \nu_k \mathbf{v}_k,\ (k = -1,0,1),\ \nu_k = (0,1,0)$$

(Eqn. 4.75) $$\mathbf{P}_{\perp} \cdot \mathbf{v}_k = \upsilon_k \mathbf{v}_k,\ (k = -1,0,1),\ \upsilon_k = (1,0,1)$$

the evolution matrix (Eqn. 4.72) can be explicitly written as

(Eqn. 4.76) $$\mathbf{U}\left(t^{(2)}, t^{(1)}\right) = \sum_{l=-1}^{1} e^{-il\phi} e^{-\delta_{l,-1}\mu_2} e^{-\delta_{l,1}\mu_2} e^{-\delta_{l,0}\mu_1} \mathbf{v}_l \tilde{\mathbf{v}}_l$$

where $\delta_{k,l} = \begin{cases} 1, & k = 1 \\ 0, & k \neq l. \end{cases}$

It should be noted that if $|\mathbf{m}_0| \gg \chi_0|\mathbf{B}|$, as it is usually the case in the ULF MRI, the integral term in Eqn. 4.68 can be safely neglected.

The initial magnetization $\mathbf{m}_0$ in Eqn. 4.68 is defined by the properties of the object (static nuclear susceptibility $\chi_0(\mathbf{r})$ and longitudinal relaxation time $T_1(\mathbf{r})$) and by the applied polarization field $\mathbf{B}_{\mathrm{p}}(\mathbf{r})$:

(Eqn. 4.77) $$\mathbf{m}_0(\mathbf{r}) = (1 - e^{-T_{\mathrm{p}}/T_1(\mathbf{r})})\chi_0(\mathbf{r}) \cdot \mathbf{R} \cdot \mathbf{B}_{\mathrm{p}}(\mathbf{r})$$

where T_{p} is the duration of the polarization field, and $\mathbf{R}$ is the rotation matrix associated with the applied spin flip pulse (if any).

Assuming that the sensor signal is proportional to the flux through the sensor pickup coil and introducing a pickup coil sensitivity vector $\mathbf{F}(\mathbf{r}) \equiv (F_x(\mathbf{r}), F_y(\mathbf{r}), F_z(\mathbf{r}))^T$, components of which are by definition flux-generated by a unit magnetic dipole placed at $\mathbf{r}$ and aligned along the corresponding axis (according to the reciprocity principle this vector is equal to the magnetic field generated by unit current in the pickup coil at the dipole position), the MRI signal can be written as

(Eqn. 4.78)

$$S(t) \propto \int_V \mathbf{F}^{\mathrm{T}}(\mathbf{r}) \cdot \mathbf{U}(t, t_0, \mathbf{r}) \cdot \mathbf{R} \cdot \mathbf{B}_{\mathrm{p}}(\mathbf{r})(1 - e^{-T_{\mathrm{p}}/T_1(\mathbf{r})})\chi_0(\mathbf{r})d^3r = \int_V K(\mathbf{r}, t)q(\mathbf{r})d^3r$$

where $K(\mathbf{r},t) \equiv \mathbf{F}^{\mathrm{T}}(\mathbf{r}) \cdot \mathbf{U}(t,t_0,\mathbf{r}) \cdot \mathbf{R} \cdot \mathbf{B}_{\mathrm{p}}(\mathbf{r})$ and $q(\mathbf{r}) \equiv \left(1-e^{-T_{\mathrm{p}}/T_1(\mathbf{r})}\right)\chi_0(\mathbf{r})$ is the contrasted spin density.

Introducing appropriate basis functions both for the measurement $\{\psi_i(t)\}_1^N$ and for the reconstructed image $\{\rho_j(\mathbf{r})\}_1^M$ the integral Eqn. 4.78 can be reduced to the matrix equation

(Eqn. 4.79) $$S_i = \sum_j K_{i,j} q_j <=> \mathbf{S} = \mathbf{K} \cdot \mathbf{q}$$

where

(Eqn. 4.80) $$S_i(t) \int_0^T S_i(t)\psi_i(t)dt,\; K_{i,j} = \int_0^T \int_V \psi_i(t) K(\mathbf{r},t)\rho_j(\mathbf{r}) d^3r dt, \text{ and}$$

(Eqn. 4.81) $$q_j = \int_V q(\mathbf{r})\rho_j(\mathbf{r}) d^3r.$$

Eqn. 4.79 then can be solved by linear algebra methods, such as for example singular value decomposition (SVD) technique [30]. Figure 4.17 illustrates this approach using simulated images. It was shown that Fourier reconstruction produces tolerable images only when $\varepsilon \ll 1$. In contrast, the direct inversion of Eqn. 4.79 applying SVD produces images with small errors independently of ε. Even at zero measurement field (i.e., $\varepsilon = \infty$), the direct reconstruction is nearly distortion-free; only the line with no precession is partially reconstructed. These simulations show that when $3 \leq \varepsilon \leq 16$ even the direct inversion method suffers from some artifacts (see middle row in Fig. 4.17). An explanation for these artifacts is that the magnetic fields of the gradient echo sequence at those values of ε are suboptimal; the signals do not contain enough information for the reconstruction—that is, the matrix **K** in Eqn. 4.79 becomes singular, illustrated by the Jacobian (Eqn. 4.67), which is equal to zero at some locations for $\varepsilon \geq 2$.

We note here that even though it was shown that direct inversion works for modest-size ($\sim 100 \times 100$) 2D images, this approach could be impractical for a full 3D image or even a high-resolution 2D image, solely due to the huge size of the matrix **K** in Eqn. 4.79.

An alternative approximate approach to correct effects of the concomitant gradients, including the blurring of the image associated with phase-encoding concomitant gradients, was developed by Myers et al. [29]. The idea is to evaluate the concomitant gradient terms $\mathbf{u}(\mathbf{r})$ (Eqn. 4.59) and $\mathbf{v}(\mathbf{k},\mathbf{r})$ (Eqn. 4.60) at some location $\mathbf{r} = \mathbf{r}_0$ and then demodulate the measurements as

(Eqn. 4.82) $$\tilde{S}(\mathbf{k}) = S(\mathbf{k}) e^{-i\mathbf{k}^T(\mathbf{u}(\mathbf{r}_0)+\mathbf{v}(\mathbf{k},\mathbf{r}_0))}.$$

The inverse Fourier transform of $\tilde{S}(\mathbf{k})$ will be corrected for concomitant gradients in the vicinity of $\mathbf{r}_0$ and a globally corrected image can be created by combining locally corrected images together. This approach to correct phase is demonstrated in Figure 4.18 using simulation data. To reconstruct the image, the FOV was divided into equally spaced square regions. The demodulated signal $\tilde{S}(\mathrm{k})$ was computed for each region, choosing $\mathbf{r}_0$ at the

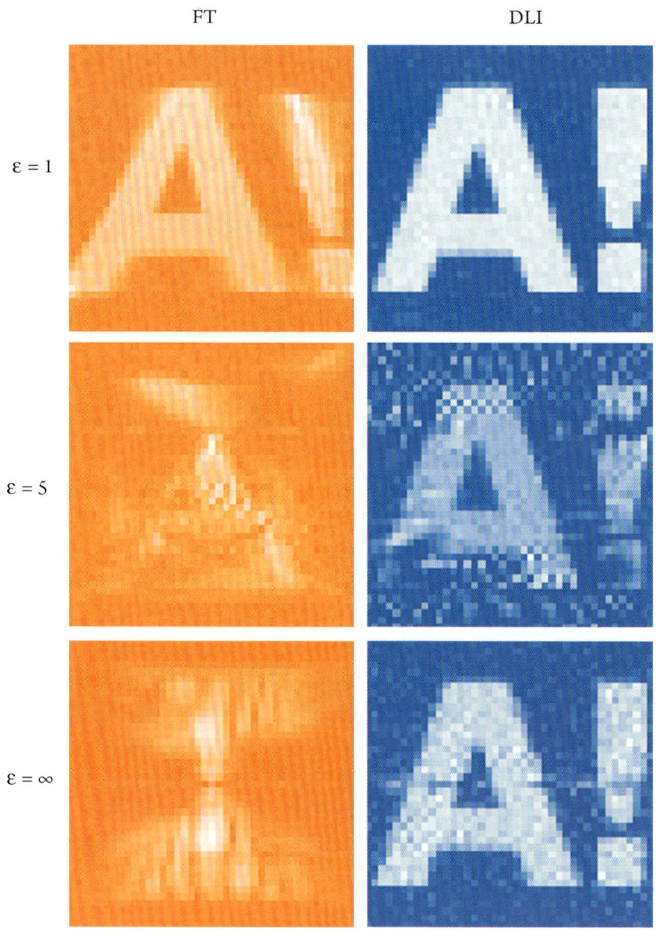

FIGURE 4.17 Examples of the reconstructed images with Fourier reconstruction (left column) and the direct linear inversion method (right column) for three values of parameter ε: top row $\varepsilon = 1$, middle row $\varepsilon = 5$, bottom row $\varepsilon = \infty$ [30].

center of that region. The blurring is eliminated and the grid lines are globally straight; the only remaining artifacts are discontinuities at the boundaries of the correction regions. These discontinuities can be further reduced using smaller correction regions, as shown on Figure 4.18B. Alternately, the post reconstruction local image-warping algorithm based on Eqn. 4.62 can be applied to illuminate these discontinuities.

One important implementation feature of this algorithm is that since each region can be reconstructed independently of the others, it could be easily adapted for parallel processing.

Concluding this section, we would like to mention that in describing the effects of the concomitant gradients we assumed that the total field (i.e., $\mathbf{B}(\mathbf{r})=\mathbf{B}_0+\mathbf{G}\cdot\mathbf{r}$) is parallel to the measurement field $\mathbf{B}_0$, which is an approximation and in general is not true. Changing the direction of the total magnetic field over the FOV during the imaging sequence (only possible at ULF) results in additional effects associated with concomitant gradients, such as Nyquist ghosting in phase-encoding dimensions. These effects are described in details in [28].

For clarity, in all other sections discussing examples of ULF MRI pulse sequences we have neglected to account for concomitant gradients.

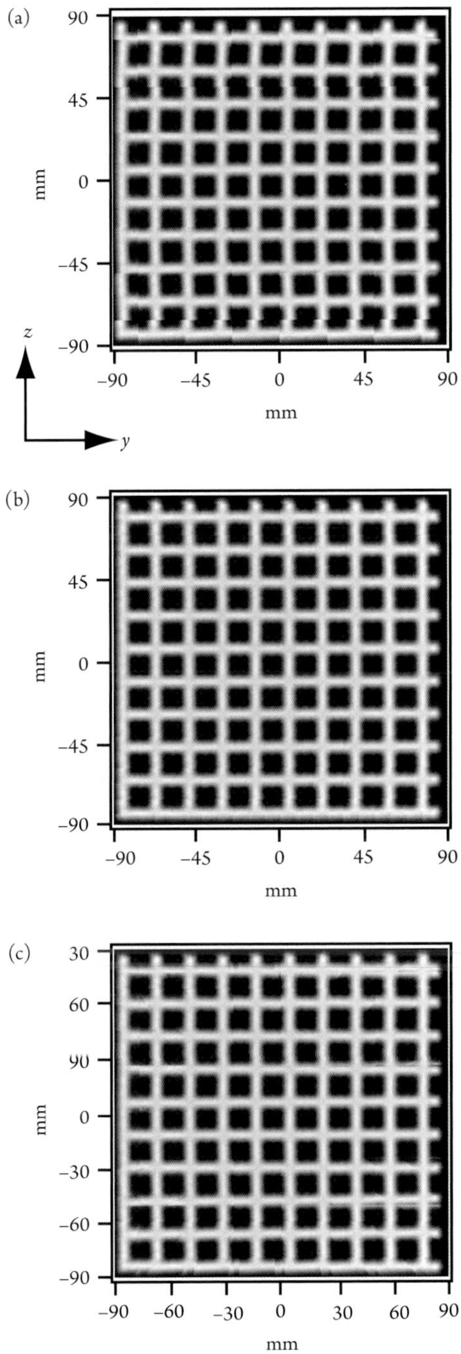

FIGURE 4.18 Phase correction algorithm. (A) 8–8 correction regions. (B) 24–24 correction regions. (C) 8–8 correction regions using local image warping.

4.3.2.2 Ghost Artifacts

Due to the low strength of the measurement field, acquisition of MRI at ULF is more susceptible to ambient fields that can result in image distortions. While these ambient fields produce only negligible effects in HF MRI, such fields can become comparable to the main MRI fields themselves in the ULF regime.

There are several sources of these ambient fields, both static and dynamic. We described that the most widely used technique to measure the NMR signal at low fields consists of polarizing the sample in a large field B_p, then switching off B_p in a time short compared to T_1 and observing the FID of the magnetization of the sample at a low-field B_m. Rapidly switching off B_p inevitably results in a transient field that arises from the currents proportional to dB/dt induced in any conductive materials (e.g., other components of the experimental apparatus and surrounding equipment).

As is the case with concomitant gradients, the orthogonal components of those stray (or ambient) magnetic fields must be accounted for and corrected at ULF to produce useful images.

One specific manifestation of the dynamic fields (that result from eddy currents induced in conducting materials in general proximity to the sample) is to change the orientation of the measurement field during the measurements.

We will endeavor to illustrate this effect using the example of 3D Fourier multiple field echo imaging. The sequence (Fig. 4.19) consists of the pre-polarization (B_p), phase-encoding (G_y and G_z), and several echo intervals created by inverting both the measurement field (B_m) and the readout gradient (G_x). Typically the measurement field is inverted to compensate for the effects of its non-uniformity and multiple echoes are used to estimate T_2 contrast. During each echo interval, one complete line of Cartesian k-space is acquired. The images are obtained for each echo and for several different polarization times.

In addition to the measurement field and the gradients presented during the phase-encoding and echo intervals, the residual field $\mathbf{B}_r$ is also present, which in general depends on time and position.

To understand the effects of the residual fields it is instructive to consider the following sequence: (1) the direction of the magnetic field is constant, aligned along a unit vector $\hat{\mathbf{b}}_1$, during the interval $t_0 \le t \le t_1$ (i.e., before the B_m field reversal shown in Fig. 4.19); (2) the direction of the field is changed in same manner from $\hat{\mathbf{b}}_2$ to $\hat{\mathbf{b}}_2$, during the interval $t_1 \le t \le t_2$ (i.e., during the B_m field reversal); and (3) the direction of the magnetic field is constant, aligned along a unit vector $\hat{\mathbf{b}}_2$ during the interval $t \ge t_2$ (i.e., after the B_m field reversal).

As we noted in the previous section, neglecting relaxation, the evolution of the nuclear magnetization $\mathbf{m}(t)$ with time can be written as

(Eqn. 4.83)
$$\mathbf{m}(\mathbf{r},t)=\mathbf{U}(\mathbf{r},t)\cdot\mathbf{m}_0(\mathbf{r})$$

where $\mathbf{m}_0(\mathbf{r})$ is the magnetization at time $t=t_0$.

The evolution matrix $\mathbf{U}(\mathbf{r},t)$ during periods (1) and (3) can be written as (see Eqn. 4.72)

(Eqn. 4.84)
$$\mathbf{U}(\mathbf{r},t)=\exp\left(\hat{\mathbf{b}}_k^{\times}(\mathbf{r})\phi_k(t)\right)=\sum_{l=-1}^{1} e^{-il\phi_k(t)}\mathbf{v}_l^{(k)}\tilde{\mathbf{v}}_l^{(k)},\ k=1,2$$

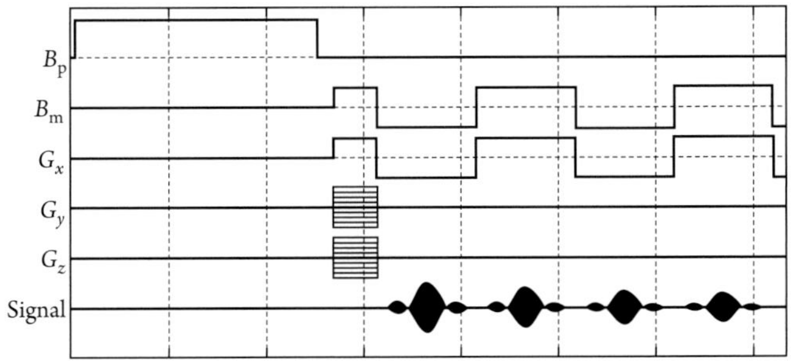

FIGURE 4.19 3D Fourier multiple gradient-echo imaging sequence.

where $\phi_2(t)=\int_{t_2}^{t}\omega(t')dt'$ and $\omega(t)=\gamma|\mathbf{B}(t)|;\{\mathbf{v}_k^{(1)}\}$ are phase integrals during periods (1) and (3) respectively and $\omega(t)=\gamma|\mathrm{B}(t)$ $\{\mathbf{v}^{(1)}\}$ and $\{\mathbf{v}_k^{(2)}\}$ are eigenvectors of the matrices $\hat{\mathbf{b}}_1^{\times}$ and $\hat{\mathbf{b}}_2^{\times}$ respectively.

To find the evolution matrix when the direction of magnetic field is not constant, as during interval (2) of the example, we define that the magnetic field rotates with angular velocity $\omega_1(t)$ around an axis aligned with a unit vector $\hat{e}_R$, in such manner that the following condition is satisfied: $\omega(t)\hat{\mathbf{b}}+\omega_1(t)\hat{\mathbf{e}}_R=\omega_{\text{eff}}(t)\left(\alpha\hat{\mathbf{b}}+\beta\hat{\mathbf{e}}_R\right)$, where a,β are constants and $\left|\alpha\hat{\mathbf{b}}+\beta\hat{\mathbf{e}}_R\right|=1$. This condition simply means that in the frame of reference following the rotation of magnetic field (see Chapter 3, Adiabatic vs. Non-adiabatic Field Rotation), the direction of the effective magnetic field is constant. In this case the resulting evolution matrix is

(Eqn. 4.85)
$$\mathbf{U}_{1,2}=\mathbf{R}_{1,2}\sum_{l=-1}^{1}e^{-il\Delta\phi_{1,2}}\mathbf{v}_l^{(T)}\tilde{\mathbf{v}}_l^{(T)}$$

where $\{\mathbf{v}_l^{(T)}\}_1^1$ is a set of the eigenvectors of the matrix $\alpha\hat{\mathbf{b}}^{\times}+\beta\hat{\mathbf{e}}_R^{\times}$;

$\Delta\phi_{1,2}=\int_{t_1}^{t_2}\omega_{\text{eff}}(t')dt'$ is the phase integral during the transition interval;

$\omega_{\text{eff}}(t)\equiv\left|\omega(t)\hat{\mathbf{b}}+\omega_1(t)\hat{\mathbf{e}}_R\right|$ is the effective Larmor frequency.

The magnetic field rotation matrix $\mathbf{R}_{1,2}=\sum_{l=-1}^{1}e^{il\Delta\phi_R}\mathbf{v}_l^{(R)}\tilde{\mathbf{v}}_l^{(R)}$, where $\{\mathbf{v}_l^{(R)}\}_{-1}^{1}$ is a set of the eigenvectors of the matrix $\hat{\mathbf{e}}_R^{\times}$; and $\Delta\phi_R=\int_{t_1}^{t_2}\omega_1(t')dt'$ is the magnetic field rotation angle.

Combining all together, the final evolution matrix for a field echo sequence can be written as

(Eqn. 4.86)
$$\mathbf{U}(\mathbf{r},t)=\sum_{l'=-1}^{1}\sum_{l=-1}^{1}Q_{l',l}e^{-il'\phi_2(t)}e^{-il\Delta\phi_1}\mathbf{v}_{l'}^{(2)}\tilde{\mathbf{v}}_l^{(1)}$$

where $\Delta\varphi_1=\varphi_1(t_1)-\varphi_1(t_2)$, and

$$Q_{l',l}=\sum_{l''=-1}^{1} e^{-il''\Delta\phi 1,2}\left(\tilde{\mathbf{v}}_{l'}^{(2)}\cdot\mathbf{v}_{l''}^{(T)}\right)\left(\tilde{\mathbf{v}}_{l''}^{(T)}\cdot\mathbf{v}_{l}^{(1)}\right),\Delta\phi_{1,2}=\int_{t_1}^{t_2}\left|\omega(t')+\omega_1(t')\hat{\mathbf{e}}_R\right|dt'.$$

Here the eigenvectors $\left\{\mathbf{v}_l^{(1)}\right\}_{-1}^{1}$ and $\left\{\mathbf{v}_l^{(2)}\right\}_{-1}^{1}$ satisfy the following relation: $\mathbf{v}_l^{(2)}\equiv\mathbf{R}_{1,2}\mathbf{v}_l^{(1)}$. In the limiting cases the coefficients $Q_{l',l}$ can be written as either non-adiabatic:

(Eqn. 4.87)
$$Q_{l',l}=\left(\tilde{\mathbf{v}}_{l'}^{(2)}\cdot\mathbf{v}_{l}^{(1)}\right)$$

or adiabatic:

(Eqn. 4.88)
$$Q_{l',l}=e^{-il\Delta\phi_{1,2}}\,\delta_{l',l},\ \Delta\,\phi_{1,2}=\int_{t_1}^{t_2}\omega(t')dt'.$$

Now we will apply this formalism to a field echo pulse sequence (as shown in Fig. 4.19). For simplicity we neglect the effects of the concomitant gradients (considered in detail in reference [28]), and assuming $|\mathbf{B}_r|\ll B_m$, the fields during the phase-encoding interval $\mathbf{B}_1$ and during the readout interval $\mathbf{B}_2$ are equal to

(Eqn. 4.89)
1) $t_0\le t\le t_1$,
$$\mathbf{B}_1(\mathbf{r})=(-B_m+(\tilde{\mathbf{g}}_{ph}\cdot\mathbf{r}))\hat{\mathbf{e}}_z$$

(Eqn. 4.90)
2) $t\ge t_2$,
$$\mathbf{B}_2(\mathbf{r})=\left(B_m+\left(\tilde{\mathbf{g}}_{rd}\cdot\mathbf{r}\right)\right)\hat{\mathbf{e}}_z$$

where $\mathbf{g}_{ph}$ and $\mathbf{g}_{rd}$ are the phase-encoding and the readout gradients. As the field during the phase encoding and the readout is approximately aligned with z-axis, the eigenvectors $\left\{\mathbf{v}_l^{(1)}\right\}_{-1}^{1}$ and $\left\{\mathbf{v}_l^{(2)}\right\}_{-1}^{1}$ are

(Eqn. 4.91)
$$\mathbf{v}_0^{(1)}=-\hat{\mathbf{e}}_z,\ \mathbf{v}_\pm^{(1)}=\frac{\left(\hat{\mathbf{e}}_x\pm i\hat{\mathbf{e}}_y\right)}{\sqrt{2}}$$
$$\mathbf{v}_0^{(2)}=\hat{\mathbf{e}}_z,\mathbf{v}_\pm^{(2)}=\frac{\left(\hat{\mathbf{e}}_x\mp i\hat{\mathbf{e}}_y\right)}{\sqrt{2}}=\mathbf{v}_\mp^{(1)}.$$

In the non-adiabatic case, the evolution matrix during the readout can be written as

(Eqn. 4.92)
$$\mathbf{U}(\mathbf{r},t)=\sum_{l=-1}^{l=1} e^{il(\omega_0 t+\Delta\varphi)}e^{il\left(\left(\mathbf{k}_{rd}+\mathbf{k}_{ph}\right)\mathbf{r}\right)}\mathbf{v}_l^{(1)}\tilde{\mathbf{v}}_l^{(1)}$$

where $\omega_0=\gamma B_m$, $\Delta\varphi=-\omega_0(t_1+t_2)$, and $\mathbf{k}_{ph}=\gamma\tilde{\mathbf{g}}_{ph}t_1$, $\mathbf{k}_{rd}=\gamma\tilde{\mathbf{g}}_{rd}(t-t_2)$ are the phase-encoding and readout k-space coordinates respectively.

In the adiabatic case, assuming that no gradients are present during the transition interval, and describing the rotation $\mathbf{R}_{1,2}$ as a combination of the rotation about the x-axis by 180 degrees, followed by a rotation about the z-axis by some angle $\Delta\phi$, we have the following expression for the evolution matrix:

(Eqn. 4.93)
$$\mathbf{U}(\mathbf{r},t)=-\sum_{l=-1}^{l=1} e^{il(\omega_0 t+\Delta\varphi')} e^{il((\mathbf{k}_{rd}-\mathbf{k}_{ph})\cdot\mathbf{r})}\mathbf{v}_l^{(1)}\tilde{\mathbf{v}}_{-l}^{(1)}$$

where $\Delta\varphi' = -\omega_0(t-t_1)-\Delta\,\varphi_{1,2} + \Delta\varphi + \pi$.

Comparing these two expressions (non-adiabatic vs. adiabatic), we see that the sign of the phase-encoding dimension is flipped relative to the readout dimension—compare $e^{il((\mathbf{k}_{rd}+\mathbf{k}_{ph})\cdot\mathbf{r})}$ in Eqn. 4.92 with $e^{il((\mathbf{k}_{rd}-\mathbf{k}_{ph})\cdot\mathbf{r})}$ in Eqn. 4.93. To paraphrase from the physical analogies presented in [31], the non-adiabatic transition forms racetrack echoes in which the precession spontaneously reverses with no change in the relative position of spins. The adiabatic transition forms "pancake" echoes in which the precession direction does not change but the relative position between leading and lagging spins is "flipped." In the intermediate case the expression for the magnetization evolution will contain both $e^{il((\mathbf{k}_{rd}+\mathbf{k}_{ph})\cdot\mathbf{r})}$ and $e^{il((\mathbf{k}_{rd}-\mathbf{k}_{ph})\cdot\mathbf{r})}$ terms.

From Eqns. 4.92 and 4.93 we see that the adiabatic and non-adiabatic cases each result in different, but artifact-free, echo images that may be analyzed in a straightforward manner. In the intermediate case the echo images contain "ghost artifacts" due to the mixing of the two behaviors. Figure 4.20 illustrates these effects using numerical simulation.

The top row in Figure 4.20 shows four reconstructed echo images (using the pulse sequence in Fig. 4.19) when the direction of the magnetic field was flipped non-adiabatically. The second row represents the adiabatic case, where we see that object position at odd-numbered echoes is flipped about the readout axis. The flipping is due to the $e^{il((\mathbf{k}_{rd}-\mathbf{k}_{ph})\cdot\mathbf{r})}$ term in Eqn. 4.93; compare to the $e^{il((\mathbf{k}_{rd}+\mathbf{k}_{ph})\cdot\mathbf{r})}$ term in Eqn. 4.92.

In the intermediate case (third row of Fig. 4.20), however, the presence of both terms $\left(e^{il((\mathbf{k}_{rd}+\mathbf{k}_{ph})\cdot\mathbf{r})}\text{ and }e^{il((\mathbf{k}_{rd}-\mathbf{k}_{ph})\cdot\mathbf{r})}\right)$ results in ghost artifacts for which the amplitude increases in each successive echo.

To illustrate how these ghost artifacts can appear in a real imaging system, we show results from a ULF MRI machine constructed to detect liquid explosives [32].The magnetic shield for this system is far closer to the sample volume than most of our other systems. The pulse sequence shown in Figure 4.19 was used, but the actual field switching falls into the intermediate case at a Larmor frequency of ~3kHz. Figure 4.21 shows the x-y-z components of the B_m field during a pulse sequence measured by a fluxgate. The elliptical nature of the vector path (right panel in Fig. 4.21) due to transient fields induced by switching the polarity of the measurement field illustrates the rotation of the magnetic field during the switching.

Illustrative echo images from the device are shown in Figure 4.22, where we used a six-echo pulse sequence. A uniform water phantom consisting of a cylinder ~250mm in diameter and 75mm deep was placed in the system, and the images shown are for one of the seven sensors used for full imaging. The bright spot in the upper right of the images

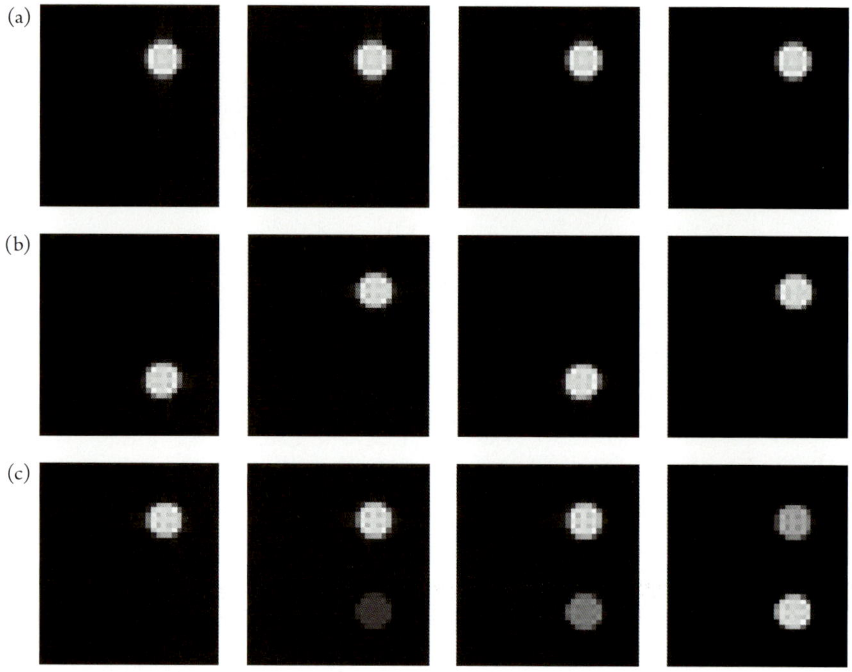

FIGURE 4.20 Top Row: Four reconstructed echo images when the direction of the magnetic field was flipped non-adiabatically. Middle Row: The adiabatic case, where we see that object position at odd-numbered echoes is flipped about the readout axis. Bottom Row: The intermediate case in which we observe ghost artifacts for which the amplitude increases in each successive echo. The horizontal coordinate corresponds to the frequency-encoded direction, and the vertical coordinate represents the phase-encoded direction.

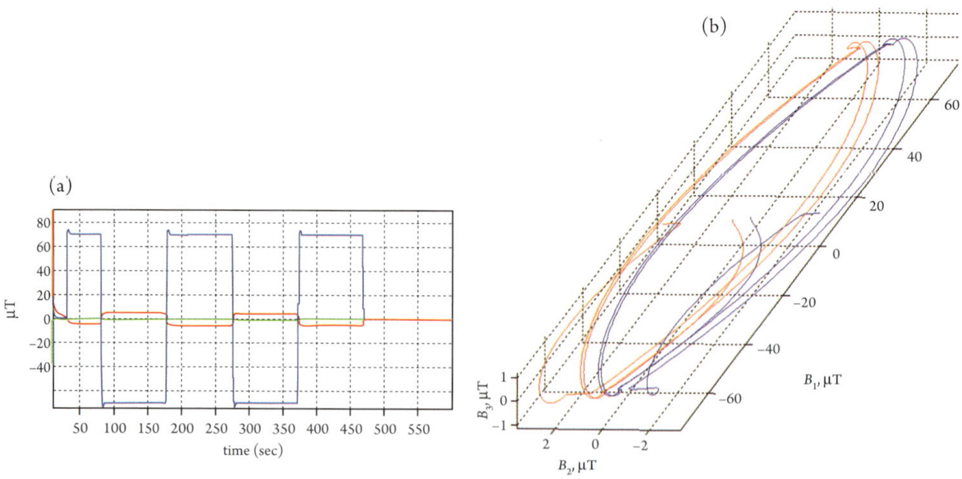

FIGURE 4.21 Actual magnetic field in the ULF MRI system from [32]. (a) Magnet field components (*x*, blue; *y*, green; *z*, red). (b) 3D representation of magnetic field vector trajectory during the transition from one polarity to the other (red line from positive to negative, blue line from negative to positive).

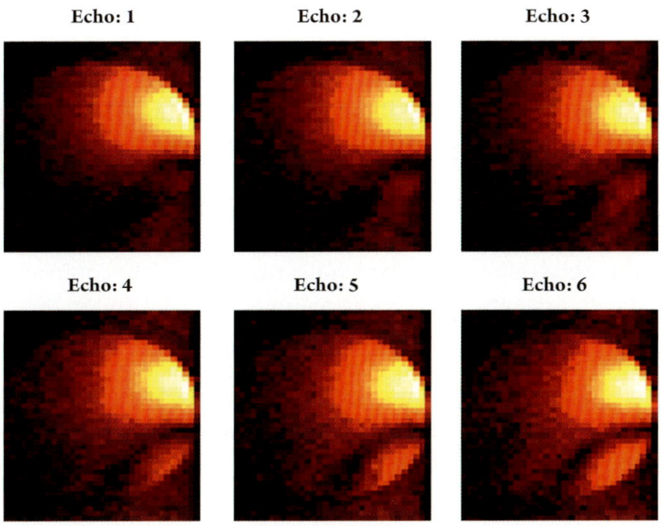

FIGURE 4.22 A uniform water phantom image. Illustrative echo images using a six-echo pulse sequence, and the images shown are for one of the seven sensors used for full imaging. The bright spot in the upper right of the images represents the sensitivity of that particular channel to the water phantom, shown clearly and accurately in the first echo. The ghost artifact appears with increasing amplitude in each subsequent echo due to the effects described above. The field of view is ~120 mm by 120 mm.

represents the sensitivity of that particular channel to the water phantom, shown clearly and accurately in the first echo. The ghost artifact in the lower right of subsequent frames appears with increasing amplitude in each subsequent echo due to the effects described above. Although it might appear much like an aliasing artifact, it is in fact the result of the residual fields from the system.

4.4 IMAGING TECHNIQUES: MAKING THE MOST OF WHAT YOU'VE GOT

ULF MRI instrumentation and imaging techniques, just as with HF MRI, are driven by the desire to maximize SNR to acquire the best-quality image possible in the shortest amount of time. Techniques such as pre-polarization, SQUID sensor detection, and averaging numerous signal acquisitions (at the expense of longer acquisition times) are all a result of this desire. While many of the approaches used in ULF MRI can confer advantages over HF (e.g., separate pre-polarization and measurement fields enable more flexible pulse sequences for some applications), ULF MRI instrumentation and pulse sequences have the extra burden of needing to compensate for the inherently lower SNR in the image and the requirement for longer acquisition and gradient-encoding times.

4.4.1 Bigger B_p Is Better (If You Are Careful)

We have already pointed out multiple times (and continue to emphasize) that one of the most obvious steps one can take to improve ULF MRI image quality is to apply the largest possible pulsed pre-polarization field to recruit additional sample magnetization. However, this approach leads to at least a couple of practical technical challenges that must be addressed. Preserving the overall benefits of the ULF approach (e.g., compatibility with MEG, contrast, ability to image through and in the presence of metal), this B_p field cannot be too large. For example, if one is using ULF MRI to image in the presence of metal, the forces induced by B_p on nearby metal must be manageable. In addition, B_p must be removed in a way that does not "undo" all of the potential advantages it might confer. The challenge is to find a technique by which a large B_p can be applied and removed in a manner that avoids introducing large amounts of noise, artifacts, or dead time in the imaging.

To illustrate the issues that need to be considered, we revisit the approaches to the B_p field removal (adiabatic vs. non-adiabatic) discussed in Section 4.2 and in detail in Chapter 3. First, consider the non-adiabatic ramp where the magnetic field is removed quickly (relative to T_1), such that spins stay aligned with B_p. If B_m is applied orthogonally to B_p, precession starts without requiring any application of a spin-flip. The pros of this approach are (1) it is conceptually simple and doesn't require a spin-flip coil and (2) the time required to perform the spin-flip (during which relaxation is occurring and signal is being lost) or any tuned RF pulses (which are sensitive to phase, etc.). This approach is also relatively fast (~10ms), so imaging data acquisition can in principle start quickly. This can be a particular advantage when T_1/T_2 is very short. The primary drawbacks of this approach are (1) it is technologically challenging to quickly turn a B_p coil off, as discussed in Chapter 2 (e.g., the large amount of energy stored in B_p must be dumped somewhere) and (2) it may induce very large transients, especially in an MSR. The transients must decay away before acquisition of meaningful signal can begin, often imposing a long deadtime. Finally, we are faced with a dichotomy that the initial B_p field is likely to be very inhomogeneous. While relaxed homogeneity requirements make the design and fabrication of B_p coils relatively simple compared to HF systems, significant inhomogeneity induces an initial distribution of orientations in the spin population that are not precisely aligned. If we begin precession from this starting condition and acquire the signal, the spins will have a large spread in their initial phase distributions. This will result in image distortions in the form of spurious echoes, not to mention loss in signal due to the misalignment of the spins.

Next, we consider the adiabatic ramp where the magnetic field is removed in such a way that the spins are rotated from the B_p axis to alignment with the B_m axis (e.g., B_p is removed slowly relative to T_1). After B_p is removed, a spin reorientation must occur to produce a measurable signal. The pros of this approach are as follows. The field homogeneity that determines the population spin orientation is determined by the B_m field, not B_p. This is because all spins in the initial population are reoriented to B_m during this process. Generating a magnetic field with a given relative homogeneity is typically far easier at relatively small fields such as B_m (typically 100μT) than for the larger B_p. Consequently, the phase spread of the spin population as it begins to precess is far smaller and distortions are minimized. The cons of this approach are that one is required to apply some form of spin reorientation (e.g., spin-flip) to initiate precession. This adds some level of complexity and requires time compared to the non-adiabatic approach. Signal is lost because of the time required to adiabatically ramp down B_p, which is by definition slow relative to T_1 and to apply spin-reorientation. We calculate that for a 100ms linear ramp from 100mT to zero field (1T/s), about 85% of the signal for gray/white matter is retained. It may be possible to further mitigate the signal loss by using programmable amplifiers to drive B_p and develop a current switch-off profile to both minimize transients and maximize residual signal. For example, we can consider a non-linear ramp with less time spent at low frequencies (where relaxation is shorter). The fraction of the signal "saved" by a nonlinear ramp compared to a simple linear ramp will depend on how T_1 depends on field, but a nonlinear ramp can

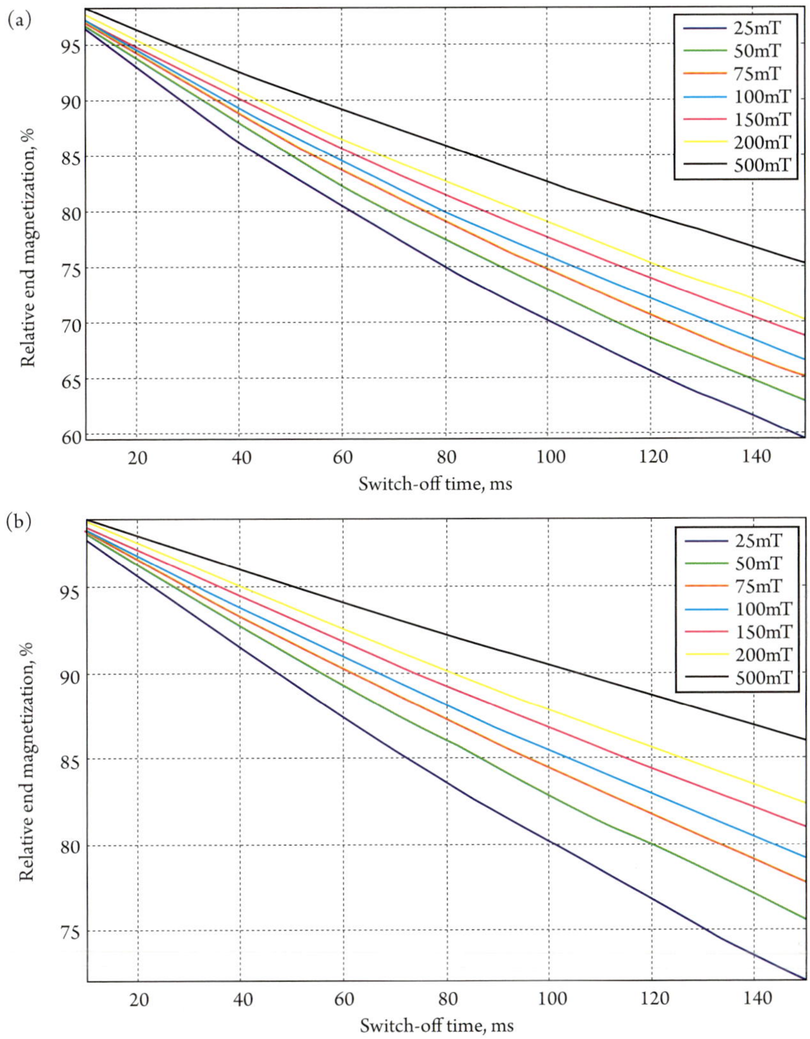

FIGURE 4.23 Estimated magnetization lost to T_1 relaxation during B_p ramp-down versus switch off time for white matter (a) and grey matter (b) for various pre-polarization field strengths.

save appreciable signal. Examples of magnetization loss as function of ramp-down time (for various ramp rates) are shown in Figure 4.23.

The practical hardware limitations of applying and removing a pulsed B_p field have already been discussed in Chapter 2. In Chapter 3 we discussed in detail imaging issues related to the method of removing B_p, which arise from transients in surrounding conducting material and phase distortions. Here we simply reiterate that while a large B_p is always best, this is only true if it increases the signal more than it increases the noise.

4.4.2 Minimize DeadTime: Projection Imaging

We have already noted that ULF MRI can differentiate T_1 contrast between some tissues and measure T_1 contrast dispersion that cannot be detected at HF (discussed further in

Section 4.5). Published values for brain tissues both at HF and ULF are shown in Table 4.2. A couple of immediately obvious points emerge from this table. There is very little change in T_2 with magnetic field even over a range from 3T to 46μT. On the other hand, T_1 changes dramatically with field. In fact, T_1 shortens with decreasing field, approaching T_2 values. A consideration at ULF is that many biological tissues are known to have T_1/T_2 values ~ 100 to 200ms at these field strengths, which is comparable to the phase-encode times used.

Consequently, signal loss due to the encoding period becomes a limitation. An alternative imaging approach is projection imaging, as shown in Figure 4.7, which may provide better results for such imaging situations. In projection imaging there is no waiting for the phase-encoding portion of a sequence. The practical downside of this approach for ULF MRI is that a current supply must be powered for not only a single readout gradient, but for all three gradients during acquisition. Our experience is that almost always introduces additional noise. In ULF MRI the noise from these current sources can be an appreciable problem, as described in Chapter 2. However, we wish to make the point that there is a lot of room for progress in ULF MRI pulse-sequence design to make more of the available signal.

4.4.3 Sensor Arrays and Parallel Imaging

We showed in Section 4.3.1.1 that even with relatively high pulsed B_p (~100mT) and excellent SQUID sensor noise of 1 fT/√Hz there is still insufficient SNR to attain 1.5 × 1.5 × 3mm^3 spatial resolution with voxel SNR≥ 30. Since t_a is already comparable to T_2 for tissue, it is not effective to increase image acquisition time due to T_2 limiting the measurable signal. Therefore the options left are averaging (which increases imaging time) or making use of one of the benefits of SQUID-based systems: the ability to build dense sensor arrays such as those used for MEG.

Arrays of sensors can be used to increase SNR or FOV or to accelerate imaging (or a combination of all these), all of which are needed to make ULF MRI competitive with HF in terms of voxel SNR and acquisition speed. Multiple sensors enlarge FOV over a single sensor because they can expand the region of sensitivity. Multiple sensors yield higher imaging SNR because MRI signal from each voxel can be acquired simultaneously by several

TABLE 4.2 Published values for brain tissue relaxation times both at HF and ULF

	3T (ms)	1.5T (ms)	46μT[(c)] (ms)
White matter T_1	1084 ± 45 [(a)], 838 ± 50 [(b)]	884 ± 50 [(a)], 646 ± 32 [(b)]	75 ± 2
T_2	69 ± 3 [(a)]	72 ± 4 [(a)]	79 ± 11
Gray matter T_1	1820 ± 114 [(a)], 1607 ± 112 [(b)]	1124 ± 50 [(a)], 1197 ± 134 [(b)]	103 ± 5
T_2	99 ± 7 [(a)]	95 ± 8 [(a)]	106 ± 11

(a) Stanisz GJ et al. (2005). T_1, T_2 relaxation and magnetization transfer in tissue at 3T. *Magn Reson Med 54*:507–512.

(b) Wright PJ et al. (2008). Water proton T_1 measurements in brain tissue at 7, 3, and 1.5T using IR-EPI, IR-TSE, and MPRAGE: results and optimization. *Magn Reson Mater Phy 21*:121–130.

(c) Zotev et al. (2009). SQUID-based microtesla MRI for in vivo relaxometry of the human brain. *IEEE Trans Appl Supercond*19(3):823–826.

sensors. An array can also allow accelerated imaging (such as SENSE, described in Chapter 1 and below) because the spatial sensitivity of the sensor array can perform some portion of encoding normally done with the gradients, and thus reduce imaging time.

4.4.3.1 Dense Sensor Arrays from Combined ULF MRI/MEG

Historically very dense arrays of SQUIDs (100–300 sensors) have been used to provide spatial sensitivity in MEG [33]. As discussed in Chapter 1 and later in Chapter 5, one of the most compelling early drivers for developing ULF MRI was that it can easily be combined with MEG to help overcome the limitation of spatial information without requiring a separate HF MRI machine. At the time of this writing, several groups (including our own) are taking advantage of the synergy in hardware to extend this work from proof-of-concept to multichannel combined ULF MRI/MEG systems [34,35]. Progress toward these systems will be described in Chapter 5. MEG is a powerful functional brain-imaging modality that provides direct imaging of neural activity with extraordinarily high (ms) temporal resolution; however, it is purely a measure of function, without any anatomical reference. In fact, the original driver for the development of ULF MRI in our group was to complement MEG by providing the "missing" anatomical reference within the same instrument [7]. Previously, our team had worked to pioneer technologies for increasing the accuracy of localizing sources of neural activity in the brain [36]. However, to provide accurate source localization, the typical MEG-measured image of neural activity was superposed on top of an MRI image of the subject's brain anatomy, acquired by a completely different instrument, with typical errors in the co-registration between the two imaging modalities of several millimeters [37,38]. Consequently, improving the localization accuracy of neural sources in MEG would be lost to the co-registration errors with the anatomy. To put this into context, regions of the human brain on opposite sides of a sulcus (or fold) are a mere millimeter apart yet can represent entirely disparate functionality. Ultimately, with the publication of the first ULF NMR results by Clarke's group, see for example [5], it became apparent that MEG and ULF MRI were possible, and our research group began to pursue ULF MRI. We naturally began the pursuit of ULF MRI with sensor arrays common to MEG systems that routinely require large (>100 sensor) arrays. The take-home message here is that applying dense sensor arrays for ULF MRI seemed a logical extension of the MEG technology.

It is interesting to note that the use of MEG-like arrays of surface coils has previously been shown in HF MRI image acceleration to provide faster imaging based on magnetic source localization such as that used in MEG [39,40]. This approach uses an inversion of the sensor data to localize the NMR signal in space as opposed to the frequency or phase signature induced by applied gradients. We note that parallel imaging may be easier to implement at ULF as opposed to HF MRI because the noise at ULF is largely independent of the sample and because SQUID sensors are not inductively coupled like tuned coils.

Our own group has investigated some of the many aspects of the benefits of array-based acquisition of ULF MRI signals. We used one parallel MRI method to acquire signals at ULF with seven channels (and validate that we were able to achieve the predicted accelerations of a factor of three). A full description of that work was published by us in reference [41]. Here we briefly review the concepts presented in that work and elaborate on ways in which one might use arrays of sensors in ULF MRI to further increase SNR and reduce acquisition time.

4.4.3.2 Image Acceleration—Sensitivity Encoding (SENSE)

Although most clinical HF MR imagers rely on a single detector (volume) coil, there are several examples of techniques for parallel imaging methods in HF MRI, including

SENSE [42], SMASH [43], and PILS [44]. While standard HF MRI uses a single large pickup (antenna or receiver) coil, parallel imaging typically relies on arrays of surface coils. At high fields these are inductive coils, and at ULF they are SQUIDs. As an introduction to the concepts of parallel MRI, we will begin by briefly outlining the SENSE approach [42].

The driving notion behind the SENSE method is to decrease the number of phase-encoding steps by a factor of R by taking fewer steps in the phase-encoding direction(s) but keeping the end values of the gradients the same. We see from Eqn. 4.23 that as long as the end values are the same, the spatial resolution will not change. Eqn. 4.38, however, tells us that taking N/R steps (instead of N steps) will reduce the FOV by a factor of R. The reduction in FOV, using normal reconstruction methods, will produce an aliased image. The SENSE reconstruction described by Preussman et al. [42] uses linear algebra and sensitivity maps for each pickup coil to reconstruct the full FOV images from the aliased ones. In the discussion below we follow the approaches described in references [41] and [45].

First let us revisit the concept of aliasing using the example in Figure 4.24. We produce a 1D image of two features using three sensor coils, as shown in the upper part of Figure 4.24. In 1D (along the phase-encode direction) the Fourier transform for a full FOV image (real part only) will look like the blue curve in Figure 4.24. Now, let us assume that we want to accelerate imaging by taking only every other step ($R = 2$). The FOV will also be cut in half ($1/R$), which causes the second object to be aliased into the first, as illustrated by the red curve. Another way of thinking about this is to envision the image signal at an aliased pixel within the reduced FOV as a superposition of up to R signals corresponding to equidistant pixels in the full FOV [41]. For example, consider the case where we have 12 pixels (in this example we will number them from left to right), as shown in the upper part of Figure 4.25. If we under-sampled by $R = 2$ (taking every other pixel in k-space), there are only six pixels in the reduced FOV image. The first pixel in the reduced FOV image would be made up of a superposition of signal from the first and seventh pixels from the full FOV image. Likewise, the second pixel in the reduced FOV image would be a superposition of information from the second and eighth pixels, and so on. For $R = 3$, the first pixel in the reduced FOV image would have information from the first, fifth, and ninth, and so on. However, we can use

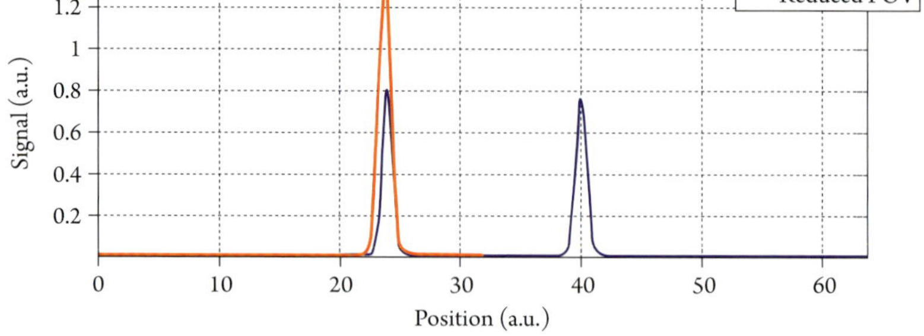

FIGURE 4.24 Top: Demonstration of 1D imaging of two objects with full FOV. Bottom: (N steps, blue trace) and an aliased reduced FOV ($N/2$ steps, red trace).

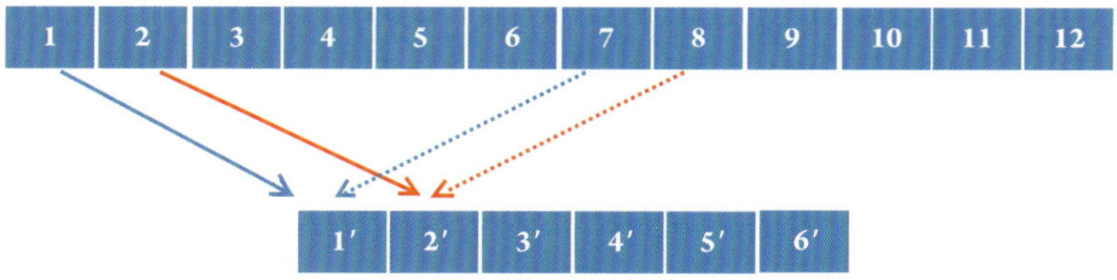

FIGURE 4.25 How 12 original pixels might be aliased in imaging accelerated by $R = 2$.

information about the sensors to help undo this aliasing. Also, we know the relationship between the aliased pixels and the pixels in the full FOV image. In the most general case (following the method of reference [46]) if we have n_c coils, and we accelerate by a factor of R, then there will be n_p pixels superposed on any pixel in the reduced FOV image, and n_p will be less than or equal to R. We know that each pixel in the individual reduced FOV coil image will contain information from multiple (R) equidistantly distributed pixels in the desired full FOV image. Additionally, these pixels will be weighted with the coil sensitivity C at the corresponding location in the full FOV.

Consider the following example. We have three coils ($n_c = 3$) and $R = 2$, which results in information from three aliased images, I. At the first pixel in the reduced FOV images there will be signal from two pixels (the first pixel and some aliased pixel):

(Eqn. 4.94)
$$
\begin{aligned}
I_1(x_1) &= C_{11}\rho_1 + C_{11'}\rho_{1'},\\
I_2(x_1) &= C_{21}\rho_1 + C_{21'}\rho_{1'},\\
I_3(x_1) &= C_{31}\rho_1 + C_{31'}\rho_{1'}.
\end{aligned}
$$

The matrix C is $n_c \times n_p$. A key feature of the SENSE method is that the sensitivity coefficients C can be derived in advance from a full FOV image acquired previously. Thus for n_c coils we will have n_c linear equations with R unknowns. As long as $n_c \geq R$ we should, in principle, be able to solve uniquely.

For any pixel in the reduced FOV image we can write

(Eqn. 4.95)
$$I_k(x_p) = \sum_{l=1}^{n_p} C_{kl}\rho_l$$

and expressed in matrix notation we have

(Eqn. 4.96)
$$\mathbf{I} = \mathbf{C}\cdot\boldsymbol{\rho}.$$

Incorporating our knowledge about the complex sensitivities at the corresponding positions for each sensor, this can be accomplished using a generalized inverse of the sensitivity matrix **C** (in the least squares method):

(Eqn. 4.97)
$$\boldsymbol{\rho} = \left(\mathbf{C}^H\mathbf{C}\right)^{-1}\mathbf{C}^H\cdot\mathbf{I}$$

where the superscript H indicates the transposed complex conjugate. In the terminology from Pruessman [42], $(C^H C)^{-1} C^H$ is an unfolding matrix used to perform signal separation.

The SENSE algorithm (Eqn. 4.97) has to be repeated for every pixel location in the reduced FOV image to finally reconstruct the full FOV image. The SENSE method works for arbitrary coil configurations, however, with a varying degree of SNR penalty (as shown in Eqn. 4.98 below). While we presented the simple 1D case for clarity, the discussion is directly extensible to 3D, in which pixels become voxels.

Thus far we have neglected noise (discussed more completely in Section 4.4.3.3), but it is instructive to briefly present the notion of SNR here to illustrate that there is some loss in SNR when using an array to perform image acceleration. The SNR is reduced by a factor of $\sqrt{R}$ because the SNR in MRI is related to the number of steps, which is reduced by R-fold in SENSE. In addition, we will see an additional SNR penalty that depends on the underlying geometry of the coil array. The encoding efficiency at any position in the FOV with a given coil configuration can be analytically described by the so-called geometry factor (g-factor), which is a measure of how easily the matrix inversion in Eqn. 4.97 can be performed.

(Eqn. 4.98)

$$SNR_R = \frac{SNR_{full}}{g\sqrt{R}}.$$

An example of SENSE reconstruction in HF MRI (from reference [46]) is shown in Figure 4.26. A description of our approach to SENSE reconstruction in ULF MRI using seven channels is found in reference [41], and an example from that work is presented in Figure 4.27. We see that with seven channels the maximum acceleration attainable, before distortions appear, is a factor of 3. The sensitivity profile of the array for the seven SQUIDs is obtained via calibration with a uniform water phantom (shown in Fig. 4.27, bottom left panel).

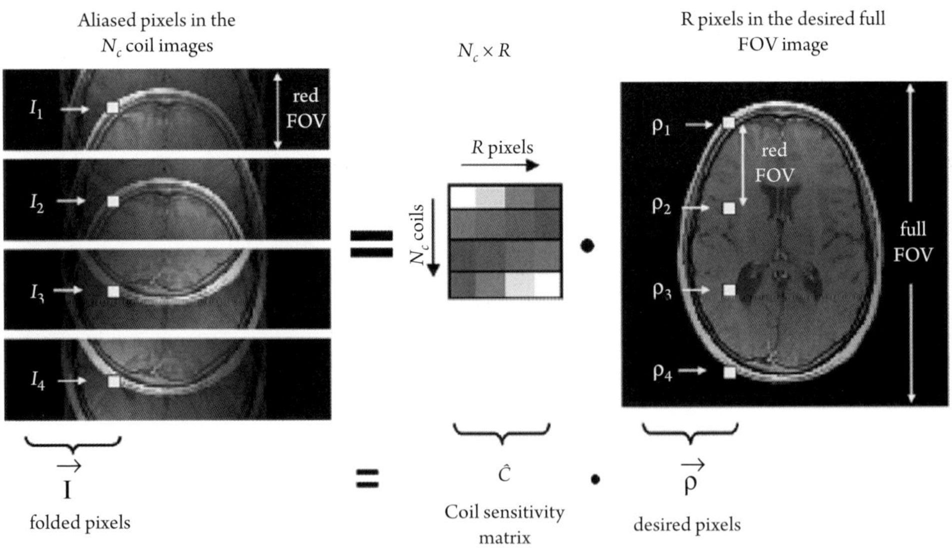

FIGURE 4.26 Illustration of the basic SENSE relation using an accelerated (R = 4) parallel MRI acquisition with N_c = 4 receiver coils. I contains the aliased pixels at a certain position in the reduced FOV coil images. The sensitivity matrix C assembles the corresponding sensitivity values of the component coils at the locations of the involved (R = 4) pixels in the full FOV image ρ. Data are from Blaimer et al., 2004 [46], with permission from Lippincott Williams & Wilkins, a Wolters Kluwer Health Business.

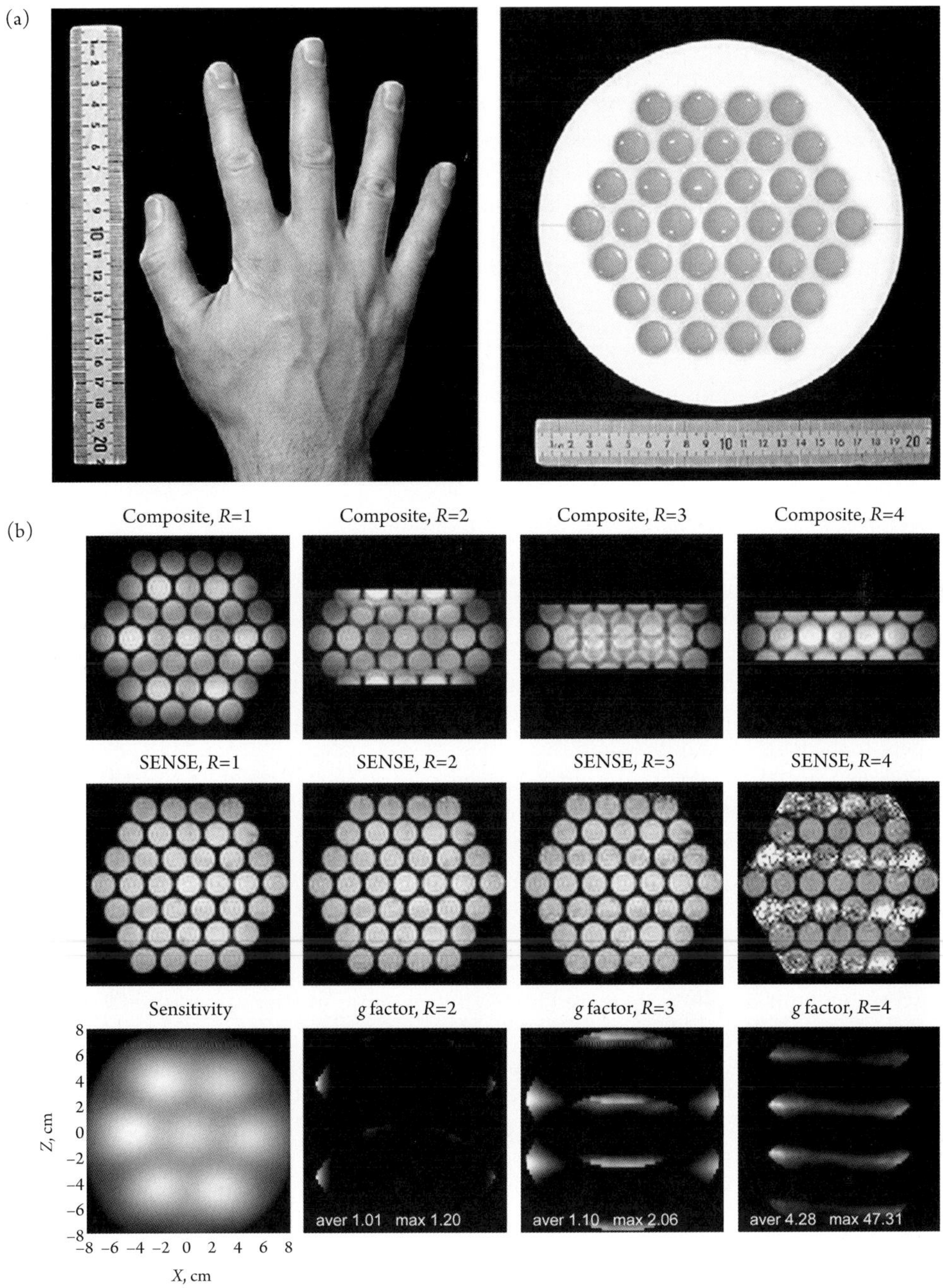

FIGURE 4.27 (a) Left is photograph of hand shown in Figure 4.15; right is photograph of the MRI phantom. (b) SENSE reconstruction of 2D phantom images for different values of the acceleration factor R. From Zotev et al., (2008) [41] with permission.

4.4.3.3 InI (The General Case of SENSE)

Clinical applications that utilize parallel MRI typically realize acceleration factors from 2 to 4. More recently [39,40], it has been shown that by using a very dense array (similar to those found in MEG and EEG) and a reconstruction method known as MR inverse imaging (InI), acceleration factors of more than 10 have been achieved, enabling fMRI with temporal resolution of less than 100ms. Although such temporal resolution is much finer than required to observe the standard hemodynamic responses in HF fMRI (typically 1–3s), ultra-fast MRI is useful for applications such as testing novel direct neuronal contrast mechanisms that might be observed with HF MRI.

InI represents a transition from the over-determined linear system in parallel MRI reconstruction (such as that for SENSE described in Section 4.4.3.1) to an under-determined one. The approach combines a very dense array (23 and 90 channels in reference [39] and 32 in reference [40]) with linear estimation. It can be shown that the parallel MRI methods such as SENSE and SMASH are specific cases of these approaches.

4.4.3.4 SNR for Parallel MRI

In the context of using a sensor array for image acceleration, one is faced with the tradeoff between faster imaging times and SNR. This is a recurring theme: one cannot minimize imaging time *and* have optimal SNR. We have shown in Section 4.3 that imaging time and SNR are inextricably coupled, independent of how many sensors one uses. On the other hand, it is also possible to use an array of MRI sensors to increase SNR (by making multiple measures of the same quantity) instead of reducing imaging time. One might naively expect that a total of N coils would result in up to $\sqrt{N}$ improvement in SNR. However, as was shown in the early work on phased arrays of surface coils in MRI [47,48], the gain in SNR strongly depends on the geometry of the coils, the type of noise present, and the weighting method employed to combine the information from coils. A simple illustration is to imagine a group of seven sensors in close-pack geometry measuring the MRI signal from some sample voxel. If we further imagine the voxel were located beneath the center sensor, it is immediately obvious that the signal measured in that sensor will be significantly larger than the signal measured in the remaining six sensors. Consequently, the SNR will not simply be increased by $\sqrt{7}$, but by some smaller value depending on the various factors mentioned.

We now return briefly to the topic of noise, which was neglected in our original discussion of parallel imaging. We are again assuming a parallel MRI system consisting of three coils. This time we do not have aliased pixels (we are not accelerating our imaging) but we do consider noise in each coil as follows:

(Eqn. 4.99)
$$\begin{aligned} I_1(x_1) &= C_{11}\rho_1 + \Delta I_1 \\ I_2(x_1) &= C_{21}\rho_1 + \Delta I_2 \\ I_3(x_1) &= C_{31}\rho_1 + \Delta I_3. \end{aligned}$$

If we do not use the array to accelerate the imaging time, then n_p (the number of aliased pixels) is 1 and C is a vector of coil sensitivities. Our composite image is found by taking a weighted average of the pixel magnitudes in the individual coil images [48]:

(Eqn. 4.100)
$$\mathbf{I} = \mathbf{C} \cdot \boldsymbol{\rho} + \Delta\mathbf{I}.$$

If **I** is measured data and **ρ** is what we are solving for, then we can use the method of maximum likelihood to solve for the values that produce a distribution that gives the observed data the greatest probability. This can be written

(Eqn. 4.101) $$l(\boldsymbol{\rho}|\mathbf{I}) \equiv \ln p(I|\boldsymbol{\rho})$$

where $p(I|\boldsymbol{\rho})$ is the probability density that given **ρ** we would measure **I**. We also need to describe the noise, which we assume here is Gaussian, zero-mean, and described by a $n_c \times n_c$ noise covariance matrix Ψ [41]:

(Eqn. 4.102) $$\Psi_{i,j} = \frac{1}{M}\sum_{m=1}^{M} n_i(m)n_j^*(m).$$

Here $n_i(m)$ is the noise value of the ith channel of measurement m and M is the total number of measurements.

In this case

(Eqn. 4.103) $$p(\rho|\boldsymbol{I}) \propto e^{\frac{-\Delta I^T \Psi^{-1} \Delta I}{2}}$$

and we can solve Eqn. 4.101 using Eqn. 4.103:

(Eqn. 4.104) $$l(\boldsymbol{\rho}|\mathbf{I}) = \frac{-(\Delta\mathbf{I})^T \boldsymbol{\Psi}^{-1}(\Delta\mathbf{I})}{2} - = -(\mathbf{I}-\mathbf{C}\cdot\boldsymbol{\rho})^T \boldsymbol{\Psi}^{-1}(\mathbf{I}-\mathbf{C}\cdot\boldsymbol{\rho})$$

to obtain

(Eqn. 4.105) $$\boldsymbol{\rho} = \left(\mathbf{C}^H \boldsymbol{\Psi}^{-1}\mathbf{C}\right)^{-1}\mathbf{C}^H \boldsymbol{\Psi}^{-1}\cdot\mathbf{I}.$$

Looking back to the SENSE equation (Eqn. 4.97), we see that noise is now included in the unfolding matrix. We can also revisit the issue of the *g*-factor describing the local noise amplification in the unfolded image in Eqn. 4.98. The noise increases in regions where the geometric relations of the coil sensitivities to a given pixel (or voxel) are not ideal. The geometry factor for a pixel p is [45]:

(Eqn. 4.106) $$g_p = \sqrt{\left[\left(\mathbf{C}^H \boldsymbol{\Psi}^{-1}\mathbf{C}\right)^{-1}\right]_{p,p}\left[\mathbf{C}^H \boldsymbol{\Psi}^{-1}\mathbf{C}\right]_{p,p}}.$$

The fact that g is a local quantity results in inhomogeneous noise in SENSE images [49].

Following the convention of reference [48], we can rewrite Eqn. 4.105 as

(Eqn. 4.107) $$\boldsymbol{\rho} = \mathbf{n}\cdot\mathbf{I}$$

to produce a composite image by taking the weighted average of the same pixel in the individual coil images:

(Eqn. 4.108) $$\textit{Composite pixel} = \sum_{i=1}^{n_c} n_i |\rho_i + \xi_i|.$$

We then maximize the SNR subject to constraints determining how the image is scaled. If we choose to scale such that the noise is constant through the composite image but lets the signal sensitivity roll off as the distance from the surface coils increases, and the noise is considered small compared to the signal, that variance is given by

(Eqn. 4.109)
$$variance = \mathbf{n} \cdot \mathbf{\Psi} \cdot \mathbf{n}$$

and thus

(Eqn. 4.110)
$$SNR = \frac{\mathbf{n} \cdot \mathbf{I}}{\sqrt{\mathbf{n} \cdot \mathbf{\Psi} \cdot \mathbf{n}}}.$$

If we then optimize the SNR to find the maximum of $\mathbf{n} \cdot \mathbf{I}$ while constraining the variance to be constant, we find the optimal SNR to be

(Eqn. 4.111)
$$SNR = \sqrt{\mathbf{I}^H \mathbf{\Psi}^{-1} \mathbf{I}}$$

or in the SENSE approach [41]

(Eqn. 4.112)
$$SNR \sim \sqrt{\mathbf{C}^H \mathbf{\Psi}^{-1} \mathbf{C}}.$$

4.4.3.5 SNR for Parallel MRI when the Voxel Is Distant

Thus far we have not specifically discussed the geometry of the array we are using. Let us now consider a specific but we hope illustrative example comparing the difference between one large pickup coil of area $3a$, or three smaller pickup coils of area a (as shown in Fig. 4.28).

Assume that the voxel being imaged is far from the coils relative to the size of the coils. We consider two limiting cases: first when the noise is totally uncorrelated, and second where the noise is highly correlated.

For **uncorrelated noise,** the single coil SNR is

(Eqn. 4.113)
$$SNR_{\text{big}} = \frac{S}{\sqrt{n}}.$$

In the case of three coils we find

(Eqn. 4.114)
$$\mathbf{\Psi} = \begin{bmatrix} n_{11} & n_{12} & n_{13} \\ n_{21} & n_{22} & n_{23} \\ n_{31} & n_{32} & n_{33} \end{bmatrix} = \begin{bmatrix} n_{11} & 0 & 0 \\ 0 & n_{22} & 0 \\ 0 & 0 & n_{33} \end{bmatrix}$$

(Eqn. 4.115)
$$SNR_{\text{three}} = \frac{w_1 s_1 + w_2 s_2 + w_3 s_3}{\sqrt{w_1^2 n_{11} + w_2^2 n_{22} + w_3^2 n_{33}}}.$$

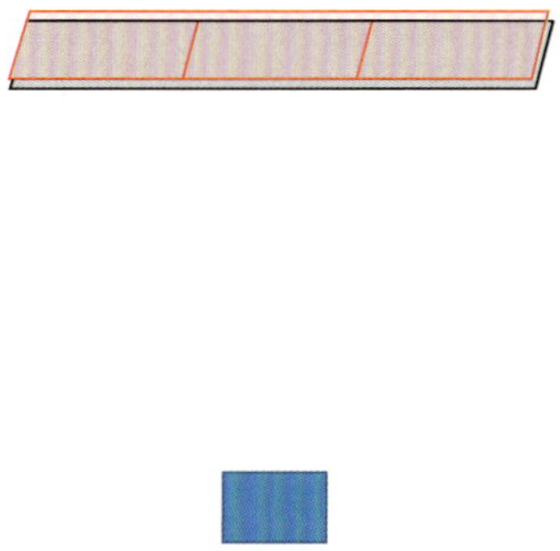

FIGURE 4.28 Array of one large coil (black border) or three small coils (red borders) with the same cumulative area, located distant from a voxel.

Since the voxel is far away we can assume the signal in all the coils is roughly the same ($s_1=s_2=s_3$) and so we can weight them all the same ($w_1=w_2=w_3$). We also consider the noise in all the coils roughly the same ($n_{11}=n_{22}=n_{33}$) to find that

(Eqn. 4.116)

$$SNR_{\text{three}} = \frac{3w_1 s_1}{\sqrt{3w_1^2 n_{11}}}$$

or more generally

(Eqn. 4.117)

$$SNR_{\text{nc}} = \frac{n_c w_1 s_1}{\sqrt{n_c w_1^2 n_{11}}} = \frac{(n_c s_1)}{\sqrt{n_c n_{11}}}$$

for n_c coils and uncorrelated noise.

Let us now consider how the SNR for three smaller coils compares to one large coil of the same area as the combined small coils (the large blue coil in Fig. 4.28). Let us assume that the signal is simply due to the flux captured (in the area covered by the coils); then the signal from one large coil is the same as $n_c \cdot s_1$ small coils (assuming they cover the same area, $s = n_c \cdot s_1$) and the numerators in Eqns. 4.113 and 4.117 are the same for a single large coil or multiple smaller coils of equal total area. But if the noise is all sensor noise (n) then one big coil has $\sqrt{n}$ in the denominator of Eqn. 4.113, but the multicoil system has $\sqrt{n_c \cdot n}$ in the denominator of Eqn. 4.117, and thus the SNR for n_c small coils is worse in performance by $\sqrt{n_c}$. On the other hand, if the noise is dominated by uncorrelated ambient noise, then the SNR will essentially be the same for both one big or many small coils because the noise collected by one large coil is the same as many small coils and the performance for one coil or many smalls is identical. This supports the general conclusion that when the voxel is far away from the sensors, it is better to have one large inductive coil than many small ones [48]. A caveat to this analysis is that the assumption that the voxel is distant from the pickup coils is rarely realized in real-world applications (see the next section).

While inductive coupling between SQUID-based sensor arrays is negligible (as opposed to HF MRI pickup coils, where the coupling can be significant), there is a consideration that is specific to pickup coils coupled to SQUID sensors that is worth mentioning. The inductive coupling between the SQUID sensor and the pickup coil will affect the performance of the array (Chapter 2). Specifically, the inductive matching between a

SQUID and pickup coils of different size will differ, which will cause specific performance characteristics to differ. For a SQUID the coupling between the flux in the pickup coil and the SQUID is

(Eqn. 4.118)

$$\Phi_s = \frac{M\Phi_p}{(L_p + L_i)}$$

where M is the mutual inductance, L_p is the inductance of the pickup loop, and L_i is the inductance of the input. While one can, in principle, optimize the SQUID for any particular coil, this isn't always practical. In our applications we purchased a standard commercially available SQUID, the CE2Blue from Supracon [50]. We routinely use this SQUID model in our systems because, at the time of this writing, it is the only commercial sensor available with an embedded cryogenic switch. For this device typical values are M = 8nH and L_i = 420nH. These values do not change with input coil. However, the input inductance does depend on the coil size and typically goes as 0.8nH × radius (in mm). On the other hand, the flux collected in the pickup coil goes as the square of the radius. So there is some additional benefit to moving to larger input coils.

However, if the noise is **correlated** such that

(Eqn. 4.119)

$$\Psi = \begin{bmatrix} n_{11} & n_{12} & n_{13} \\ n_{21} & n_{22} & n_{23} \\ n_{31} & n_{32} & n_{33} \end{bmatrix} = \begin{bmatrix} n_{11} & \alpha n_{11} & \alpha n_{11} \\ \alpha n_{11} & n_{11} & \alpha n_{11} \\ \alpha n_{11} & \alpha n_{11} & n_{11} \end{bmatrix}$$

where $0 \le \alpha \le 1$, then we find

(Eqn. 4.120)

$$SNR_{\text{three}} = \frac{w_1 s_1 + w_2 s_2 + w_3 s_3}{\sqrt{n_{11}\left(w_1\left(w_1 + \alpha w_2 + \alpha w_3\right) + w_2\left(\alpha w_1 + w_2 + \alpha w_3\right) + w_3\left(\alpha w_1 + \alpha w_2 + w_3\right)\right)}}$$

(Eqn. 4.121)

$$SNR_{\text{three}} = \frac{w_1 s_1 + w_2 s_2 + w_3 s_3}{\sqrt{n_{11}\left(w_1\left(w_1 + \alpha(w_2 + w_3)\right) + w_2\left(w_2 + \alpha(w_1 + w_3)\right) + w_3\,\alpha(w_1 + w_2)\right)}}.$$

Again, if the voxel is far away we can assume the signal in all the coils is roughly the same ($s_1 = s_2 = s_3$) and so we can weight them all the same ($w_1 = w_2 = w_3$).

(Eqn. 4.122)

$$SNR_{\text{three}} = \frac{3w_1 s_1}{\sqrt{n_{11}\left(3w_1^2(1 + 2\alpha)\right)}}$$

(Eqn. 4.123)

$$SNR_{\text{three}} = \frac{3s_1}{\sqrt{3n_{11}(1 + 2\alpha)}}.$$

Or more generally

(Eqn. 4.124)
$$SNR_{n_c} = \frac{n_c s_1}{\sqrt{n_c n_{11}\left(1+\left(n_c-1\right)\alpha\right)}}.$$

As we approach 100% correlated α = 1 and

(Eqn. 4.125)
$$SNR_{\text{three}} = \frac{s_1}{\sqrt{n_{11}}}$$

we find that if the noise is 100% correlated we get no improvement from having more coils. In reality the noise will be somewhere between totally uncorrelated and 100% correlated. For example, with the seven-channel system of Zotev et al. [41] we found up to 20% noise correlations.

If the noise is correlated ambient noise, multiple coils provide even less benefit, because the noise appears in all the sensor channels. It is also worth noting that when the sensors (pickup coils) are relatively distant from the MRI signal source (that is, the pickup coils are small relative to the distance from the voxel of interest) an array of many such small coils is not effective for image acceleration because the sensitivity profile for each sensor is about the same.

4.4.3.6 SNR for Parallel MRI when the Voxel Is Close

We now consider the more realistic, and complex, case of the MRI voxel of interest being close to the pickup coil (separation between voxel and pickup relative to size of the pickup), as shown in Figure 4.29. In such cases, the weighting can make a significant difference. For example, when a voxel is in very close proximity to the pickup, a single large coil will suffer from a net cancellation of signal (that is, within the area of the pickup coil the flux lines going into the plane of the coil are effectively cancelled by those coming out of the plane). However, a small pickup is more likely to measure a larger net signal because the flux lines into and out of the sensor plane are unlikely to balance (be symmetrical).

In Figure 4.29, the signal is distributed between three small coils as $s_1 = -s$, $s_2 = s$, and $s_3 = -s$. We can weight the signals by $w_1 = w_3 = -w_1$ and $w_2 = w_1$, thus resulting in a measurable signal. In the large coil there is no weighting, so the net signal is zero. Thus the SNR might be $\geq\sqrt{n_c}$ when we are up close. This is true whether the noise is correlated or uncorrelated.

To summarize, when the voxel is distant (relative to coil size) we cannot expect to get much improvement from an array versus a single coil of comparable size, but this depends strongly on the type and origin of the noise, the coil size, and distance [51]. However, when the voxel is close to the pickup we can expect SNR to improve by $\geq\sqrt{n_c}$ by using smaller coils over larger coils.

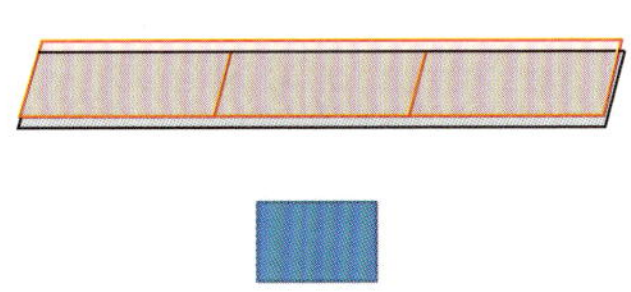

FIGURE 4.29 Array of one large coil (black border) or three small coils (red borders) with the same cumulative area, located near a voxel.

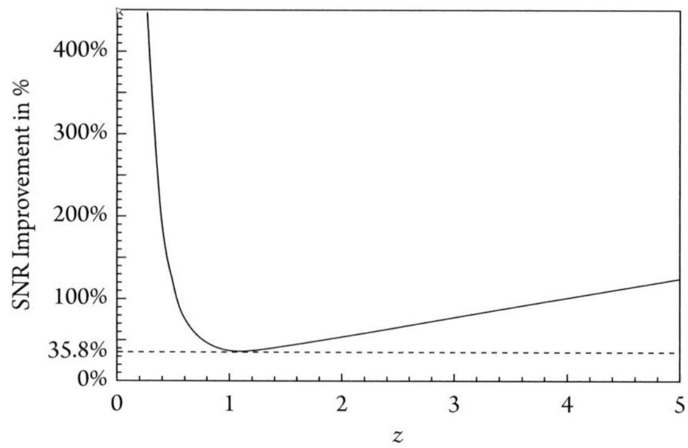

FIGURE 4.30 Improvement in SNR for the ideal array over a simple circular loop of diameter $d = 1$. The improvement is shown along the main axis of the loop as a function of the distance in the z-direction. From Wang et al. [51], used with permission from IEEE.

Wang et al. [51] consider the hypothetical situation of the signal from an "ideal" infinite array versus the "ideal" single coil (of finite size) for a dipole source placed at a given depth in a conducting media. In this case (shown in Fig. 4.30), the significant benefit realized by having many small coils at close distances is clearly seen and arises because of the weighting. When the coil diameter is comparable to the distance to the voxel, there is only ~36% improvement in SNR even compared to an infinite (in number of channels and area covered) array. As the source moves deeper (further away from the pickup loop) the SNR slowly improves. The final caveat is that the SNR improvement will be smaller for a finite array.

4.5 ON THE PLUS SIDE

While low SNR, longer acquisition, and reduced T_1 time at low fields are obvious limitations, there are some advantages to ULF MRI, some of which we shall now discuss. The first is the *unique MRI contrast* arising from the overlap of the Larmor frequency with the msec-sec dynamics of molecular or physiological processes. These enhanced contrast mechanisms are not accessible by fixed-field MRI or conventional field-cycling methods [15,52,53]. They include T_1 dispersion (with [54,55] and without [52,56] contrast agents) and resonant contrast produced by overlapping the Larmor frequency with biomagnetic processes of interest [57]. The second is the *flexible instrumentation that is compatible with a variety of applications precluded by HF approaches.* This includes imaging through or in the presence of metal [58,59], compatibility with imaging modalities like MEG [7,22], and the ability to reduce, remove, or reorient magnetic fields for applications such as portable or bedside MRI using novel pulse sequences. Third is the *potential for lower-cost MRI instrumentations.* As liquid helium (LHe) supplies and rare earth magnet material become more costly and scarce, the expense of field generation for HF MRI will likely continue to increase. SQUID-based systems require only tens of liters of LHe, and systems can employ recycling [60] or cryocoolers [61] to dramatically reduce LHe consumption. As the technology of atomic magnetometers advances, there is also some potential for ULF MRI [62] that does not require any cryogens. Finally, *ULF MRI instrumentation has the potential to be lightweight and portable.* Typical ULF MRI instrumentation (neglecting passive magnetic shielding for the moment) is

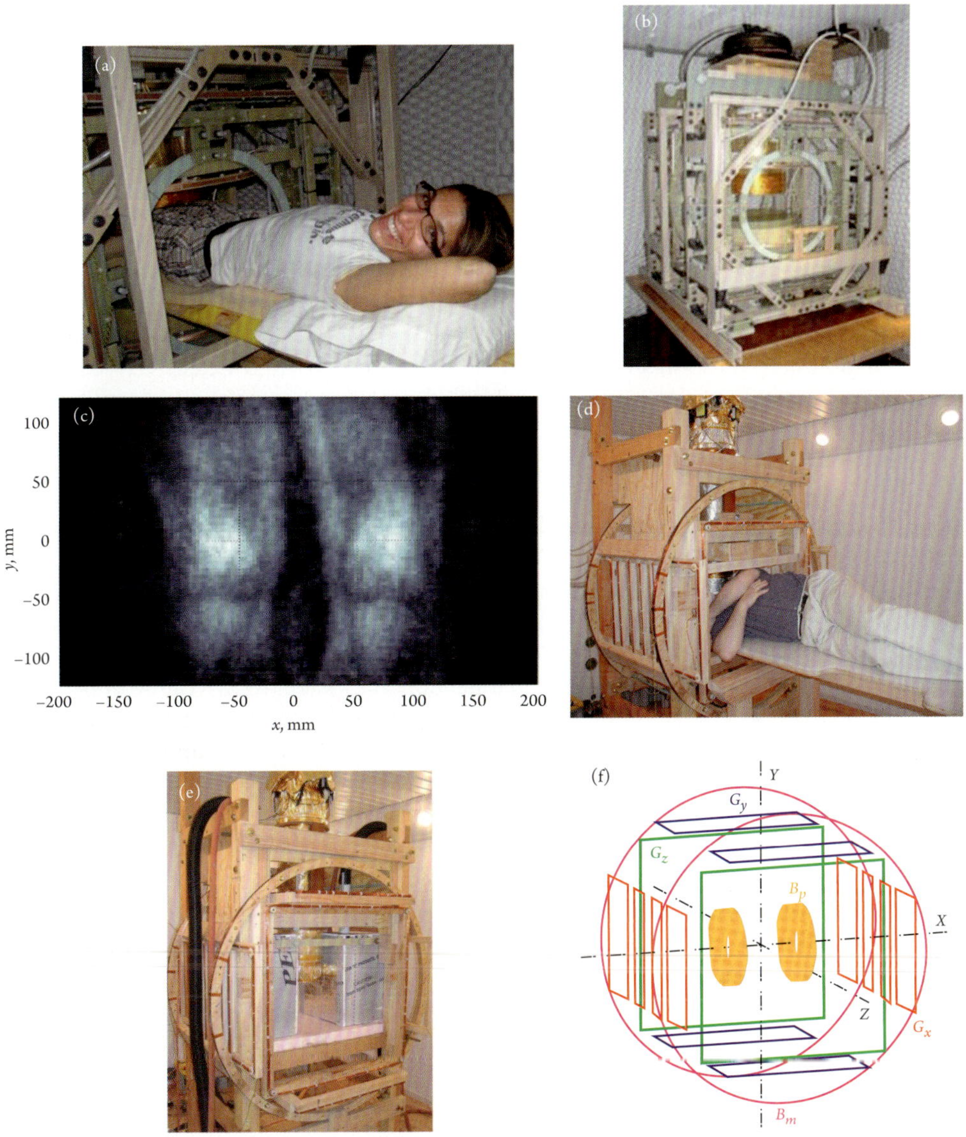

FIGURE 4.31 An example of ULF MRI hardware. Subject positioning (a), apparatus (b) and ULF MRI of the human knees (c). Subject positioning (d), apparatus (e) and coil schematic (f) for a ULF MRI and MEG system for scanning the human brain. Data are adapted from reference [32].

orders of magnitude lighter than HF systems. For example, the systems shown in Figure 4.31 can be moved by two people (order of 200 pounds), whereas the weight of a 3T imager (GE Signa EXCITE 3T High-Field MRI)! is on the order of 27,000 pounds HF MRI imagers also require not only specialized equipment to move, but also specially constructed buildings and magnetic shielding, which contributes to the extraordinarily high cost of these installations. While the combination of ULF MRI with MEG will always require an MSR, it is possible that ULF MRI alone can work without such a room.

At the time of this writing a number of technical obstacles must be overcome to realize a practical clinical ULF MRI device: (1) image quality and speed must improve; (2) adequate CNR must be achieved; (3) technical requirements such as the use of an expensive magnetically shielded room must be relaxed; (4) pulsed pre-polarization must be achieved without large dB/dt; and (5) the consumption of cryogens must be eliminated or greatly reduced. We have already discussed most of these challenges, and note that minimizing (or even eliminating) the consumption of rare cryogens is technologically available today but has not been implemented by our team. If the other issues can be effectively addressed, we believe there are significant opportunities for ULF MRI to address applications that traditional MRI cannot.

Figure 4.31 shows two ULF MRI systems designed by our team at Los Alamos. The design and application of these systems has been discussed extensively elsewhere (e.g., [4,7,63]) and in Chapter 2, but we present them here to establish a physical frame of reference for the instrumentation scale, and begin the discussion of the potential benefits of ULF MRI.

What may be immediately noticeable is the simplicity of the hardware for field generation, which is produced by wire-wound coils on wood or fiberglass forms. The magnitude of the measurement fields is ~10 to 100μT, and typical gradients are in the ≅μT/cm range (60Hz/cm for protons), produced with modest (<1 Amp)current. The approximate diameter of the measurement field coils shown in Figure 4.31 is ≅1m. In both cases the sensor systems shown (described in Chapter 2) consist of seven second-order SQUID gradiometers passively cooled by ~10 to 30 liters of liquid helium. The system shown in the upper panel of Figure 4.31 produces ~70mT pulsed pre-polarization field at the coil surface. The B_p coil uses a Fluorinert-based coolant and operates at room temperature. The system in the bottom panel attains ≅30mT pre-polarization field at the center of the sampling volume, using resistive liquid nitrogen-cooled coils. Both systems pulse at ≅1Hz duty cycle and can be easily de-energized. The ability to de-energize the systems is an important difference between ULF and HF imagers because de-energizing the field makes them safe for venues like the operating room, intensive care unit, or field hospital and greatly simplifies their transport. This is in contrast to traditional HF superconducting or permanent magnet-based systems.

Any practical MRI machine must address the issue of magnetic shielding. Shielding serves two purposes: to protect patients and staff from the strong magnetic fields (especially in HF systems) and to isolate the sensors from external magnetic noise (especially in ULF systems). The system in the bottom panel of Figure 4.31was designed to perform both MEG and ULF MRI and thus is operated in a high-quality mu-metal shielded enclosure to enable clean acquisition of the low-frequency MEG. This system was used to acquire the images shown in Figure 1.1 in Chapter 1 and the MEG/MRI image shown in Figure 4.1. The system shown in the top panel of Figure 4.31 was designed to be mobile but still operate at rather low frequencies (≤4kHz), and thus was built to operate inside a smaller two-layer mu-metal shield approximately 2m on each side. While this system was designed for the inspection of liquids in an airport [32], it also produces promising anatomical images (an image of the knees acquired with this system is shown in Fig. 4.31, top right). If MEG is not required, and one wishes to acquire only ULF MRI, it is likely that by increasing the Larmor frequency modestly (perhaps near 20kHz) it may be possible to operate with only an RF shield. Eliminating the requirement of a mu-metal shield reduces both the system weight and cost rather dramatically. ULF MRI systems operating with only an RF shield have been reported [5,61]. However, these still generally require several-mm-thick aluminum eddy-current shields. For a truly light and portable MRI system, a practical shielding system has yet to be fully demonstrated. One possibility that, to our knowledge, has not yet been tested is an "active" shield, such as those used in MEG [64].

Although the spatial resolution of ULF MRI remains less than conventional clinical MRI (typically 3mm vs. 1mm), the potential for imaging in the presence of metal and open and inexpensive MRI systems that would be suitable for rural clinics or emergency rooms, intensive care units, and the operating room remains quite promising.

4.5.1 Flexible Field Orientation and Strength

A key feature of the ULF MRI system design is that by using such simple and relatively low-power equipment to generate the magnetic fields, it is possible to reorient the magnetic fields in any direction. While this has yet to be fully exploited, one can envision numerous applications that such a flexible field enables. For example, projection imaging is one of the earliest approaches to MRI [1]. In the most common approach to projection imaging, various lines in *k*-space are acquired by reorientation of the magnetic field gradients, as shown in Figure 4.7. While HF MRI is limited to reorienting the gradients because the main magnetic field cannot be rotated (and rotation of the sample is typically impractical), it is relatively simple to build three orthogonally oriented B_m coils for ULF MRI that could enable the magnetic field direction to be manipulated in any direction. This could also be useful in applications with helmet-shaped arrays of sensors, where not every sensor is optimally sensitive to a single precession direction. Another example is the technique of magnetic resonance electrical impedance tomography (MREIT) [65,66]. As the approach is currently performed in HF MRI systems, only the component of current that produces magnetic field along the main magnetic field of the scanner can be imaged.

Mathematical and current injection methods have been devised to work around this limitation, but simply being able to reorient the direction of the measurement magnetic field would be more direct and accurate, especially in situations where the assumption of tissue isotropy is not valid. Thus rotation of the magnetic field would enable the direct acquisition of other components. For these reasons, it may be advantageous to create a MREIT system using ULF MRI [67] (discussed further in Chapter 5). ULF MRI enables both rotation of the main magnetic field axis to capture off-axis components and the ability to "overlap" the Larmor frequency with either applied or inherent currents for a "resonant" approach to imaging, in a physiologically relevant regime of frequencies (Hz to kHz). This is entirely unique to the ULF approach. In addition, the current noise, an artifact to which MREIT is extremely sensitive, produced at ULF will be orders of magnitude less than the spurious currents produced in subjects by HF MRI gradient and RF coils.

One of the most interesting arguments for the benefit of the flexible fields of ULF MRI is that the strength of any of the magnetic fields can be easily varied, which also varies the Larmor frequency. This leads to the ability to use the frequency (or field) variability of T_1 in materials of interest as a form of contrast, so-called T_1 "frequency dispersion." The value of this has been shown in many striking examples at higher field [9,14,56,68,69], although the fixed field of the scanner in traditional MRI is an issue. Clarke et al. have recently shown the advantage of T_1 contrast in discriminating between certain tissues at ULF, including benign and cancerous prostate tissue at ULF [52,70], for which there is little or no measurable difference at HF. This may lead to unique and exciting applications of ULF MRI. We have also shown significant dispersion between brain tissues between HF and ULF [15]. However, the true power of the approach remains to be practically demonstrated and validated. The potential promise of unique contrast and/or dispersion contrast warrants its own discussion and is presented in Sections 4.5.3 and 4.5.4, and in Section 4.5.5, where we discuss the relative tradeoffs in SNR and CNR for ULF MRI.

The low fields of ULF and the flexibility to turn fields completely off present a variety of benefits. One benefit of being able to completely turn off all magnetic fields is that a ULF MRI system could be transported or used in situations where rigorous environmental control is difficult. One could envision a "pallet"-sized MRI machine (assuming that shielding can be made manageable) that could be mobile for field applications (i.e., battlefield MRI) and bedside MRI in hospitals, where moving patients presents many drawbacks, from morbidity to the increased staff required. The low magnetic fields used during readout enable imaging to be performed in the presence (or even through) metal [58,59], as we discuss in the next section (4.5.2).

4.5.2 Susceptibility Artifacts, RF Screening, and Imaging in the Presence of Metal

We have defined the magnetizing (polarizing) magnetic field as B_p, measured in units of Tesla. When the magnetic fields pass through materials, as is typically the case in MRI, one may need to consider what part of the local field inside the material originates from the magnet and what field results as a consequence of the material itself. The most common and general definition for a magnetic field in any substance is given by

(Eqn. 4.126)
$$B=\mu_0 \cdot (H+M)=\mu_0 \cdot H(1+\chi_v)$$

where μ_0 is the magnetic permeability of free space, H is the "magnetic field strength," M is the magnetization, and χ_V is the volume magnetic susceptibility, a dimensionless quantity that describes the contribution to the total magnetic flux density present, made by a substance when subjected to a magnetic field. When there is no material (e.g., vacuum) χ_V is 0 and B and H will be the same. But inside a material, B will be affected by the magnetic susceptibility of the material. Moreover, as Eqn. 4.103 shows, the influence of the magnetic susceptibility of a material will only increase with field strength.

Traditional MRI, especially in clinical applications, uses very high magnetic fields (1.5 or 3T or even higher) for which the effect of susceptibility must be considered. For example, one consequence of susceptibility variations is that all objects placed in the magnetic field will disturb the field homogeneity, causing local magnetic field gradients. When two adjacent regions have very different susceptibility (for example, tissue next to a void, such as would be found in the lungs or chest cavity), a spatial variation of the magnetic field will arise in areas close to the border between the two materials. This leads to magnetic field gradients that distort the image via frequency changes, or alterations in T_2^*. In the human body, which consists of a large number of different tissue types and organs of different shape and susceptibility, the local field distribution can be very complex. In practice, shim gradients, of linear or higher order, are locally optimized for each measurement in order to minimize magnetic field inhomogeneities in the studied region. At ULF such distortions due to differences in tissue are greatly reduced. An example of the challenges caused by susceptibility differences at HF is seen in the typically poor image quality of lungs. Hyperpolarized gases have been suggested to improve the signal for lung imaging, to improve the low signal. Because the susceptibility artifact is greatly reduced at ULF, the use of hyperpolarized gases combined with ULF MRI appears to be a very promising approach for lung imaging [71].

Materials with "somewhat" positive susceptibility are said to be paramagnetic or, if the susceptibility is large, ferromagnetic. In these cases, when placed in an external field, the magnetic field within the material is strengthened. If the magnetic susceptibility is negative, the material is said to be diamagnetic. For example, water is diamagnetic with $\chi_V = -9.05 \times 10^{-6}$ at 37°C [72] (in SI units). Nonmagnetic metals such as titanium and aluminum are paramagnetic with $\chi_V = 182 \times 10^{-6}$ [73] and 22×10^{-6} [74], respectively, as is oxygen gas ($1 \times 9\ 10^{-6}$[74]). Iron, with a large susceptibility of $\chi_V = 1011 \times 10^{-6}$ [73], is ferromagnetic. Most tissues are diamagnetic and have susceptibility values between –11 and –7ppm, which is quite close to that of water ($\chi_V = -9.05 \times 10^{-6}$ at 37°C). Within soft tissues the susceptibility values are very similar and therefore the susceptibility-induced field gradients are small. Blood ($\chi_V = -7.9$ppm [75]) and air ($\chi_V = 0.36$ppm) have susceptibilities that differ substantially from the susceptibility of soft tissue; hence, larger magnetic field gradients can be found near these interfaces [73].

In most cases, the image distortions associated with susceptibility differences at HF are considered undesirable and must be minimized and corrected as much as possible. However, there is one notable exception: the basis of the most common form of fMRI depends on a susceptibility difference arising from the fact that hemoglobin in blood is diamagnetic when oxygenated but paramagnetic when deoxygenated. While this difference is small, it produces changes in the overall susceptibility of red blood cells associated with oxygenation [72]. The changes in local magnetic field associated with susceptibility as a function of O_2 content then produce measurable changes in T_2^*. Since it has long been hypothesized that changes in blood flow and blood oxygenation are related (albeit indirectly) to neural activity, these small changes in susceptibility have allowed BOLD fMRI to become a dominant technique in functional brain imaging and mapping. Since these susceptibility effects scale with magnetic field, the trend in fMRI, as with anatomical MRI, has been toward the highest magnetic fields possible. Common volume magnetic susceptibilities relevant to anatomical and functional imaging are shown in Table 4.3.

While susceptibility is a boon to functional imaging, it can pose challenges for other aspects of anatomical imaging as the magnetic field is increased. For example, cosmetics containing paramagnetic materials are well known to produce these artifacts [76]. Such susceptibility-derived effects can result in dephasing and frequency shifts of nearby spins. This results in artifacts in the MR image, primarily a loss of signal but also a distortion of the image, as seen in Figure 4.32. In this example we see the effects of an uncorrected susceptibility artifact associated with a mechanically produced hair oil [77]. An example of an even more pronounced artifact from hair products containing pigments made from

TABLE 4.3 Susceptibilities (SI) at 37-C

Material	χ_V
Water	$-9.05 \cdot 10^{-6}$
Whole blood* (deoxygenated)	$-7.9 \cdot 10^{-6}$
Oxygenated red blood cells	$-9.42 \cdot 10^{-6}$
Deoxygenated red blood cells	$-6.07 \cdot 10^{-6}$
Omniscan gadolinium contrast agent	$+11.55 \cdot 10^{-6}$

Data are from reference [72] except *, which is from reference [75].

paramagnetic iron oxide can be found in [78]. The maximum spatial distortion due to a susceptibility change Δ_χ at the boundary between two different materials is [75]

(Eqn. 4.127)
$$\Delta x \approx \frac{\Delta \chi B_{\mathrm{m}}}{G_{\mathrm{r}}}$$

where G_{r} is the readout gradient. Thus, for a given susceptibility difference $\Delta\chi$, the distortion can be minimized by lowering the measurement field B_{m} and/or raising the gradient G_{r}. Swapping the frequency-encode and phase-encode directions modifies the susceptibility artifacts without eliminating them.

The presence of any metal (or other conducting material, ferromagnetic or not) causes large distortions in the magnetic field and significant artifacts. Metals (and other conductors) cause magnetic field (and image) distortions as a result of both the susceptibility and induced currents. The range of signal loss depends on the metal and on the pulse sequence (spin echo, gradient echo). For example, spin-echo (SE) sequences are less prone to susceptibility artifacts than gradient-echo sequences. In SE, the 180-degree refocusing pulse corrects the susceptibility-induced dephasing of spins (which belongs to T_2^* effects). Short echo times allow less time for dephasing and reduce signal loss. The local change in precession frequency gives rise to image distortion along the frequency-encoding direction [58]. These artifacts can make imaging even in the presence of small amounts of metal challenging, and the challenge grows with increasing field strength. Nevertheless, at the time of this writing standard clinical MRI systems routinely utilize 3T magnets; some human systems have attained 7T and small animal imagers even higher fields. The strategy for imaging in these HF systems is to rigorously screen for and exclude metal.

ULF MRI may provide an alternative for cases where susceptibility artifacts are sufficiently large to prevent attaining quality images at HF, or where it is not possible to rigorously exclude metal. For example, the image of the hand with the metal rod shown in Chapter1, Figure 1.1, would not be possible in HF. Even with pulsed pre-polarization at 0.1T, using adiabatic ($\cong$100ms) ramp-down, dB/dt_{max} is $\cong$ 1T/s, an order of magnitude

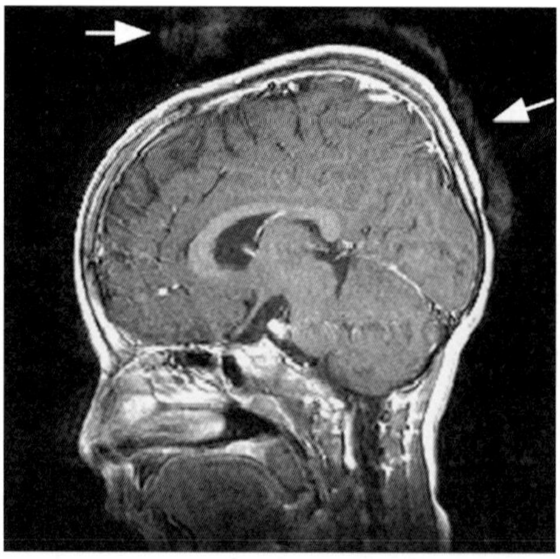

FIGURE 4.32 Susceptibility artifact at high field. In this example we see the effects of an uncorrected susceptibility artifact (indicated with arrows) associated with a mechanically produced hair oil. Figure is reproduced with permission from [77].

lower than found for standard 1.5T systems [79]. The force on metals is also reduced by an order of magnitude, which is conducive to imaging in situations where metal might be present in the subject or environment. In addition, the heating of metal is also virtually eliminated since RF pulses are not required. In typical HF systems, metals can easily be heated to dangerous levels by RF. Furthermore, even with the relatively low conductivity of tissue and blood, the RF used in HF MRI can deposit significant amounts of energy into the subject, which presents a safety consideration. Even if time-varying magnetic fields are used at ULF, the energy deposited in the human body via the RF excitation scales quadratically with field strength; consequently, the specific absorption rate (SAR, or energy deposition) is also greatly reduced. On the other hand, in applications where one needs to ramp B_p down quickly, the dB/dt can produce sufficient local currents (and associated potentials in tissue) to stimulate neural responses, although the total energy deposited into the tissue remains small.

An excellent demonstration of the benefit of ULF MR over HF MRI for imaging in the presence of metal is also presented in the work of John Clarke's group [58] (Fig. 4.33). In that work, images of water-filled grid-phantoms containing a $1.5 \times 10 \times 15\text{mm}^3$ titanium bar were collected at 7T and at 66μT. Figures 4.33A and 4.33D show photographs of the phantom, while Figures 4.33B and 4.33C show images acquired at 7T. In Figure 4.33B the frequency-encoding gradient was oriented perpendicular to and in Figure 4.33C it was parallel to the titanium bar. The orientation of the sample relative to the RF coil remained the

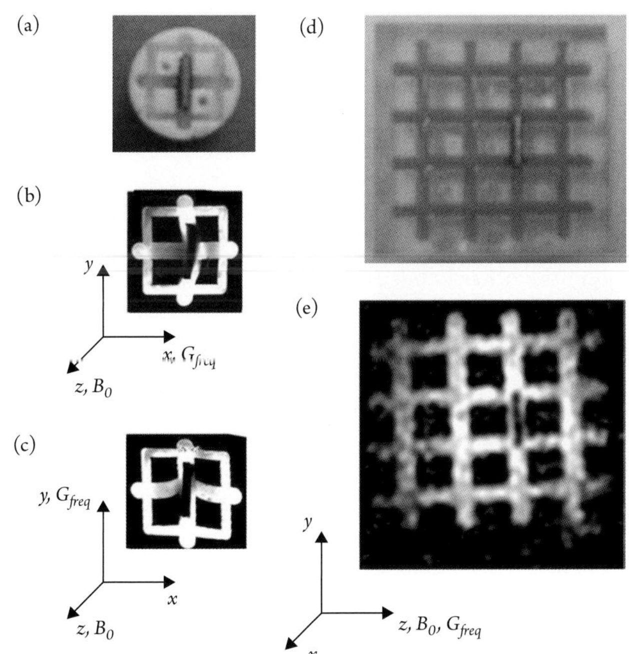

FIGURE 4.33 Comparison of MRI in the presence of metal between ULF and HF MRI. A and D show photographs of the phantom, while B and C show images acquired at 7T. In B the frequency-encoding gradient was oriented perpendicular to and in C it was parallel to the titanium bar. E shows an image of the phantom with titanium rod acquired at B_m = 66μT with a readout gradient of 110μT/m oriented along the z-axis (the configuration that produced maximum distortion at high field). Data are from reference [58].

same. Using the imaging parameters $B_0 = 7T$, $G_r = 40$ mT/m and the susceptibility difference between water and titanium

$$\Delta\chi = (182 - (-9)) \cdot 10^{-6} \approx 191.10^{-6}$$

one can use Eqn. 4.126 to predict a maximum distortion of 3mm, which is clearly observed in the images (reported to have 0.2mm spatial resolution). This example also illustrates the effect of the orientation of the readout (frequency-encode) gradient with respect to the object. We see that placing the axis of the object along (parallel to) the direction of the readout gradient somewhat reduces the distortion.

Figure 4.33E shows an image of the phantom with a titanium rod acquired at $B_m = 66\mu T$ with a readout gradient of 110μT/m oriented along the z-axis (the configuration that produced maximum distortion at HF). The image distortion is negligible, as expected from Eqn. 4.126 (which predicts a 0.3mm distortion for this case, well below the ~1mm calculated image resolution).

We have seen that conductors produce strong distortions at HF MRI, but another effect that arises when we image in the presence of metal is that the conductor causes RF screening (that affects both the RF pulse and the NMR signal itself). The effect can be understood in the context of the skin depth (discussed also in Chapter 1), the value in a conductor at which the RF field falls to $1/e$ of the surface value:

(Eqn. 4.128) $$\delta = (\pi\mu_0\mu\sigma f)^{-1/2}$$

where μ_0 is the permeability of free space, μ and σ are the relative permeability and electrical conductivity of the material, and f is the frequency in Hz. Most of the time we use $\mu = 1$.

For example, copper = 5.96×10^7 and aluminum = 3.5×10^7 at 20°C. Thus, at the 1.5T of a common clinical scanner (64MHz) the depth is ~8 or 11μm for copper or aluminum, respectively. On the other hand, a typical ULF frequency of 4 kHz would result in a skin depth of ~1or 1.3mm for copper or aluminum. To put this into context, if we imagine wrapping some sample in household aluminum foil (16μm thick) and trying to image that sample, in a 1.5T imager the foil will absorb more than 75% of the RF signal produced by the imager on the way into the sample and also absorb more than 75% of the signal coming out of the sample. In contrast, that same foil will absorb less than 1% of the signal in the 4kHz ULF MRI system! A more extensive list of materials and skin depths is given in Chapter 1.

As described in [58] and the references therein, if metal is located within the sample, the resultant RF inhomogeneity can result in a signal diminution or enhancement, particularly near the metal. These artifacts dominate the susceptibility artifacts for metals with high conductivity and low susceptibility (e.g., copper or aluminum), whereas for materials with low conductivity and high susceptibility, such as titanium, these current-induced artifacts are small compared to susceptibility artifacts. If the sample or part of the sample is completely enclosed in a metal container, screening of both the applied RF field and the detected RF NMR signal is the dominating effect. Consider another practical example: the typical wall thickness of an aluminum can is ~200μm [58,80]. A sample inside such an aluminum can would be impossible to image in a clinical MRI scanner (~99.99999 signal loss at 1.5T); however, there have been demonstrations of imaging inside such cans [32,58] at ULF (<15% signal loss at 4kHz).

This becomes relevant not only for imaging in the presence of medical implants but also for a recent application of ULF MRI to examine liquids for security screening [32,81], where the ability to image through a variety of consumer packaging, including metal cans, becomes critical. Our team demonstrated that the NMR signal from water can be measured through up to 2mm of copper [59].

4.5.3 Contrast

Contrast in physiological MRI can be most simply defined as the difference between two tissue types in some measurable parameter space, such as T_1 or T_2. While the specific parameters may vary, contrast provides the foundation of any imaging modality. MRI is sensitive to NMR parameters such as relaxation, just as density or atomic number (Z) differences form the contrast in x-ray imaging or how materials absorb light is the basis of photography. The variation between parameters such as T_1 and T_2 in different materials (i.e., tissues) provides the powerful and unique information that forms the foundation of MRI images. For example, T_1 contrast is a basic tool in medical MRI. Differences in T_1 between tissues (studied at a fixed magnetic field) are routinely used for applications such as detection and characterization of brain lesions, studies of the gray/white matter junction in cortex, and detection of cancer (to name just a few).

We have already discussed the observation that contrast in MRI varies with field (frequency) and prospects for enhanced contrast at low fields. The table in Section 4.4.2 shows some values of T_1 for brain tissue at various magnetic fields. Table 4.2 shows that, as is well known in MRI, T_1 and sometimes T_2 change as a function of field. T_1 for brain and other tissues changes rapidly as a function of magnetic field over the ULF regime from μT to 100mT. For example, T_1 for gray matter changes from ~100ms at 46μT to ~1s at 1.5T. In fact, as the magnetic fields decrease, T_1 approaches T_2 [15]. Consequently, it may be an advantage to "turn the knob"(if one is able to) on the imaging field to optimize the contrast.

The underlying reason why T_1 changes with magnetic field is that the number of resonant protons available to transfer energy to the lattice changes with magnetic field. Specifically, only magnetic field fluctuations at the Larmor frequency can cause T_1 relaxation, and the frequency of these field fluctuations depends strongly on the molecular dynamics. The water molecules, which contain the protons that are the major source of the MRI signal, are typically free to move, are lightly bound to macromolecules (as is the case for most water in soft tissue), or are strongly bound, like hydrated solids [82]. Another way this is described for NMR is in terms of "correlation time" τ_c, or how much time a proton spends interacting with the macromolecules around it.

Figure 4.34 shows qualitatively the spectral density of protons as a function of Larmor frequency [83]. We can see that for structured water protons such as those in tissue (medium range of τ_c), as the magnetic field strength increases there are fewer protons available to transfer energy efficiently to the lattice. This is why the T_1 time in tissue is lengthened as the field increases (or shortens as the magnetic field is decreased). Figure 4.35 further presents the time scales of the NMR fluctuations from various molecular processes and compares them to proton Larmor frequency [84]. As one can see, HF MRI (in the 60–120MHz range) would largely derive any contrast from intramolecular motion only, whereas at ULF, relaxation will be a function of (and thus able to probe) numerous other processes.

The variation in relaxation times as a function of frequency and material can provide opportunities to enhance contrast. There are numerous examples of situations where T_1 differences between materials can be more pronounced at low fields than at high. There are already data to indicate that T_1 differences exist between tissue types and between

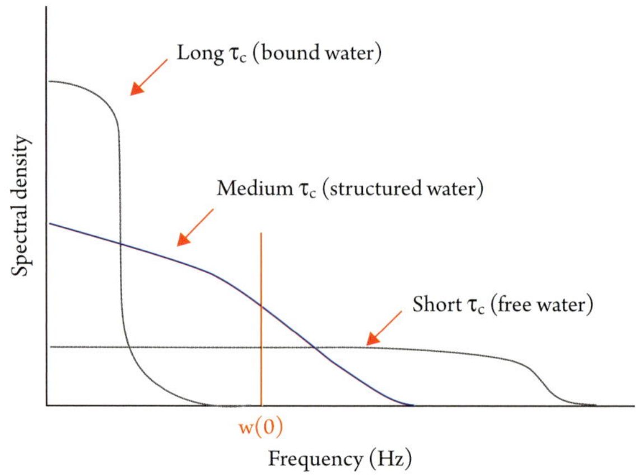

FIGURE 4.34 Qualitative example of the spectral density versus frequency for water. Adapted from reference [83].

normal and cancerous tissue, and that contrast may be enhanced at fields ≤100mT [69]. It has been proposed that these contrast differences, or the ability to vary contrast, which is easy to achieve at ULF because fields can vary so easily, may render the method superior to HF MRI for some applications even if the SNR is reduced, because the CNR is better [52].

We will briefly discuss here two recent examples put forth by John Clarke's team. In the first, using an agarose gel phantom designed to mimic tissue properties, it was shown that T_1 contrast between two phantom tissue types was flat from 100Hz to 10kHz and then had a dramatic T_1 dispersion until there appeared essentially no contrast past 10MHz [52]. These results are summarized in Figure 4.36 from that work. In this example, it would appear that ULF is essential to obtain any image contrast at all for these tissue phantoms.

In more recent work [70], Clarke's group showed that for excised prostate tissue samples, there was a significant intrinsic T_1 contrast between healthy and cancerous tissue at 132μT. They found that T_1 progressively decreases as the percentage of cancer increases, and that ULF MRI may be a viable noninvasive method for the detection of cancer even with reduced SNR compared to HF MRI. These encouraging results will need to be validated with *in vivo* studies but provide compelling arguments for continued efforts in ULF MRI.

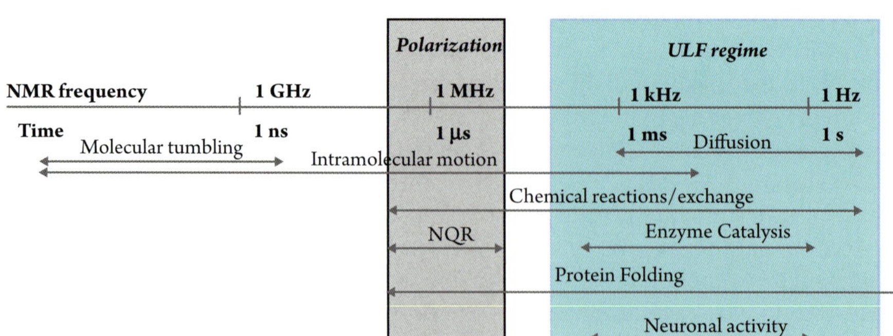

FIGURE 4.35 Timescales of the NMR fluctuations versus proton Larmor frequency. From reference [84].

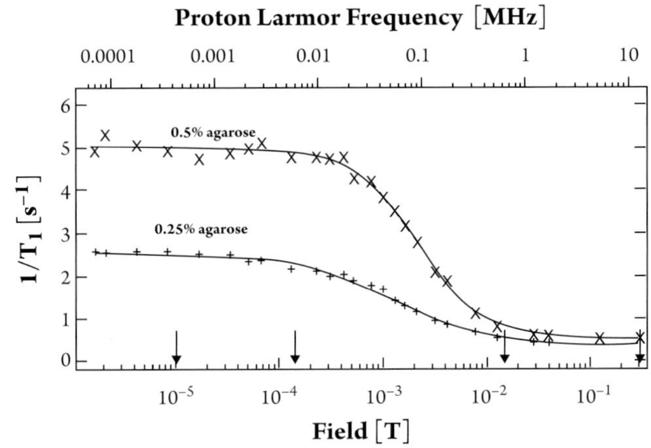

FIGURE 4.36 T_1 dispersion in agarose gel. Data are from reference [52].

The issue of SNR versus CNR is a topic we will return to in Section 4.5.5, but first let us consider using the variation in T_1 as a function of magnetic field, or what is known as T_1 dispersion as a form of contrast.

4.5.4 DispersionContrast: Measuring T_1 at ArbitraryField

In conventional MRI the change in T_1 as a function of magnetic field cannot be easily exploited, because the main field of the magnet is fixed. Thus the tissue contrast (the T_1 difference between various tissue types) is "fixed" at the field of the magnet, typically 1.5 or 3T. We have already introduced the idea that there is no ideal field at which T_1 contrast is maximized for all tissue types. This is further illustrated Figure 4.37, which shows T_1 as a function of magnetic field for a variety of tissue types. For these reasons there are several groups that are pursuing what is known as "field-cycling" MRI, in which some method of changing the main field of the scanner is implemented to exploit these changes in tissue contrast (see, for example, references [9,85] and the references therein). Similar to ULFMRI, most of these methods involve pre-polarization, but the readout fields are still in the tens of mT and detection is by conventional inductive coils.

The motivation in both ULF and field-cycling MRI is that it appears T_1 contrast is often higher at lower fields than commonly used in clinical imagers. The contrast between normal and tumor tissue in the breast actually changes sign between 0.1MHz and 10MHz.This variability argues for another possible parameter for imaging contrast: "dispersion contrast," in which the image is constructed on the basis of how contrast changes as a function of field, not simply a single contrast value at a fixed field.

For example, T_1 changes dramatically as a function of magnetic field for tissues with high protein concentrations, due to couplings between the protons and quadrupolar ^{14}N in protein molecule backbones [56,68]. This field-dependent T_1 contrast (also called "nitrogen dips") has been used to enable imaging of tissues with varying protein concentrations [56] and may be useful for the study of changes in protein, such as demyelination in multiple sclerosis. Myelin has substantial protein content, and nitrogen dips have been observed in white matter [86], so a reduction of myelin associated with lesions should correspond to a reduction in protein content detectable with T_1

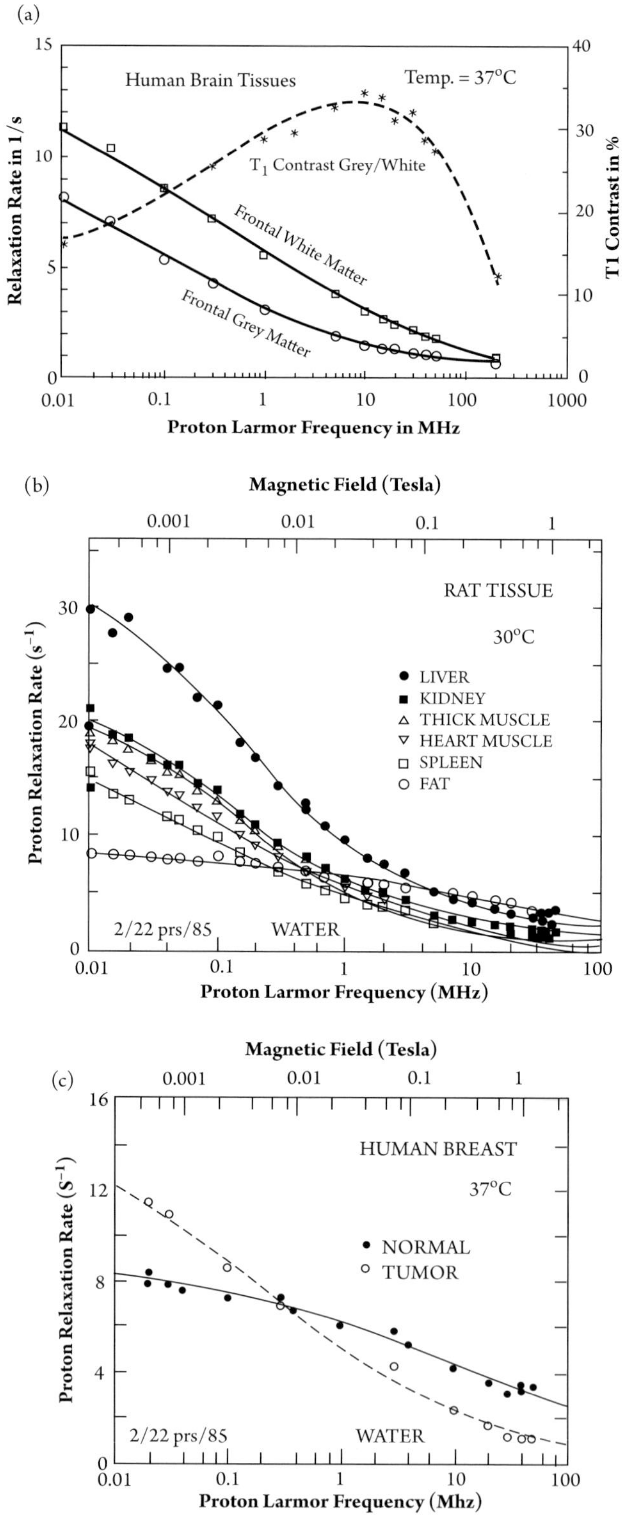

FIGURE 4.37 (a) T_1 dispersion in human brain gray vs. white matter. From reference [14]. (b) T_1 dispersion for various tissues of a rat. From reference [68]. (c) T_1 dispersion at 37°C for human breast tissue normal vs. invasive duct adenocarcinoma. From reference [68].

dispersion imaging. An example of nitrogen dips in frog muscle, acquired by our team using a field-cycling NMR relaxometer, is shown in Figure 4.38. Ungersma et al. [56] used this approach in field-cycling MRI to produce "protein-weighted" images of the human wrist by producing an image where T_1 in muscle was reduced due to the cross-coupling (at the minimum of a nitrogen dip) and another image far from the dip (and with longer T_1). Since most nonmuscular tissues (e.g., fat) do not exhibit such dispersion, an image weighted to the presence of tissue with high protein content is produced by subtraction of these two images.

As an aside, these nitrogen dips caused by coupling between ^{1}H and ^{14}N are also referred to as "cross relaxation" or "double resonance" and occur at the nuclear quadrupole resonance (NQR) frequency of the nitrogen nuclei. NQR is a method that has been studied extensively in the context of detection of explosives and drugs (see, for example, reference [87]), many of which have strong NQR signatures. T_1 dispersion of the proton NMR signal has been used to read out the NQR signature in materials such as the explosive TNT, where often the proton NMR signal is higher than the NQR signal itself (see, for example, reference [88]).

Dispersion contrast (e.g., producing images based on how T_1 varies at differing field strengths) is generally not possible in conventional HF MRI, where magnetic field strength is fixed. By using methods commonly employed in ULF MRI (pulsed fields and variable-strength electromagnets), T_1 can be sampled over a wide range of frequencies, and this T_1 contrast dispersion can be used as an imaging parameter. In the field-cycling MRI at somewhat higher fields (discussed earlier in this section), typically the bore of the magnet is taken up by an additional magnet used to vary the main field; thus the sample region is restricted and the frequency range achievable is limited. The ULF approach should be able to reach a wider range of frequencies, including very low frequencies (<1kHz). When the T_1 dispersion behavior of water was recently revisited using SQUID-based ULF MRI [53] capable of attaining Hz-level Larmor frequencies, a previously unreported and dramatic dispersion due to a very slow exchange process at ~100Hz was discovered. We believe that many other similarly interesting effects remain to be discovered at ULF.

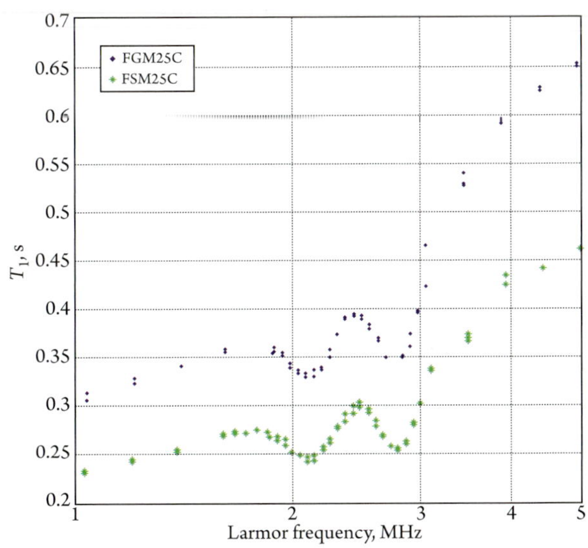

FIGURE 4.38 Nitrogen dips from NMR T_1 measurements from the sartorius and gastocnemius muscle of a frog.

The pre-polarization approach of ULF MRI also enables measurement of T_1 at the pre-polarization field and readout at essentially any field between B_p and B_m. In one implementation, used to inspect liquids by relaxometry [84], we showed that by measuring T_1 in the pre-polarization field (≅2MHz) using different polarization times, while measuring T_2 at the much lower measurement field (≅2kHz), we could discriminate between many different liquid types. For the material identification studies our team has pursued, the relaxation dispersion provides unique information that can be used to tell liquids apart.

4.5.5 CNR: A Cautionary Tale

Although we have discussed the fact that the ULF regime may offer enhanced or even unique contrast compared to HF MRI, we cannot leave the reader with the impression that greater T_1 contrast always leads to a more informative image. It is crucial to examine this question: When does the improved contrast (that *may* be) observed at ULF provide sufficient differentiation to compensate for the reduced signal? When using ULF MRI to exploit contrast it is important to consider not just curves like this in Figure 4.37 that show contrast as a function of field, but also the CNR. Very often contrast may be enhanced at ULF, but when the lower SNR is factored in, the HF image still contains more diagnostic information.

An accurate comparison of both SNR and CNR between ULF and HF instruments would require a detailed analysis of the acquisition system and details of the protocol being used. Comparing the efficacy of two totally different systems to resolve tissue depends on many factors such as noise, voxel size, pulse sequence being used, etc. However, for the sake of illustration, let us consider the case where all other factors are equivalent between the systems except T_1 and SNR. We will then use CNR as the figure of merit for our comparison.

Recalling the discussion in Chapter 1, for two different tissues types A and B,

(Eqn. 4.129)
$$\mathrm{CNR} \propto \frac{S_\mathrm{A} - S_\mathrm{B}}{\sigma}\left(t_{Seq}\right)^{1/2}$$

where the signal is $S_\mathrm{A} = S{\cdot}\exp(-R_\mathrm{A}t)$, and $R_\mathrm{A} \equiv 1/T_{1\mathrm{A}}$. For any two such tissues there will be some optimal evolution time when the difference in signal, S_A–S_B, between them is maximized. Here we are assuming that we polarize to full recruitment of spins before we start to acquire the signal and we neglect differences in proton density between tissue.

(Eqn. 4.130)
$$\mathrm{CNR} \propto \frac{S}{\sigma}\left[\exp\left(-R_\mathrm{A}t\right) - \exp\left(-R_\mathrm{B}t\right)\right].$$

This optimal time for contrast is then

(Eqn. 4.131)
$$t_c = \frac{\ln R_\mathrm{A} - \ln R_\mathrm{B}}{R_\mathrm{A} - R_\mathrm{B}}.$$

Let us consider some simple examples to help illustrate what Eqn. 4.130 means. First, consider gray matter and white matter in the human brain. From the gray/white matter data shown in the left panel of Figure 4.37 [14], we can see that the contrast difference actually appears to peak around 10MHz (~0.25T). One might infer from this result that it would be better (from the point of view of maximizing contrast between these two tissues) to produce an image at 0.25T than 3T (~128MHz). However, it is not so simple when we examine the whole picture.

At 10MHz (from Fischer et al. [14]) we see that $R(\text{gray}) = 1.5$ and $R(\text{white}) = 3$, whereas at 128MHz (taking the values from Wright et al. [89]), $R(\text{gray}) = 0.62$ and $R(\text{white}) = 1.19$. Let us initially assume that the SNR is the same for both cases (call it 1) for the same voxel. In this case, as illustrated in Figure 4.39, the difference in maximum contrast is indeed clearly better for the 10MHz case at earlier acquisition times. However, the contrast evolves, and it would seem that all one has to do is wait a bit longer and the contrast at 128MHz will be nearly as good. But a complicating factor is that as we wait for the contrast to reach its maximum, the signal is dying away. Recall we have neglected T_2 relaxation for this discussion. For both these tissue types, T_2 doesn't change strongly with field. But if T_2 effects dominate, waiting longer may not be an option. This is true for both low and high fields.

Now let us revisit the assumption that the SNR at 0.25T is the same as that at 3T. As we know, the SNR at ULF is unlikely to be as high as that at HF, so our initial assumption of equal SNR is most likely unrealistic. For the purpose of the illustration, let us now naively assume that the SNR will be ~10 times better at 3T (because B_0 is ~10 times higher) at the time of maximum contrast (again neglecting T_2 effects).

In this case you are much better off using a 3T because the CNR will be higher. While our simple exercise again points to the popularity of 3T machines over 0.25T devices, we also raise the importance of completely analyzing the application before concluding which approach provides the greatest CNR. In summary, the main lesson from this exercise is that simply looking at T_1 values alone might be quite misleading.

However, let us now return to the example from John Clarke's work with the agarose phantom [52] discussed in Section 4.5.3 and shown in Figure 4.36. Based on these data, one sees that at ULF (1,000Hz) $R_A = 2.5$ and $R_B = 5$ (for 0.25% and 5% agarose gels respectively), and by ~12MHz the differences between R_A and R_B are nonexistent. In such cases the CNR is always better at ULF, but only if the SNR is high enough to produce a useful image.

Another way to think about this is to consider the ability to resolve the tissue contrast information in the image. Let us consider the probability distribution for measuring each

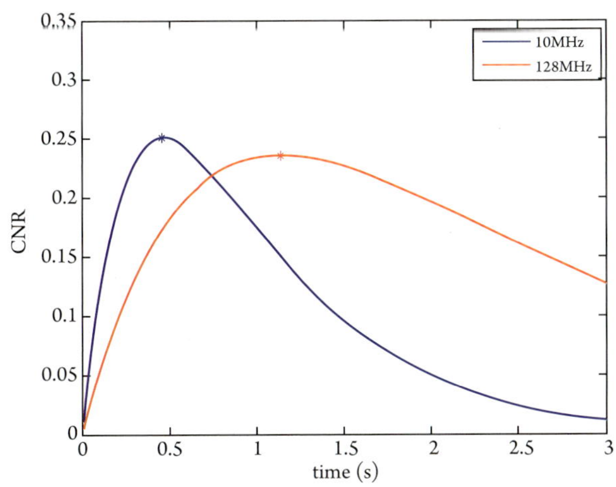

FIGURE 4.39 Plot of gray vs. white matter contrast between 10MHz and 128MHz assuming the same SNR in either case, and neglecting T_2.

of two tissue types, as shown in Figure 4.40. The separation between the peaks is related to the maximum difference in signal, which occurs at time t_c when the greatest contrast has evolved:

(Eqn. 4.132)

$$\Delta \propto \left[\exp(-R_A t_c) - \exp(-R_B t_c)\right].$$

The width of these peaks is related to the SNR by

(Eqn. 4.133)

$$\sigma = \frac{1}{SNR}.$$

Returning to the example of white and gray matter, at 3T this would be $\Delta = 0.235$. One can envision two peaks separated by this value. We estimate that the SNR for such a 3T image would be ~30 (based on the 3T brain images we have acquired); consequently, the width of the peaks $\sigma = 0.03$. One can easily conclude these tissues would be easy to resolve. On the other hand, at 0.25T $\Delta = 0.25$ (a bit better), but if we expect an SNR 10 times lower due to polarization, then the width is $\sigma = 0.3$. These tissues will be hard to resolve.

Of course, one can also consider T_1 dispersion itself as a form of contrast, but such an analysis of CNR should always be taken into account to understand the relative benefits and whether or not the loss in signal is truly compensated.

4.5.6 Safety Considerations in Various Settings

The MRI safety concerns, and their scaling with magnetic field, associated with induced currents and ohmic heating have been discussed in Chapter 1. In addition to the ohmic heating, there is a serious safety consideration associated with the force applied by large magnetic fields on ferromagnetic materials that can attract metal in the vicinity of the field, potentially with great acceleration. Even an object as small as a hairpin can be accelerated to speeds as high as 40mph (18m/s) by the time they enter the bore of the magnet, creating a serious hazard. Although the actual instances of MRI accidents appear underreported [90,91], every year there are numerous examples of objects attracted into the bore of an MRI magnetic field. In Pennsylvania alone, between 2004 and 2008 it was

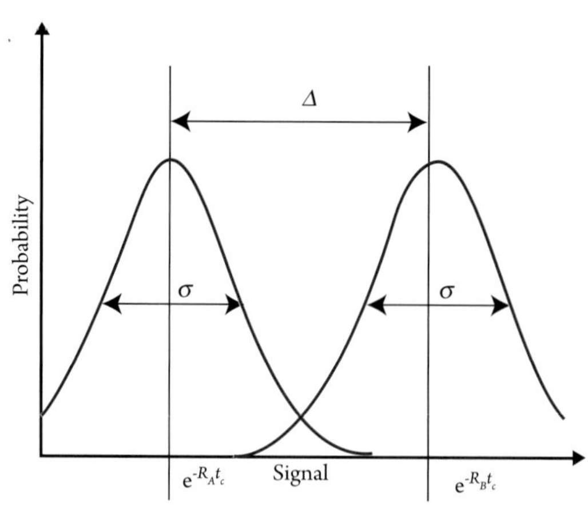

FIGURE 4.40 Signal vs. probability to illustrate the signal separation issue with CNR.

reported that some 27 items became projectiles in the vicinity of a HF MRI machine (with another 16 ferromagnetic items brought into the MRI scanner room without becoming projectiles, and 5 ferromagnetic items that were almost brought into the MRI scanner room) [92]. A modest extrapolation of these numbers indicates that there must be hundreds of such incidents per year nationwide. Several instances have become high profile in the media, including the attraction and discharge of a police officer's gun [93] and the tragic death of a child hit by an improperly introduced oxygen tank in the MRI room [94]. Modern magnet design has enabled systems in which the fields from the magnet can fall off rapidly with distance, but at best the nominal field strength still falls off as $1/r^3$, and as an attracted object begins to be pulled toward the MRI it very quickly becomes uncontrollably accelerated.

This reality has multiple consequences, including the following: (1) HF MRI must entail rigorous prescreening of subjects for MRI; (2) it limits those eligible for MRI scans, and (3) the use of any magnetic materials in proximity to the magnet is severely restricted (including surgical instruments, medical monitoring equipment, and life support). For example, anyone with metal from medical implants (nerve stimulators, pacemaker, aneurysm clips, implanted electrodes associated with epilepsy surgery) or extensive dental work will not be imaged at many MRI centers for safety reasons [95]. In such cases information must be gained from the less informative CT imaging. Moreover, anyone with an unknown history (accident victims) may not be able to undergo an MRI as it isn't know whether metal will be present, or a set of screening x-rays may be required.

While the pulsed pre-polarization fields of ULF MRI present considerations associated with dB/dt (as we discussed in Section 4.2.1), these values are typically much lower than to produce unwanted effects. Further, the low field strengths of ULF MRI greatly reduce the hazards associated with the movement or heating of metal.

4.6 CONCLUSIONS

In this chapter we have discussed the pros and cons of ULF MRI. The primary message we wish to convey is that there is a good reason that HF MRI is the dominant medical imaging technology. There are some situations (e.g., imaging in the presence of metal, or the compatibility with MEG) where ULF MRI may be the only option. ULF MRI also offers an opportunity to exploit differences in contrast that appear unique. There will certainly be some cases (e.g., anatomical imaging of nonpathological brain tissues) where the CNR may not compensate for the loss of SNR at ULF, at least not with our current understanding and instrumentation. There will likely be other cases and tissue types (for example, those shown by John Clarke's group [52]) for which CNR uniquely exists. There is also the potential at ULF to exploit not just contrast at a fixed field but also the variation in contrast as a function of field (dispersion), and this dispersion might also provide unique diagnostic information. However, one must always give careful consideration to CNR when considering the potential diagnostic quality of the images.

We must also remember that there are applications and environments in which it is simply not possible to use HF MRI due to any one of a number of reasons, including size and weight, large and potentially dangerous magnetic fields, and cost. In these cases, ULF MRI may provide a valuable alternative, even if the inherent image quality does not compete with HF MRI. In Chapter 5 several applications based on the advantages of ULF MRI will be presented, and this will enable us to delve further into the pros and cons of ULF MRI.

REFERENCES

1. Lauterbur PC (1973). Image formation by induced local interactions: examples of employing nuclear magnetic resonance. *Nature 242*: 190–191.
2. Detre JA, Alsop DC (1999). Perfusion fMRI with arterial spin labeling (ASL). In: Moonen CTW, Bandettini PA (Eds.), *Functional MRI*. Heidelberg: Springer-Verlag, pp.47–62.
3. Ogawa S, Lee TM, Nayak AS, Glynn P (1990). Oxygenation-sensitive contrast in magnetic resonance image of rodent brain at high magnetic fields. *Magn Reson Med 14*: 68–78.
4. Zotev VS, Matlachov AN, Volegov PL, et al. (2007). Multi-channel SQUID system for MEG and ultra-low-field MRI. *IEEE Trans Appl Supercond 17*(2): 839.
5. Clarke J, Hatridge M, Mossle M (2007). SQUID detected magnetic resonance in microtesla fields. *Annu Rev Biomed Engin 9*: 389–413.
6. Seton HC, Hutchinson JMS, Bussel DM (1997). A 4.2 K receiver coil and SQUID amplifier used to improve the SNR of low-field magnetic resonance images of the human arm. *Meas Sci Tech 8*: 198–207.
7. Zotev VS, Matlashov AN, Volegov PL, et al.(2008). Microtesla MRI of the human brain combined with MEG. *J Magn Reson 194*: 115–120.
8. Vesanen PT, Nieminen JO, Zevenhoven KCJ, et al. (submitted). *Hybrid ultra-low-field MRI and MEG system based on a commercial wholehead neuromagnetometer.*
9. Lurie et al. (2010). Fast field cycling magnetic resonance imaging. *Comptes Rendus Physique 11*: 136–148.
10. Ljunggren S (1983). A simple graphical representation of fourier-based imaging methods. *J Magn Reson 54*: 338.
11. Twieg D (1983). The k-trajectory formulation of the NMR imaging process with applications in analysis and synthesis of imaging methods. *Medical Physics 10*(5): 610–621. doi:10.1118/1.595331. PMID 6646065.
12. Callaghan PT (1991). *Principles of Nuclear Magnetic Resonance Microscopy*. Oxford Science Publications.
13. http://www.ebyte.it/library/educards/mri/K-SpaceMRI.html
14. Fischer HW, Rinck PA, Van Haverbeke Y, Muller RN (1990). Nuclear relaxation of human brain gray and white matter: Analysis of field dependence and implications for MRI. *Magn Reson Med 16*: 317–334.
15. Zotev VS, Matlashov AN, Savukov IM, et al. (2009). SQUID-based microtesla MRI for in vivo relaxometry of the human brain. *IEEE Trans Appl Supercond 19*(3, pt 1): 823–826.
16. McDermott R, et al. (2002). Liquid-state NMR and scalar couplings in microtesla. *Magnetic Fields Science 295*: 2247.
17. Guidance for Industry: Guidance for the Submission of Premarket Notifications for Magnetic Resonance Diagnostic Devices, Document issued on November 14, 1998, http://www.fda.gov/downloads/MedicalDevices/DeviceRegulationandGuidance/GuidanceDocuments/ucm073818.pdf
18. *Criteria for Significant Risk Investigations of Magnetic Resonance Diagnostic Devices*, July 14, 2003.
19. Mößle M, Han S-I, Myers WR, et al. (2006). SQUID-detected microtesla MRI in the presence of metal. *J Magn Reson 179*: 146–151.
20. Matlachov AN, Volegov PL, Espy MA, et al. (2004). SQUID detected NMR in microtesla magnetic fields. *J Magn Reson 170*: 1–7.
21. Myers WR (2006). *Potential Applications of Microtesla Magnetic Resonance Imaging Detected Using a Superconducting Quantum Interference Device.* Ph.D. thesis http://escholarship.org/uc/item/19x7q88x#page-9
22. Magnelind PE, Gomez JJ, Matlashov AN, et al.(2011). Co-registration of interleaved MEG and ULF MRI using a 7-channel low-Tc SQUID system. *IEEE Trans Appl Supercond 21*(3, pt. 1): 456–460.
23. Senft A, Franz K, Ulrich CT, et al. (2010). Low field intraoperative MRI-guided surgery of gliomas: A single-center experience. *Clin Neurol Neurosurg 112*(3): 237–243.
24. NEMA reference volume coils. *NEMA Standards Publication MS 1-2008: Determination of Signal-to-Noise Ratio (SNR) in Diagnostic Magnetic Resonance Imaging.*
25. NEMA Standards Publication MS 6-2008. Determination of Signal-to-Noise Ratio and Image Uniformity for Single-Channel Non-Volume Coils in Diagnostic MR Imaging. http://www.nema.org/download.cfm?isRedirect=false&docTypeId=0&docId=20611&filename=/ms6_final_website.pdf

26. Myers W, Slichter D, Hatridge M, et al. (2007). Calculated signal-to-noise ratio of MRI detected with SQUIDs and Faraday detectors in fields from 10 lT to 1.5 T. *J Magn Reson 186*: 182–192.
27. Weisskoff RM, Cohen MS, Rzedzian RR (1993). Nonaxial whole-body instant imaging. *Magn Reson Med 29*: 796–803.
28. Volegov PL, Mosher JC, Espy MA, Kraus RH Jr (2005). On concomitant gradients in low-field MRI. *J Magn Reson 175*: 103.
29. Myers WR, Moßle M, Clarke J (2005). Correction of concomitant gradient artifacts in experimental microtesla MRI. *J Magn Reson 177*: 274–284.
30. Nieminen JO, Ilmonieni RJ (2010). Solving the problem of concomitant gradients in ultra-low-field MRI. *J Magn Reson 207*: 213–219.
31. Abragam A (1961). *Principles of Nuclear Magnetism.* Oxford University Press, Oxford, England.
32. Espy M, Flynn M, Gomez J, et al. (2010). *Superconductor Science and Technology 23*(3): pp.034023 (8pp)
33. Hamalainen M, Hari R, Ilmoniemi RJ, et al. (1993). Magnetoencephalography—theory, instrumentation, and applications to noninvasive studies of the working human brain. *Rev Mod Phys 65*(2): 413–497.
34. Nieminen JO, Vesanen PT, Zevenhoven KCJ, et al. (2011). Multichannel SQUID system for combined MEG and ultra-low-field MRI. Presented at the Superconductivity Centennial Conference, The Hague, Netherlands.
35. Matlashov AN, Burmistrov E, Magnelind PE, et al. (2012). SQUID-based systems for co-registration of ultra-low field nuclear magnetic resonance images and magneto encephalography. *Physica C 482*: 19–26.
36. Volegov P, Matlachov A, Mosher J, et al. (2003). Noise-free magneto encephalography recordings of brain function. *Phys Med Biol 49*: 2117–2128.
37. Adjamian P, et al. (2004). Co-registration of MEG with MRI using bite-bar fiducials and surface matching. *Clin Neurophys 115*: 691.
38. Poghosyan V, Ionnides AA (2007). Precise mapping of early visual responses in space and time. *Neuroimage* 35(2): 759–770.
39. Lin F-H, et al. (2006). Dynamic magnetic resonance inverse imaging of human brain function. *Magn Reson Med 56*(4): 787–802.
40. Lin F-H, et al. (2010). K-space reconstruction of magnetic resonance inverse imaging (k-InI) of human visuomotor systems. *Neuroimage 49*: 3086–3098.
41. Zotev VS, Volegov PL, Matlashov AN, et al. (2008). Parallel MRI at microtesla fields. *J Magn Reson 192*(2): 197–208.
42. Pruessmann KP, Weiger M, Scheidegger MB, Boesiger P (1999). SENSE: Sensitivity encoding for fast MRI. *Magn Reson Med 42*(5): 952–962.
43. Sodickson DK, Manning WJ. (1997). Simultaneous acquisition of spatial harmonics (SMASH): fast imaging with radiofrequency coil arrays. *Magn Reson Med 38*(4): 591–603.
44. Griswold MA, Jakob PM, Nittka M, Goldfarb JW, Haase A (2000). Partially parallel imaging with localized sensitivities (PILS). *Magn Reson Med 44*: 602–609.
45. Hellstrandh S, Stenvall D (2003). Implementation and evaluation of sense in 3d mri. Master's thesis, Linkopings universitet, Linkoping, Sweden.
46. Blaimer M, Breuer F, Mueller M, Heidemann RM, Griswold MA, Jakob PM. SMASH, SENSE, PILS, GRAPPA: how to choose the optimal method. *Top Magn Reson Imaging 15*(4): 223–236.
47. Roemer PB, Edelstein WA, Hayes CE, Souza SP, Mueller OM (1990). The NMR phased array. *Magn Reson Med 16*: 192–225. doi:10.1002/mrm.1910160203
48. Hayes CE, Roemer PB (1990). Noise correlations in data simultaneously acquired from multiple surface coil arrays. *Magn Reson Med 16*: 181–191. doi:10.1002/mrm.1910160202
49. Pruessmann KP, Weiger M, Boesiger P (2001). Sensitivity encoded cardiac MRI. *J Cardiovasc Magn Reson* 3(1): 1–9.
50. http://www.supracon.com
51. Wang J, Reykowski A, Dickas J (1995).Calculation of the signal-to-noise ratio for simple surface coils and arrays of coils. *IEEE Trans Biomed Eng 42*(9): 908–910.

52. Lee S, Mossle M, Myers W, et al. (2005). SQUID-detected MRI at 132 μT with T1- weighted contrast established at 10 μT-300 mT. *Magn Reson Med* 53: 9–14.
53. Hartwig S, Voigt J, Scheer H-J, et al. (2011). Nuclear magnetic relaxation in water revisited. *J Chem Phys* 135: 054201. doi:10.1063/1.3623024
54. Alford JK, Rutt BK, Scholl TJ, et al. (2009). Delta relaxation enhanced MR: Improving activation-specificity of molecular probes through R1 dispersion imaging. *Magn Reson Med* 61: 796–802.
55. Magnelind PE, Savukov IM, Araya YT, et al. (2009). Super paramagnetic nanoparticle contrast agents in ultra-low field MRI. Presented at the 50th ENC, March 29–April 3, Pacific Grove, California.
56. Ungersma S, Matter N, Hardy J, et al. (2006). Magnetic resonance imaging with T1 dispersion contrast. *Magn Res Med* 55: 1362–1371.
57. Kraus R, Volegov P, Matlachov A, Espy M. (2008). Toward direct neural current imaging by resonant mechanisms at ultra-low field. *Neuroimage* 39: 310–317.
58. Mößle M, Han S-I, Myers WR, et al. (2006). SQUID-detected microtesla MRI in the presence of metal. *J Magn Reson* 179: 146–151.
59. Matlachov AN, Volegov PL, Espy MA, et al. (2004). SQUID detected NMR in microtesla magnetic fields. *J Magn Reson* 170: 1–7.
60. http://catalog.gwrinstruments.com/viewitems/all-categories/helium-liquefiers-systems?
61. Eom B, Penanen K, Day PK, et al. (2009). Development of cryogen-free ultra-low field MRI instrument. *US Proc Intl Soc Mag Reson Med* 17:
62. Savukov IM, Zotev VS, Volegov PL, et al. (2009). MRI with an atomic magnetometer suitable for practical imaging applications. *J Magn Reson* 199(2): 188–191.
63. Zotev VS, Matlashov AN, Volegov PL, et al. (2007). SQUID-based instrumentation for ultra-low-field MRI. *Supercond Sci Technol* 20(11): S367–S373.
64. Kelha VO, Pikki JM, Peltonen RS, et al. (1982). Design, construction, and performance of a large-volume magnetic-shield. *IEEE Trans Magn* 18: 260–270.
65. Woo EJ (2007). Recent development of magnetic resonance electrical impedance tomography toward high-resolution conductivity imaging. Proceedings of the 2007 Joint Meeting of the 6th Int. Symp. on Noninvasive Functional Source Imaging of the Brain and Heart and the Int. Conf. on Functional Biomedical Imaging, NFSI and ICFBI 2007, 201–204.
66. Zhang X, Yan D, Zhu S, He B (2008). Noninvasive imaging of head-brain conductivity profiles. *IEEE Eng Med Biol* 27(5): 78–83.
67. Magnelind P, George J, Gomez J, et al. (2011). Towards functional magnetic resonance imaging at ultra-low fields. Presented at the Superconductivity Centennial Conference, The Hague, Netherlands, 18–23.
68. Koenig SH, Brown RD (1984). Determinants of proton relaxation rates in tissue. *Magn Reson Med* 1: 437–447.
69. Koenig SH, Brown RD III (1987). *Relaxation in Tissue, NMR Spectroscopy of Cells and Organisms*, Vol. II, ed. Gupta EK. Boca Raton: CRC Press, pp. 75–114.
70. Busch S, Hatridge M, Mößle M et al. (2012). Measurements of T_1-relaxation in ex vivo prostate tissue at 132 μT. *Magn Reson Med* 67(4):1138–1145. doi:10.1002/mrm.24177. Epub 2012 Jan 31.
71. Venkatesh AK et al. (2003). MRI of the lung gas-space at very low-field using hyperpolarized noble gases. *Magn Reson Imag* 21(7): 773–776.
72. Spees et al. (2001). Water proton MR properties of human blood at 1.5 Tesla: Magnetic susceptibility, T1, T2, T2*, and non-Lorentzian signal behavior. *Magn Reson Med* 45: 533–542.
73. Carlsson A (2009). Susceptibility effects in MRI and 1H MRS The spurious echo artifact and susceptibility measurements, Ph.D. thesis, Department of Radiation Physics, University of Gothenburg, Gothenburg, Sweden.
74. http://hyperphysics.phy-astr.gsu.edu/hbase/tables/magprop.html
75. Schenk (1996). The role of magnetic susceptibility in magnetic resonance imaging: MRI compatibility of the first and second kind. *Med Phys* 23(6): 816–850.

76. Eschera K, Shellockb FG (2013). Technical Note: Evaluation of MRI artifacts at 3 Tesla for 38 commonly used cosmetics. *Magn Reson Imag*, available online 3 January 2013.
77. Kaur P, Kumaran SS, Tripathi RP, et al. (2007). Protocol error artifacts in MRI: Sources and remedies revisited. *Radiography 13*: 291–306.
78. McKinstry III RC, Jarrett DY (2004). Magnetic susceptibility artifacts on MRI: A hairy situation. *AJR Am J Roentgenol* 182: 532.
79. Butala NB, Shehada RE, Costandi PN, et al. (2011). Maximum dB/dt and switching noise in 1.5T MRI scanners for safety evaluation of active implantable medical device. *Proc Intl Soc Mag Reson Med 19*:
80. http://answers.yahoo.com/question/index?qid=20081020152525AArUCDt
81. Espy M, Flynn M, Gomez J, et al. (2009). Applications of ultra-low field magnetic resonance for imaging and materials studies. *IEEE Transactions on Applied Superconductivity 19*(3; pt.1): 835–838.
82. http://www.revisemri.com/questions/misc/shorter_t1_tissues
83. http://www.revisemri.com/questions/misc/longer_t1_high_field
84. Espy M, Matlashov A, Volegov P (2013). SQUID-detected ultra-low field MRI. *J Magn Reson* 127–141. doi:10.1016/j.jmr.2013.02.009
85. Matter NI, Scott GC, Grafendorfer T, et al. (2006). Rapid polarizing field cycling in magnetic resonance imaging. *IEEE Trans Med Imag 25*(1): 84–93.
86. Koenig SH, Brown RD 3rd, Spiller M, Lundbom N (1990). Relaxometry of brain: why white matter appears bright in MRI. *Magn Reson Med 14*: 482–495.
87. Miller JB, Barrall GA. Explosives detection with nuclear quadrupole resonance: An emerging technology will help to uncover land mines and terrorist bombs. http://www.americanscientist.org/libraries/documents/2005317163027_306.pdf
88. Blinc R, Seliger J, Arcon D, et al. (2000). H-14N double resonance of TNT from a land mine. *Physica Status Solidi A180*(2): 541–545.
89. Wright PJ, Mougin OE, Totman JJ, et al. (2008). Water proton T1 measurements in brain tissue at 7, 3, and 1.5T using IR-EPI, IR-TSE, and MPRAGE: results and optimization. *Magn Reson Mater Phy 21*:121–130.
90. Potpourri of MRI Safety Statistics: http://mrimetaldetector.com/blog/2008/11/potpourri-of-mri-safety-statistics/
91. Potpourri of MRI Safety Statistics: http://www.psqh.com/novdec07/imaging.html
92. Safety in the MR Environment: Ferromagnetic Projectile Objects in the MRI Scanner Room: http://patientsafetyauthority.org/ADVISORIES/AdvisoryLibrary/2009/Jun6%282%29/Pages/56.aspx
93. Beitia A, Meyers S, Kanal E, et al. (2002). Case report: spontaneous discharge of a firearm in an MR imaging environment. *AJR Am J Roentgenol 178*(5):1092–1094. Available online at http://www.ajronline.org/content/178/5/1092.full
94. Chen DW (2001). Boy, 6, dies of skull injury during MRI.NY Times [online]. 2001 Jul 31 [cited 2009 Mar23]. Available online at http://www.nytimes.com/2001/07/31/nyregion/boy-6-dies-of-skull-injuryduring-mri.html?n=Top/Reference/Times%20Topics/Subjects/C/Children's%20Health.
95. Tagliati M, Jankovic J, Pagan F, et al., National Parkinson Foundation DBS Working Group. (2009). Safety of MRI in patients with implanted deep brain stimulation devices. *Neuroimage* 47(Suppl 2): T53–T57.Cea sit, quiate que nem et, officatustet denime cuptas plaboru ptatquas nia eos volorro videbit

CHAPTER 5

APPLICATIONS IN ULF MRI

We have thus far discussed many important features of ULF MRI, and established (we hope) at least most of the background required for one to assess whether ULF MRI would be beneficial to a specific application. We focused largely on the technical issues that surround acquisition of magnetic resonance images and the differences between ULF and traditional HF MRI. We will now briefly explore a variety of applications of ULF MRI currently being pursued, and also speculate about other possible applications that may whet your appetite to pursue ULF MRI and help to advance this exciting new field. In this chapter we will outline preliminary efforts and considerations for (1) multimodal imaging of human brain anatomy and function; (2) new approaches to image human brain function enabled by ULF MRI; and (3) applying relaxometry to differentiate materials. We will end the chapter with a few observations to, we hope, pique your curiosity.

5.1 MULTIMODAL IMAGING OF HUMAN BRAIN ANATOMY AND FUNCTION: MEG AND ULF MRI

EEG and MEG are at present the only noninvasive imaging techniques that can passively and noninvasively measure the consequences of neural activity on the timescale at which neurons communicate (sub-millisecond to tens of milliseconds). Unlike other techniques, such as fMRI and positron emission tomography (PET), MEG and EEG are "direct" measurements of neural activity, or at least neural activity with signals that are measurable at some distance from cortex. EEG and MEG measure such neural activity in the brain through detection of the electrical potentials present at the surface of the head (EEG) [1] or the magnetic fields just above it (MEG) [2]. In contrast, the signals measured by fMRI and PET directly result from blood flow, oxygenation, and metabolism, which have been hypothesized to be associated with neural activity [3,4].

Although the inverse problem that converts the measured signals to localized sources of activity is ill-posed for both MEG and EEG, model-based source localization approaches that apply well-founded constraints (for example, number, strength, and direction of sources relative to cortex) have become sufficiently reliable as to accurately localize event-related potentials in cognitive studies and guide surgical decisions [5].

EEG source localization requires that the considerable influence of the shape and conductivity of the volume conductor, particularly the skull, be accurately modeled in the inverse solution. Magnetic fields are less distorted by the resistive properties and shape of the skull and scalp. While the debate is still active, MEG is often regarded as having less ambiguous spatial localization [2,6] and is a powerful and well-regarded method for noninvasive studies of neural activity in the human brain, and a powerful diagnostic tool for diseases such as epilepsy [7]. We also note that MEG and EEG are most sensitive to different orientations of neuronal current sources; however, Mosher et al. clearly demonstrated that the proverbial "radial" (or tangential) sources when one assumes an ideal spherical head are not realistic in practice due to the residual asymmetry of a realistic head model [8].

MEG localization of small discrete cortical sources requires co-registration with anatomical images, typically acquired by MRI, to localize function relative to anatomical features and landmarks. Anatomical geometry of the skull and of cortical soft tissue may be employed to improve the accuracy of forward modeling procedures and to constrain inverse procedures, which can also enhance the accuracy of source localization [2,9].

Virtually all clinical MEG instrumentation remains exclusively based on the SQUID because of the sensitivity required to measure the minute magnetic fields produced by neural activity, nT to fT. There have been promising demonstrations of MEG using the atomic magnetometer [10]; however, a clinical device has yet to be demonstrated at the time of this writing. Highly sensitive SQUID detectors are incompatible with conventional HF MRI, which is acquired at magnetic fields typically 1.5T and higher. As an aside, there has been excellent progress with combining EEG with HF MRI. However, the HF MRI-induced currents remain a significant confound to acquiring EEG in MRI scanners—for example, ballistocardiogram artifacts from the EEG lead moving in the field due to blood pulsating. There will be no such effects at ULF because the fields are lower. Also, MEG does not require leads and closed loops like EEG. Nevertheless, combined EEG and fMRI is being widely adopted despite the challenges. While we will not discuss in detail the merits of MEG versus EEG, we simply point out that the ability to combine MEG and MRI (or even fMRI) may add similarly valuable information as EEG combined with MRI. And, as we shall discuss in Section 5.2, many of the motivating factors for combined EEG and fMRI are relevant for combined MEG and fMRI as well. It is likely that the only approach to combining MEG and MRI in a single device will have to be through ULF MRI, and even the potential for easier integration of EEG with MRI via ULF approaches may bear fruit by providing enhanced coverage of neural activity.

In present clinical applications, the anatomical (HF) MRI and functional MEG data must be acquired in two separate systems. This introduces a "co-registration" process for the datasets that can introduce source localization errors ranging from 2 to 10mm [11,12], depending on the approach. Hence, there is a strong desire in the neuroscience community for improved approaches to co-register MEG/MRI data and enhance the potential of MEG.

In the decades since their discovery, it seemed that MEG and MRI were divergent technologies—requiring the lowest possible magnetic field environment for the former and the highest possible magnetic fields for the later. However, even as MRI reached to higher and higher magnetic fields, researchers never lost interest in the possibility of low-field MRI for inexpensive systems [13]. In early 2000, as we discussed in Chapter 1, Clarke et al. at UC Berkeley pioneered the combination of pre-polarization with SQUID detection at very low Larmor frequencies (~ few kHz) [14], recording the first-ever MR images of plants, and human forearm and fingers at fields as low as 132μT (5.6kHz) [15]. When it appeared that SQUID-based ULF MRI was possible, the ability to combine MEG and MRI in a single imaging session was a logical next step. Such efforts were first pursued experimentally by our group at Los Alamos National Laboratory (LANL). The motivation was that using the same SQUID arrays for simultaneous detection of both MEG and the anatomical MRI would improve the data co-registration and eliminate the requirement for two costly devices.

In 2004 our team obtained the first proof-of-principle results in recording simultaneous MEG and MRI signals [16,17]. Figure 5.1 shows the somatosensory evoked magnetic response from the human brain recorded simultaneously with the free induction decay (FID) signal at 268Hz (red curve), and in the absence of the NMR (blue curve). These experiments illustrate that simultaneous recording of such signals is very difficult to perform because of the large low-frequency noise arising from the applied magnetic field needed for the NMR precession. This noise was dominated by micro-vibrations of the SQUID gradiometer in the NMR field. In later experiments MEG and MRI signals were recorded sequentially and the external field and gradients were zeroed during the MEG recording. This approach greatly reduced the noise during the MEG without appreciably compromising the experimental goal of data co-registration to a single coordinate system.

We published the first-ever ULF MRI of the human brain in 2008 [18]. MRI was recorded by a flat array of seven axial second-order gradiometers at 46μT measurement field using liquid nitrogen-cooled pre-polarization coils that generated a 30mT field. The image resolution we reported was $3 \times 3 \times 6\text{mm}^3$ and a single scan took ~15 minutes. Six scans were averaged to improve the SNR of the images up to about 30. Auditory evoked magnetic field signals were recorded immediately after the ULF MRI session was finished. Data co-registration was not possible because the subject moved between recording of the ULF MRI and MEG, to achieve better coverage of the MEG signals. However, these results demonstrated that a SQUID-based system could be used for both ULF MRI of the human brain and MEG. The data are shown in Figure 5.2.

Co-registration of auditory evoked magnetic field mapping and ULF MR imaging was performed by our team in 2010 [19], using interleaved data recorded in a single session. This set of measurements enabled the MEG map to be accurately superposed with the MRI. The co-registration error of the different coordinate systems was assessed to be less than 1mm. However, due to transients that resulted from switching the fields for the MRI protocol, MEG measurements could not begin until the transients decayed sufficiently. This typically required several seconds per acquisition. The pulse sequence and data from this experiment are shown in Figure 5.3. Although we did not rigorously pursue the origin of

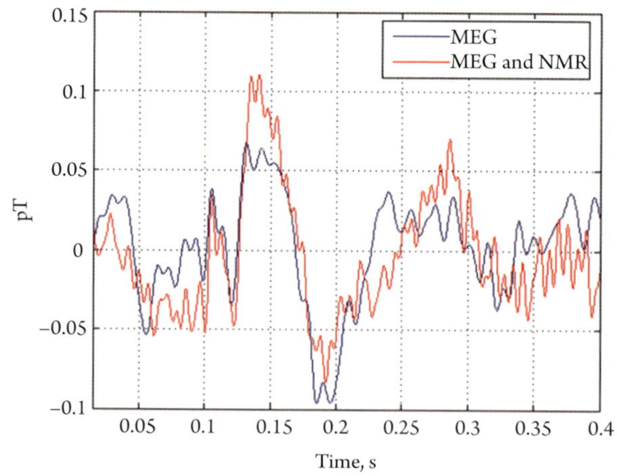

FIGURE 5.1 Comparison of the somatosensory response for MEG only (blue) and MEG and simultaneous NMR (red). The high-frequency oscillations in the MEG and NMR data are from microphonics in the SQUID moving in the 268.5Hz measurement field. Data are adapted from Matlachov AN, Volegov PL, Espy M, et al. (2005). Instrumentation for simultaneous detection of low field NMR and biomagnetic signals. *IEEE Trans Appl Supercond 15*(2): 676–679.

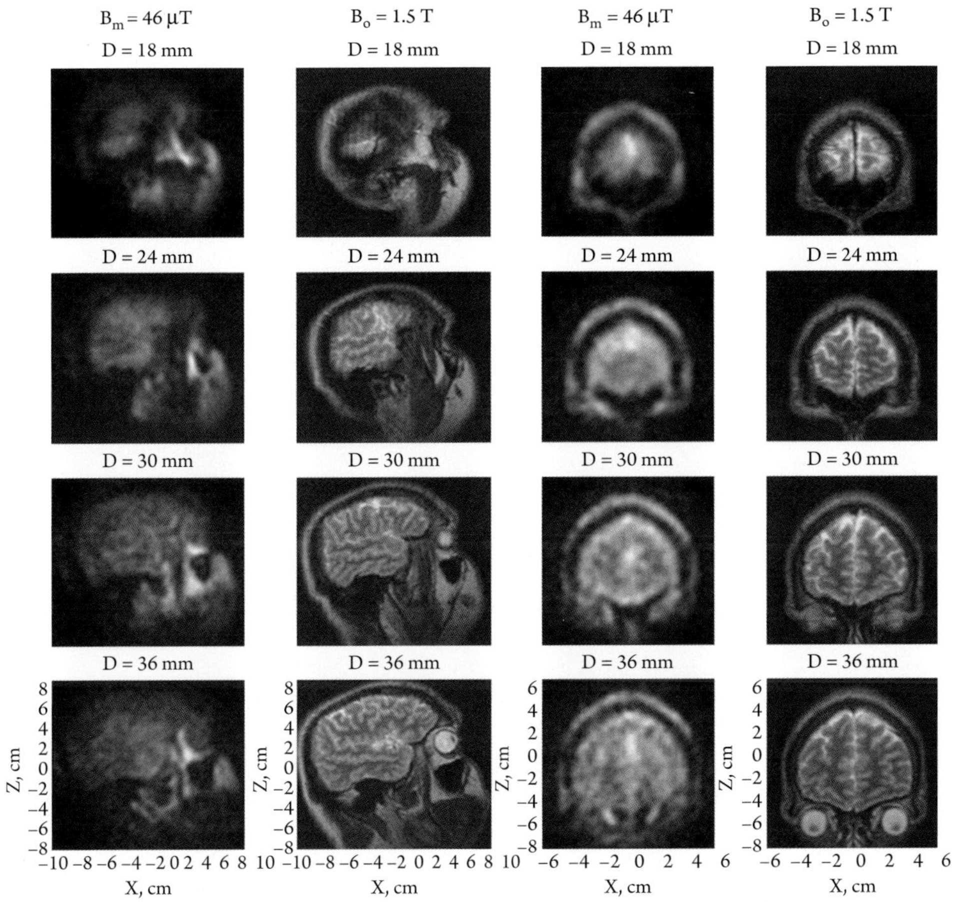

FIGURE 5.2 The first ULF MRI of the human brain and comparable images at HF. Data are from Zotev VS, Matlachov AN, Volegov PL, et al.(2008). Microtesla MRI of the human brain combined with MEG. *J Magn Reson 194*(1): 115–120, with permission from Elsevier.

these transient fields, a likely source was eddy currents arising from the walls of the magnetically shielded room (MSR). A MSR is typically required for MEG to reduce low-frequency magnetic field noise that interferes with the acquisition of the brain signal. For example, the MSR used in our combined MEG/ULF MRI experiments consisted of two alternating layers of aluminum and μ-metal. The effects of pulsed fields within an MSR have been studied by colleagues in Finland [20]. It is an interesting potential confound for combined MEG/ULF MRI systems that the requirement for shielding imposed by the MEG both reduces the noise and poses an additional challenge to the MRI. In addition to the eddy current-induced transient magnetic fields that interfere with the MEG signal, the mu-metal may become magnetized by the pre-polarization field, which can distort the ULF MRI image. Nieminen et al. described a novel self-shielded pre-polarization coil as a potential method to mitigate these effects [21].

While the data thus far have indicated "proof-of-concept" for a combined MEG and MRI device, clinical MEG instruments must have a large array of SQUID sensors. Large sensor arrays are required in MEG to facilitate the accuracy and reliability of solving the inverse problem of source localization: thus, the more SQUIDs the better. Most clinical

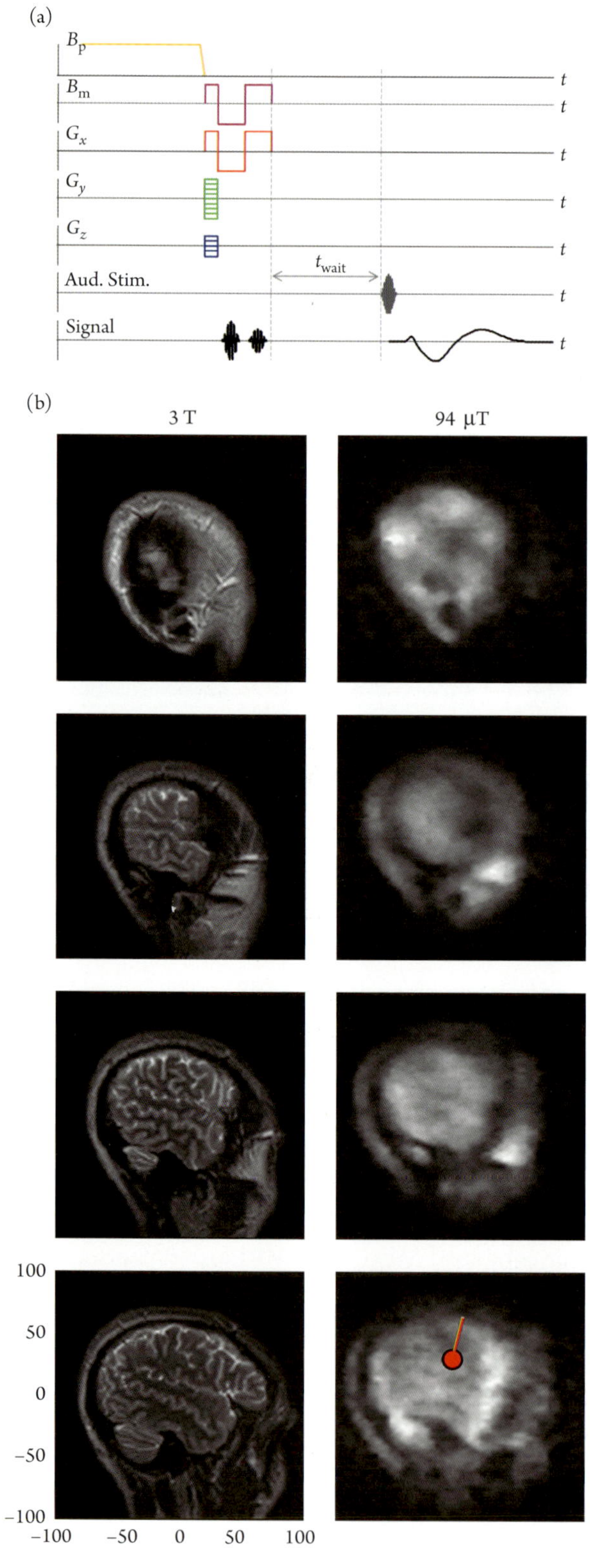

FIGURE 5.3 (Upper) MEG interleaved ULF MRI pulse sequence. (Bottom) MRI at 3T (left) and 94μT (right). The red arrow indicates the dipole for the auditory signal as it was located to the ULF MRI. From Magnelind et al. [19], with permission from IEEE.

MEG systems have large SQUID arrays with as many as 306 sensors. Thus it is critical that the number of MEG channels needs to increase from what has been demonstrated thus far in combined devices. These large SQUID sensor arrays can be used for image acceleration [22,23], which is likely critical to improving the acquisition speed (by using the spatial sensitivity of the array to reduce the required number of imaging steps) and quality of the ULF MRI.

Two groups, at the time of this writing, are actively studying the technology and methods of combining MEG and ULF MRI in a single device. These include our group at LANL and the European MEGMRI project [24]. While both groups have approached the problem from an MEG starting point (which is logical since MEG is a much more mature technology), it is important to recognize that a combined MEG and ULF MRI system is not just an upgraded conventional MEG machine. Adding ULF MRI capability to MEG implies not only the addition of coils for generation of fields and gradients, but also designing a system with SQUID-based sensors capable of tolerating the magnetic fields generated by the ULF MRI sequence. This has been (and continues to be) one of the most challenging requirements in a combined MEG/ULF MRI system in which the SQUIDs should work immediately after being exposed to a pre-polarizing field of up to 0.2T. Furthermore, as we discussed above, virtually all reliable MEG signal acquisition must be performed in a MSR. This adds the potential confound in MEG/ULF MRI systems of large transient magnetic fields arising from eddy currents induced in the MSR, which persist even long after the polarization field is removed.

The LANL and MEGMRI systems are somewhat similar; both leverage commercial MEG cryostats, MSRs, and basic measurement and gradient coil hardware. Photographs of both systems are presented in Figure 5.4.

At LANL we have adopted the approach of separately optimized magnetometers for imaging and MEG and an external liquid nitrogen-cooled B_p (normal conducting, see Chapter 2) coil. Our colleagues use a combination of magnetometer and planar gradiometers in the array and a self-shielded superconducting coil. A detailed description of our preliminary system design is found in [25]. A brief description of their system is found in [26], and a more complete one is expected in [27]. Although neither system is completed at the time of this writing, preliminary data from the MEGMRI system are presented in Figure 5.5.

None of the brain images acquired to date meets the general criterion of being "clinically relevant" in terms of ability to resolve key features of anatomy (e.g., cerebellum) or with respect to acquisition time. However, combined ULF MRI/MEG systems will only improve as the technology and methods are advanced. One should also not lose sight of the fact that the objective of ULF MRI is not to compete with HF MRI purely in terms of image quality; rather, it is for ULF MRI to provide a capability that HF MRI cannot have, such as combined MEG and MRI acquisition. A key area of progress that is essential to achieving better ULF MRI is (stronger) pre-polarization. As pre-polarization fields increase, it will be a continuing challenge to design SQUID sensors that can survive and rapidly recover in the proximity of dynamic fields inside the MSR. At the same time, there may be gains in the area of noise reduction. Achieving 100mT pre-polarization and 1fT/$\sqrt{\text{Hz}}$ noise will lead to images that are quite improved over any demonstrated thus far [28].

The time required to acquire an image of a given quality is, as previously demonstrated, inexorably tied to the strength of the pre-polarization field and the number of sensors available to acquire the MRI signal. The large number of sensors required in MEG sensor arrays therefore appears naturally synergistic with image acceleration in ULF MRI. For example, the sensor population for the initial hybrid LANL design (shown in Fig. 5.6) consists of 16

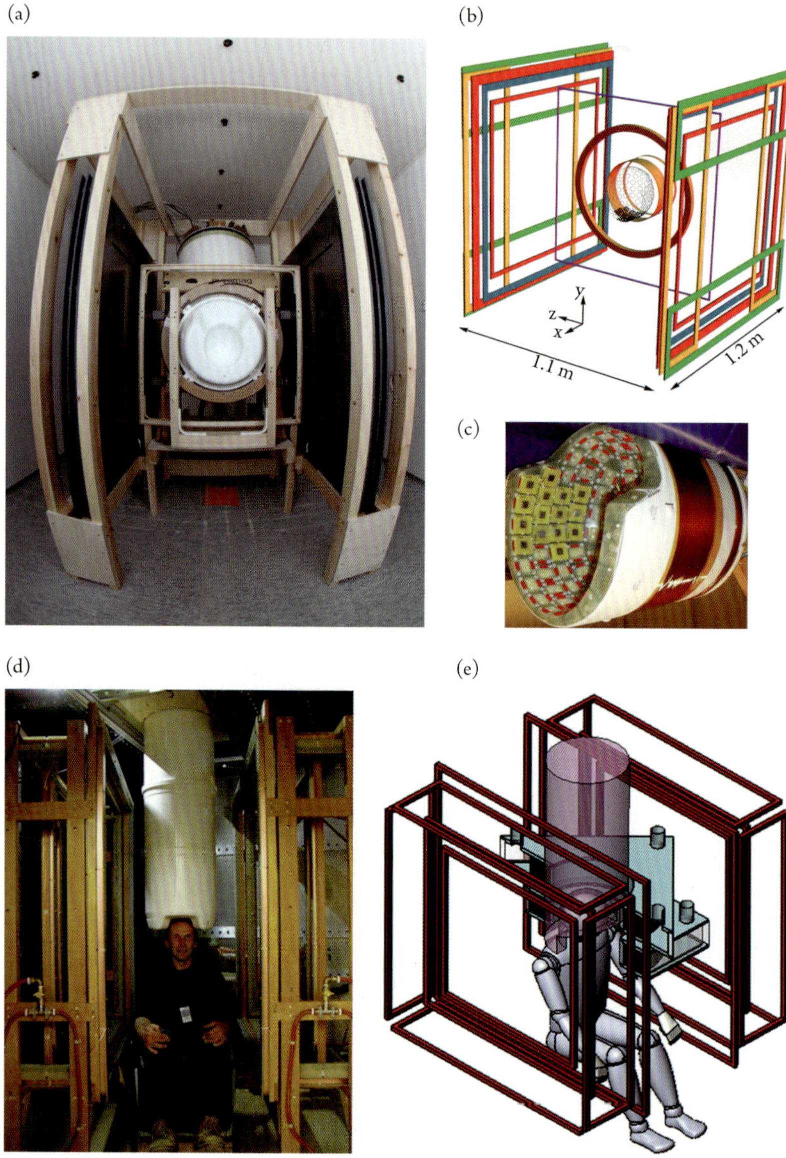

FIGURE 5.4 Photographs (left) and schematics (right) of the combined MEG and ULF MRI systems. (a)-(c) are from the MEGMRI consortium hybrid system, from [21] with permission from Elsevier. (d) and (e) LANL system.

clusters of four $8 \times 8\text{mm}^2$ magnetometers (64 total) for MEG, with each cluster surrounded by a 40mm circular Nb wire-wound pickup coil for MRI detection [25] (see Fig. 5.6). The sensor layout reflects the geometry of a Neuromag 122™ [29] cryostat that we refurbished for this application. In the future, it will be possible to populate all positions with MEG clusters and MRI channels. Finally, there remains significant room for improvement in the pulse sequences. Thus far most systems have relied on simplistic imaging hardware (for example, battery-driven) to reduce noise and minimize cost. But this leads to inefficient

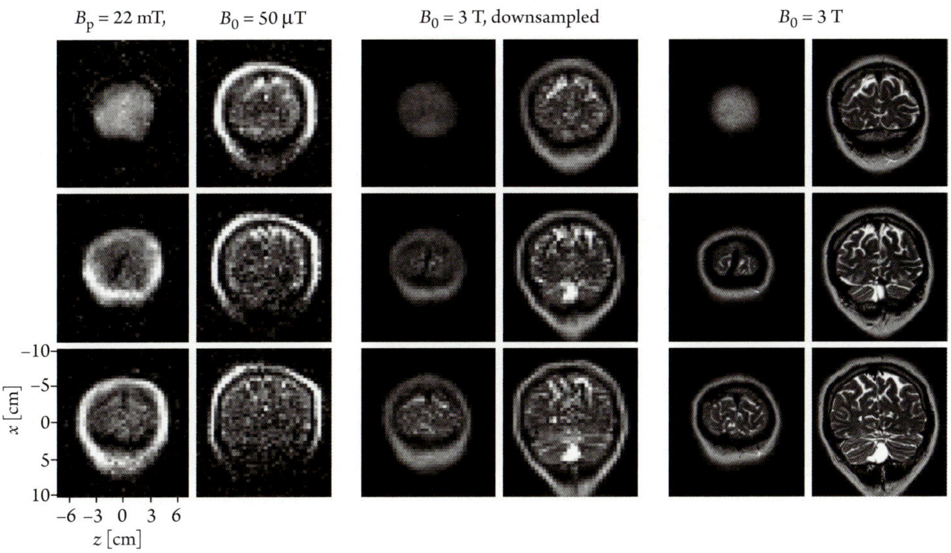

FIGURE 5.5 (Left) Coronal slices of the human brain acquired with the hybrid MEGMRI device. B_p and B_m were 22mT and 50μT, respectively. Total imaging time was 92 minutes, with eight averages. (Center) $T2$-weighted HFMR image of the same subject obtained at 3T. The resolution of the HF MR image was reduced to match that of the ULF MR image. (Right) HF MRI of the same subject at 3T with high resolution. For more details, see [26]. Images courtesy of Dr. Jaakko Nieminen, Aalto University.

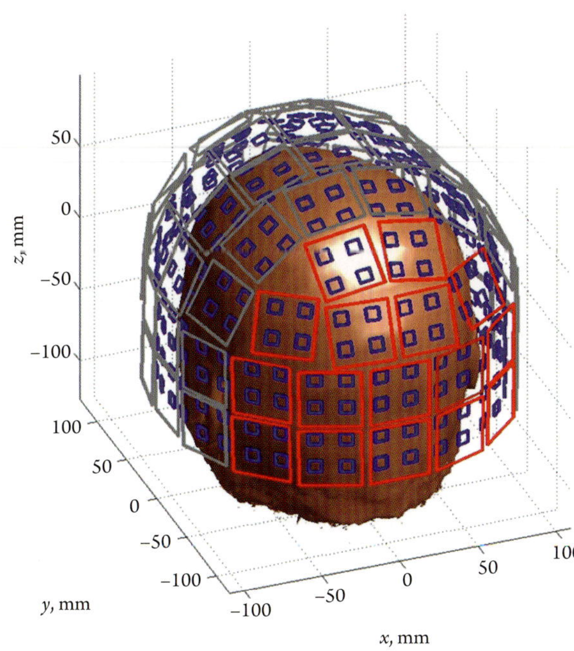

FIGURE 5.6 Layout of MEG (blue squares) and MRI (red squares) sensors in the LANL system. The initial coverage is of occipital cortex and can be upgraded to a total of 244 MEG and 61 MRI positions. Image is adapted from [25].

pulse sequences (i.e., Fourier imaging instead of projection). We briefly revisit some of these considerations below in the context of combined MEG and MRI systems.

The remainder of the discussion in this section is based largely on the hardware currently under construction in our laboratory at LANL. This serves to provide a concrete foundation from which we present real-world experience and practical challenges and solutions. However, the ultimate design and performance of combined MEG and MRI systems will almost certainly evolve as the promise of the approach is more fully appreciated and further research efforts are stimulated.

Our focus is toward the specific application, and we refer the reader to Chapter 2 for a more in-depth and general discussion of ULF MRI hardware.

5.1.1 Pre-polarization in the MSR

The generation of the pre-polarization field appears, at first glance, to be quite straightforward. Typically the requirement is for a pulsed magnetic field of ~0.1T or more to be on for ~1s (several T_1 times for tissue) and then off for a similar amount of time for the signal acquisition. We have already highlighted that, unlike in traditional HF MRI (where B_p is generated by superconducting or large permanent magnets), the B_p field in ULF MRI can be very inhomogeneous, can be pointed in any direction, and can change field strength to optimize contrast for various applications or tissue. While the benefits of this flexibility at ULF are clear, there are some challenges of which one must be aware: (1) cooling and energy removal are considerations for any pulsed field magnet and (2) the removal of the B_p field will generate transient currents in conducting surfaces such as MSR walls and other conducting materials in or near the system (in general, the ramp-up of B_p produces negligible impact on images because it is slower and far from the measurement period). These eddy currents can be long relative to the T_2 of the material being imaged, resulting in a loss of measurable signal while waiting for the eddy currents to decay to a level at which SQUID sensors can measure the signal of interest. In addition, as we already noted, the pre-polarizing pulses may also magnetize the walls of the MSR and induce field drift inside the MSR that will distort imaging gradients and shift the Larmor frequency in such a fashion that the image will be irreparably distorted (see Chapter 3).

The European MEGMRI consortium (see Fig. 5.4, upper) has decided upon a strategy that utilizes a self-shielded coil [30] that minimizes the effects of transients. The results appear very effective and encouraging. Further, if this magnetic field coil is made superconducting as they have designed, it can be integrated into the cryostat and resistive losses are effectively eliminated while the cooling is elegantly handled [26,27]. A practical downside to this approach is that the superconducting filaments in the magnet wire can trap significant flux at high current. In the present MEGMRI consortium design the trapped flux leads to remnant magnetization, which produces image distortions that challenge conventional image reconstruction. At the time of this writing pre-polarization is limited to a relatively modest 24mT. However, there are potential solutions being considered (for example, a non-adiabatic "demagnetizing" pulse that would reduce magnetization without affecting spins) that will likely resolve current limitations and enable the fields to be significantly increased.

We recently implemented a new and reasonably successful approach in some of our instruments to compensate for the various field transients. The transient pulses received by the SQUID sensors have an exponential decay shape that includes both high- and low-frequency components in the total spectral content. The higher-frequency components decay more rapidly than the lower frequencies. Our solution was to design a second electronic feedback to the sensor that is frequency-dependent, which makes the sensors much less sensitive at lower frequencies and thereby increases the sensor dynamic range for low-frequency signals. This approach has proven to work well in ULF MRI, where the signal of interest is of significantly higher frequency (in our implementation) than in MEG. The implementation maintains the SQUIDs within their dynamic range by compensating for the transients so that the SQUIDs are able to operate within 10ms of B_p ramp-down, even when operating inside rather small MSRs [31].

This approach was not, however, implemented in our interleaved MEG and ULF MRI measurements, where we simply waited for the transients to die away. The difference between the frequency range of the MEG signal (~1–1,000Hz) and the frequency at which we typically acquire the ULF MRI signal (~4–40kHz) is a key consideration for this decision. The second feedback loop described would limit sensitivity to the MEG low-frequency components. While the goal of transient mitigation for MRI only is primarily to keep the SQUIDs within their dynamic range, for MEG and ULF MRI one also needs to be able to deconvolve the transients from the signals of interest. It would seem that the best strategy for interleaved MEG and ULF MRI inside the MSR would be to avoid producing the transients in the first place.

We have thus far only attempted ULF MRI with the second feedback strategy and a slow (0.5s) adiabatic ramp-down using the system shown in Figure 5.4, which is housed in a two-layer MSR. We have been able to attain pre-polarization fields of 20mT using this strategy. To achieve higher pre-polarization fields in combined MEG and ULF MRI, while imaging tissue with short T_2 times, more aggressive mitigation of transients will be required. Thus, a self-shielded coil as described in [30], the use of an external compensation coil, or appropriate pulse shaping of the B_p ramp-down will be needed.

Finally, the memory of permeable materials (such as those used in MSRs) results in an increasing magnetization of the MSR with repeated application of pulsed pre-polarization fields. This is one artifact that can be nullified or accounted for by application of various pulse-sequence strategies, including alternating the direction of the pre-polarization pulse or applying "dummy" pulses in the opposite polarity to prevent magnetization from building up in the permeable material.

Before we leave our discussion of pre-polarization it is also worth mentioning that others have demonstrated the possibility of using the pre-polarization field shape itself to encode image contrast [32].

5.1.2 Future Directions in Combined MEG/ULF MRI

With the vast bulk of research and development effort in the field aimed at improving the ULF MRI technology, there has not yet been sufficient time for application of combined MEG/ULF MRI to advance neuroscience or functional brain studies. This may represent one of the greatest attractions to this field: the opportunities for both technological advances and scientific discovery are myriad. The potential for new techniques, application, and discovery is vast indeed. In addition to the mundane cost benefit of combining two imaging modalities (MEG and MRI) into a single instrument, the scientific benefits of combined anatomical and functional imaging for studies of the human brain have been extensively discussed [33,34]. For example, investigating the dynamics in the human brain requires studies that provide *both* excellent temporal and spatial resolution. Resolving activity such as synchronous oscillations requires at least ~2.5ms temporal resolution, while spatially resolving different areas of visual cortex requires ~5mm spatial resolution or better. A key to understanding how the human brain works will be the ability to infer both causality (when) and connectivity (where) between neurons during processing. Many neural behaviors, such as synchronous oscillations, or any activity that depends on the initial state of the neuron, will not be phase-locked to the stimulus and will require single trial analysis. The very best currently available noninvasive experimental methods, used singly or in combination, have significant limitations that constrain investigation of neural activity to large synchronous (or at least semi-synchronous) populations and/or repeated (averaged) sampling. Furthermore, modern techniques can measure neural activity either localized in space (e.g., fMRI) or precisely characterized in time (e.g., MEG and EEG), but not both. One limited approach to measure neural activity highly resolved in both space and time is to tightly couple the spatial (anatomical) and temporal measurements (for example, using spatial filters based on anatomical knowledge). Sadly, such approaches preclude investigating any long-range (or even moderate-range) communication and signaling. We remind the reader again that the combination of fMRI with EEG is one approach that may help resolve some of these issues, but to leverage MEG with fMRI will likely require a ULF approach.

In the next section we will see that ULF MRI may provide a unique window into neural activity that when combined with MEG can indeed provide a new insight into the spatio-temporal activity of the human brain that may make the combination far more powerful than the sum of its parts.

5.2 NEW APPROACHES TO IMAGE HUMAN BRAIN FUNCTION UNIQUELY ENABLED BY ULF MRI

5.2.1 MEG and Flow-Based fMRI at ULF

Functional MRI relies on a connection between cerebral blood flow, metabolism, and oxygenation with neuronal activity [35] to provide ~1mm spatial resolution of function. Typically the temporal resolution is 3 to 4s (1s for event related tasks). The hemodynamic signal lags the neural activity, taking ~3s to peak. There is evidence that fMRI reflects information about neuronal firing rates or oscillatory power in the same region under normal conditions [36]. However, the detailed relationship between the fMRI signal and the neuronal response is not well understood. Thus, while providing excellent localization, fMRI provides only modest insight into neural system dynamics. Applications with clinical consequences such as diagnostics and surgical planning need paradigms in which the neural correlates of the fMRI signal have been validated using combined electrophysiological and imaging approaches [37]. Toward this end, there has been great effort and progress at combined EEG and fMRI (see [38] and references therein for a relatively recent overview).

Thus far, however, information is primarily combined from separate instruments because of the instrumentation limitations discussed above. But there needs to be the strongest correlation possible between the sources defined by the different methodologies. Many cognitive paradigms are most effective during the first presentation: learning, recognition, studies involving deception or confederate studies, and many experimental designs where judgments must be made. Clinical symptoms are often not reproducible—for example, epileptic activity is seizure-dependent and schizophrenic observation can be hallucination-dependent.

The most commonly used form of fMRI is based on the different magnetic susceptibilities of oxyhemoglobin and deoxyhemoglobin. These levels change as a function of brain activity, giving rise to blood oxygen level-dependent (BOLD) fMRI. BOLD fMRI is widely employed because of its high sensitivity and easy implementation. However, the BOLD effect increases with magnetic field, typically requiring large magnetic fields (>1T).

Thus the BOLD approach to fMRI will probably not work at ULF. However, fMRI is also routinely performed at high fields using arterial spin labeling (ASL) techniques such as flow-sensitive alternating inversion recovery (FAIR) [39–41]. ASL methods differentiate the net magnetization of endogenous arterial water flowing proximally to the region of interest from the net magnetization of tissue. fMRI based on ASL is possible at ULF, as the effect is not field-dependent. We have recently demonstrated flow-based imaging at ULF using FAIR [42]. Because the electrophysiological brain response is faster than the hemodynamic one, it may be possible to interleave the acquisition such that the MEG and fMRI are acquired for the brain response to the same event. Interleaved data will provide for direct comparison of electrophysiological and hemodynamic brain activity obtained during a single collection. While single-collection EEG/fMRI is being widely adopted, single-collection MEG/fMRI is possible only at ULF.

5.2.2 Direct Neural Current Imaging

Although the ability to combine MEG and MRI into a single device is one approach to improving the performance and perhaps increasing the utilization of MEG, it is ultimately still combining two separate imaging modalities. Currently, there is no single modality for imaging human brain function that provides both temporal and spatial resolution sufficient to meet many pathology diagnostic needs, to plan intervention, or to address many important questions in neuroscience (such as connectivity between populations of neurons, the role of feedback, or oscillations in cognition). One could arguably claim that researchers have been searching for this "silver bullet" of imaging brain function for nearly a century, since Adrian and Matthews reported "localizing" the electrical activity noninvasively recorded from the brain in the occipital lobes using a technique related to modern EEG [43]. Today, with many research efforts around the world focused on this goal, it remains elusive. ULF MRI is among the newest tools in the arsenal of technology to image human brain function. In addition to the multimodal approach, there are at least two uniquely ULF approaches that we present here. The search for a modality capable of direct measurement and imaging of neural activity in the human brain embarked on an exciting new path at the close of the 20th century when researchers proposed that magnetic fields resulting from neuroelectrical activity could interact with a spin population, through phase shifts and dephasing [44–46]. Shortly thereafter, we presented the possibility that resonant interactions between the neural magnetic fields and the spin population were possible in the ULF regime [47], and this was followed by a theoretical and methodological exploration by Cassara et al. [48,49]. Together, the prospect of acquiring an image of neural activity based on the interaction between the neural magnetic fields and the spin population has been called "direct neural current imaging," or DNI (or nc-MRI). DNI promises the tomographic certainty of volumetric fMRI, with temporal resolution in direct relation to neural activation. One reported experimental measurement of DNI at HF based on the enhanced dephasing resulting from neural currents [50] has been vigorously debated in the neuroimaging community [51]. It is widely held that the authors did not convincingly differentiate between a neural effect and the orders-of-magnitude-larger "susceptibility artifact" caused by the BOLD signal. A key strength of DNI at ULF is that the confounding susceptibility artifact is virtually nonexistent. Moreover, the overlap between proton Larmor frequency at ULF and the frequency band of cortical neural activity permits resonant absorption by the population of proton spins of magnetic energy supplied by the cortical activity.

We reported the observation of this effect in phantoms, in which we measured the interaction of a weak current ($\sim 10\mu A$) with the ULF NMR signal both by resonance and dephasing [47,52]. The frequency spectrum of neural activity spans the range from a few Hz to a few kHz, at most, and the Larmor frequency for proton spins overlaps with this neural frequency spectrum only in the ULF regime (recall that $\omega_L = 4$kHz, the highend of the neural frequency spectrum, for $B \approx 100\mu$T). Consequently, "resonant absorption" can occur only at fields below 100μT, may enable measurement of the DNI effect, and could provide a tool to directly measure neuronal population oscillations and other frequency-dependent neural population phenomena.

The general premise for DNI measurements is that neural currents produce a magnetic field that locally perturbs the proton spin dynamics. While we have a reasonable expectation that the perturbing field originating from neural currents will have spatial scales on the order of ~10μm and timescales of ~1 to 10ms, and we know the signal from neurons can be detected far from the head in MEG, the actual spatiotemporal nature of the local field resulting from the complex and widespread activity of neurons in the brain on the scale that the spin population samples during a DNI protocol is very difficult to model, although has been estimated [49]. A successful demonstration of ULF DNI not only could provide a unique tomographic modality for imaging brain function, but will ultimately provide a new understanding of the local magnetic field distribution in the brain that results from the superposition of an extraordinarily complex set of fields resulting from intracellular and intercellular currents with poorly understood spatiotemporal distribution and synchronization.

The interaction of the neural fields with the spin population will induce both population phase changes and resonant absorption of energy at the Larmor frequency. While this interaction occurs independent of the details of the spatiotemporal distribution of the neural fields, those details will ultimately determine whether ULF DNI generates a measurable effect. We have discussed how B_m can readily be adjusted over a 1 to 100μT range (or more) with corresponding proton frequency $\omega_L = 40 \sim 4{,}000$Hz, thereby enabling us to select the proton ω_L at which we measure the ULF MRI. The power spectra for neural activity extends to a few kHz [53,54], over a similar range. Local field potentials reflecting mostly cooperative activity in neural populations are generally thought to extend from 10 to 90Hz [55]. The exact shape of any given neural activity spectrum will depend strongly on the stimulus causing the cortical activation.

We describe the interactions with a simple formalism that will allow us to compare "typical" phase changes resulting from the interaction and the effect of resonant absorption. Summarizing the approach described in [47], we can describe the effect of external magnetic fields, $\mathbf{B}(\mathbf{r},t)$, on the spin population by using a rotating reference frame aligned with the measurement field B_m (aligned with the z-axis) and rotating at the frequency $\omega_L = \gamma B_m$. Assuming $\gamma|\mathbf{B}(\mathbf{r},t)|\Delta t \ll 1$ (which is true for the neural generated fields), where Δt is the observation time, one can show [47] that the component, B_z, of the *neural* field aligned with B_m (the MRI field, defining the z-axis) will cause the precession frequency of the spin to vary according to $\omega_L + \Delta\omega = \gamma(B_m + B_z)$, and this will result in a phase shift:

(Eqn. 5.1)
$$\Delta\varphi_{||} = \int_0^t \gamma B_z(t')dt'$$

or

(Eqn. 5.2)
$$\Delta\varphi_{||} = \gamma \overline{B_z(\mathbf{r},t)}\Delta t.$$

Any component of the neural field, B_{xy}, that is off-axis relative to B_m will have the effect of tipping the spins away from or toward B_m (depending on the spatial synchrony the neural field with the spins) and this will also have an effect on the magnitude.

(Eqn. 5.3)

$$\Delta\varphi_{\perp}=\int_{o}^{t}\gamma B_{xy}(t')e^{i\omega_0 t'}dt'$$

or

(Eqn. 5.4)

$$\Delta\varphi_{\perp}=\gamma\left|\overline{B_{xy}(r,t)e^{i(\omega_0-\omega)t}}\right|\Delta t$$

Bars denote the time average over the observation time Δt. Rotation about the z-axis, $\Delta\phi_{||}$, is the underlying effect that has been widely proposed as the basis for DNI in HF MRI [45]. The magnitude of this effect is independent of the measurement field strength and is proportional to the mean value, over Δt, of the neural-generated magnetic field projected on B_{m}. Magnetic fields originating from neural activity will thus induce little net phase differences in the spin population if such activity produces zero-mean fields over the observation window (typically a few tens of milliseconds or more) [56,57].

Rotation about an axis orthogonal to B_{m} is responsible for the "resonant effect" $\Delta\varphi_{\perp}$, uniquely observable with ULF NMR because of the overlap in frequency of the neural fields with ω_{L}. This effect is proportional to the component of neural magnetic fields orthogonal to B_{m} averaged with a sinusoidal function at ω_{L}. If we now focus on the component of $\mathbf{B}(r,t)$ rotating about the z-axis at ω, we can write

(Eqn. 5.5)

$$B_{\perp}(r,t)=B_{\perp}e^{-i(\omega t+\varphi)}$$

and

(Eqn. 5.6)

$$B_{\perp}=\sqrt{B_x^2+B_y^2}$$

which gives

(Eqn. 5.7)

$$\varphi_{\perp}=\gamma\left|\overline{B_{\perp}e^{i(\omega_m-\omega)^t}}\right|\Delta t$$

at resonance, $\omega=\omega_L$, and Eqn. 5.7 can be simplified to

(Eqn. 5.8)

$$\Delta\varphi_{\perp}=\gamma\left|\overline{B_{\perp}}\right|\Delta t.$$

For nonresonant external fields $|\omega-\omega_{\mathrm{L}}|\Delta t\geq 2\pi$ and $\Delta\varphi_{\perp}$ becomes very small.

The ULF techniques allow $\mathbf{B}_{\mathrm{m}}$ to be chosen such that ω_{L} overlaps with a portion of the neural activity spectrum, resulting in significant rotation of the magnetization vector through resonant interactions. The resonant interaction only occurs when the Larmor frequency of the spin population overlaps with the frequency (or some portion thereof) of the neural activity; thus, ULF approaches are required. There is no component of the frequency spectrum of neural activity that extends to the >42MHz frequencies of HF MRI.

In [47], we experimentally demonstrated detection of the resonant interaction between magnetic fields designed to simulate those arising from neural activity, with a proton spin population in ULF (μT) NMR experiments (without imaging). We demonstrated through the use of current phantoms that, in the case of correlated zero-mean current distributions such as one might expect for many types of neural activity, resonant interactions will produce larger changes in the observed NMR signal than dephasing. The current phantoms were chosen to test the feasibility of detecting resonant interactions that may lead to direct and tomographic imaging of neural activity in the human brain using MRI techniques at

ULF. In addition, we established an approach that is sensitive to magnetic field distributions local to the spin population in cortex at the Larmor frequency of the measurement field. As we have often pointed out, the Larmor frequency at ULF can be readily manipulated by varying B_m, and SQUID sensors provide extraordinary sensitivity independent of frequency; consequently, one can also envision using ULF DNI to image the frequency distribution of the local fields in cortex. Finally, we note that while it is unlikely that ULF DNI can provide the temporal resolution of MEG or EEG, ULF DNI is completely compatible with simultaneous acquisition with MEG. The ULF DNI in such a multimodal approach would provide a robust constraint for solving the MEG inverse problem. The MEG would in turn provide temporal interpolation of the tomographic neural activity measured by the ULF DNI. Such a system may enable noninvasive exploration of the correlation between local fields induced by neural activity in cortex and more "distant" measures of brain activity such as MEG and EEG.

Experimental efforts to measure the ULF DNI have not provided definitive evidence of this effect, but relatively simple modeling efforts [49,52] would lead us to understand that the present state of ULF MRI with pre-polarization on the order of 100mT and SQUID noise of $\sim 1\mathrm{fT/Hz^{1/2}}$ is still an order of magnitude (or more) away from where we need to be to experimentally measure these effects. However, the payoff could be tremendous.

5.2.3 Magnetic Resonance Electrical Impedance Tomography (MREIT) at ULF

Recent work indicates that changes in electrical impedance at frequencies below 100Hz may provide another approach for imaging function [58,59]. Therefore one can seek, instead of direct endogenous current imaging as proposed for DNI, to image the electrical property changes caused by neural currents but using much larger exogenous (external) currents. These approaches may also lend themselves to observation by ULF MRI where distributions of applied currents can be imaged (MREIT) at ULF. Additionally, we raise the possibility that the resonant interaction between the *applied* current and the spins may be employed to selectively measure the change in the applied current. There is a close relation between DNI and MREIT, with the difference being the origin and nature of the current (endogenous current in one case and exogenous in another). Although speculative, the impact that successful DNI or MREIT-based demonstration of fast neural imaging would have on brain research cannot be overstated.

Electrical impedance tomography (EIT) has been shown to be a powerful tool that provides dynamic measures of tissue conductivities, but it is limited by low spatial resolution surface voltage measurements and the need to solve an ill-posed inverse problem [60]. Researchers have produced cross-sectional images of conductivity distribution inside the human body by means of EIT, with promising applications such as providing tissue impedance for EEG/ECG source analysis, detecting cancer and stroke [61], and assessing lung structure and fluid burden [60]. Conventional EIT reconstructs conductivity images from boundary current–voltage data [60, 62–65] measured from an array of surface electrodes attached on some portion of the body. Time-varying (sinusoidal) currents in the frequency range from near DC to ~1MHz are injected through electrodes, and the voltages induced by the currents passing through the resistive tissue are measured at other electrodes. The voltages at the injection electrodes are usually discarded due to electrolyte polarization effects. The boundary current–voltage dataset is used to reconstruct images of the internal conductivity and permittivity distributions.

Combining EIT with MRI adds the dimension of tomographic *in situ* measurement of local magnetic field perturbations produced by the currents applied in EIT from which a conductivity map can be deduced. In this way, MREIT can provide high-spatial-resolution images of electrical conductivity without the need to solve the ill-posed current-source problem in traditional EIT. In principle MREIT can provide spatial resolution for conductivity images comparable to the resolution of the MRI. Just as anatomical MRI has been driven to ever-higher fields by the lure of better spatial resolution, MREIT is most commonly performed at high magnetic fields, >1T.

MREIT is a relatively recent noninvasive imaging modality in which magnetic resonance current density imaging (MRCDI) is combined with EIT. The first demonstrations of MREIT [66–68] showed that MRI could be used to measure the magnetic flux density induced by exogenous current injection. MREIT is measured by applying a current source via surface electrodes during a regular spin-echo MRI sequence (see, for example, [69]). During MRI, the injected current produces phase changes that can be computed from the MRI phase differential images [70]. The magnitude of the phase changes depend on the strength and duration of the applied current. The current density J can be computed from B based on Ampere's Law, $J = \nabla \times B/\mu_0$; however, all three components of $B = (B_x, B_y, B_z)$ must be measured. However, MRI measures only the component of B that is parallel to the direction of the field B_m, and as we have repeatedly said, this field cannot be changed for traditional HF systems. Obtaining all three components would require that the object under study be rotated twice inside such a scanner. Early attempts to obtain the conductivity, σ, from J in this fashion [67,68,71–73] have been reported, but the methods are difficult and impractical (especially for human subject applications).

Recent efforts have focused on reconstructing the conductivity image from only one component of the magnetic field (usually referred to as B_z) that is parallel to B_m [68,74,75] using multiple injection currents [76]. It was also suggested that MREIT based on MRCDI with injection currents at the Larmor frequency may provide even more information, including orthogonal components of B, without rotation [77]. There have been recent successful demonstrations of MRCDI with injection currents at the Larmor frequency in conventional MR machines (1.5 or 3T) [78,79]. However, the Larmor frequency for these systems is tens to hundreds of MHz (128MHz for 3.0T). Such a regime is far from physiological processes (e.g., propagation of EEG responses through tissues) and far from the optimal contrast of tissues for most clinical and research uses [61,80]. Finally, the current levels needed to obtain all MREIT images to date have been too large to safely apply to the human head (3mA was the smallest applied MREIT current reported, applied to the human knee [81]). While the MREIT signal depends on a variety of parameters, it is widely reported that a minimum of 1 mA will be required [82–85].

Combining EIT with ULF MRI would enable the direct measurement of all three magnetic field components needed to solve for J (without requiring sample rotation) since the field direction in a ULF system can be readily changed in both orientation and strength. Furthermore, the low and tunable measurement field enables overlap with the frequency of injected currents in a "resonant method" in a physiologically interesting regime. This can open the door for probing the msec-sec dynamics of molecular or physiological processes not accessible by fixed-field or conventional field-cycling MRI. ULF MRI enables the Larmor frequency to be varied over interesting regimes of tissue impedance contrast <10kHz that will almost certainly reveal entirely new contrast mechanisms [86–88] based on T_1 dispersion and resonant contrast produced by overlapping the Larmor frequency with biomagnetic processes [47] or the injected currents in MREIT.

We could imagine that ULF MREIT could ultimately provide a fast, inexpensive, and noninvasive technology for continual monitoring of a patient's neurological status, allowing for accurate diagnosis and treatment planning with multiple disorders, including epilepsy [89], acute stroke [90], traumatic brain injury [91], and vasospasm [92].

5.2.3.1. Current Status of ULF MREIT

Our group has made progress in demonstrating preliminary measurements of MREIT in a phantom at ULF [42]. A static (DC) current is passed through electrodes and the induced magnetic field adds to the measurement field to generate a detectable phase-shift of the MR signal. We were able to measure both phase-shift and resonant effects of applied 5 to 10mA DC and AC currents using an MRI readout of 94μT ($\omega_L \sim$ 4,000kHz).

The interaction of the applied current with the spin population will induce both population phase changes and resonant absorption of energy at the Larmor frequency, as we discussed in Section 5.2.2 on DNI. Again we are discussing the interactions between an external magnetic field, $B(r,t)$, on the spin population using a rotating reference frame aligned with the measurement field B_m and rotating at the Larmor frequency $\omega_L = \gamma B_m$. Assuming $\gamma|B(r,t)|\Delta t \ll 1$, where Δt is the observation time, one can show that the evolution of the magnetization due to the external field $B(r,t)$ can be described as a rotation $\Delta\phi_{||}$, or phase-shift, about B_m (the z-axis) and a tipping $\Delta\phi_\perp$ about an axis orthogonal to B_m [93]:

(Eqn. 5.9)
$$\Delta\varphi_{||} = \gamma \overline{B_z(\mathbf{r},t)}\Delta t$$

(Eqn. 5.10)
$$\Delta\varphi_\perp = \gamma\left|\overline{B_\perp e^{\imath(\omega_L-\omega)}}\right|\Delta t.$$

Bars denote the time average over the observation time Δt. While in Section 5.2.2 (Eqns. 5.2 and 5.7) we were discussing $B(r,t)$ as neural in origin, the above statements are also true for $B(r,t)$ arising from applied currents. The rotation about the z-axis, $\Delta\phi_{||}$ (the underlying effect that has been widely proposed as the basis for direct neural current imaging in HF MRI) [45], also describes the phase-shift observed in MREIT. The magnitude of this effect is independent of the measurement field strength and is proportional to the mean value, over Δt, of the applied magnetic field projected on the B_m axis (which is typically the z-axis). Eqn. 5.10 describes the tipping of magnetization about an axis orthogonal to B_m by magnetic fields at the Larmor frequency, ω_L. By resonant absorption one can measure the effects of $B(r,t)$ orthogonal to B_m, without requiring object rotation. It should also be noted that the resonant signal also contains information about the relative phase of the applied current. In the experiment described in [47] and Section 5.2.2 we detected the NMR signal produced by resonant absorption in a water phantom. In that work we were able to detect μA-level currents (~3μA/mm^2), which approaches the expected levels of 0.3 to 1.5μA/mm^2 for 1mA EIT injection in the brain (from [59] and scaled from [94]). We also reported using ULF MRI that detection of a 10μA DC current could clearly be seen in the image [52] (based on dephasing). These demonstrations give a positive indication that resonant MREIT is possible.

The seven-channel instrumentation used to demonstrate MREIT at ULF is shown in Figure 5.7 and has been described in detail elsewhere (see, for example, [18,19,95,96]) and Chapters 2 and 4 of this book. While this system has afforded great versatility, it was not designed or optimized for MREIT. Consequently, the demonstration described below leaves significant room for improvement.

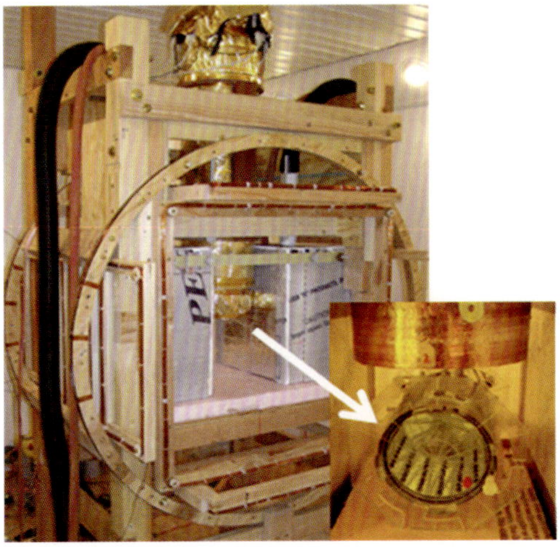

FIGURE 5.7 LANL system for simultaneous MEG/ULF MRI and EGI MREIT phantom in the system (*inset*). The depictured setup is for gradient-echo imaging when the orthogonality of B_p and B_m is used.

We used a phantom provided to us by colleagues at Electrical Geodesics Inc. (EGI), who were collaborators on the work shown here. The typical phantom is an acrylic cylinder tank approximately the size of the average adult human head (Fig. 5.8). One hundred twenty-eight standard EEG Ag/AgCl electrodes are hermetically placed into the holes uniformly arranged on the lateral surface in eight rows and sixteen columns for recording voltages. External current is injected through four MREIT electrodes with lead approach angles at 90 degrees to B_0 to minimize artifacts.

The cylinder is filled with saline with conductivity close to that of cerebrospinal fluid. Agar gel insertions of smaller size and lower conductivity (cylindrical and rectangular rods) or biological samples can be placed inside the cylinder in arbitrary positions [97].

An example of the gradient-echo sequence used for MREIT is shown in Figure 5.9. In this case, B_p and B_m were orthogonal and B_p was ramped down non-adiabatically and the precession was initiated by turning on the B_m field. However, we also intend to investigate a spin-echo approach in which we adiabatically ramp down the B_p field with the B_m field

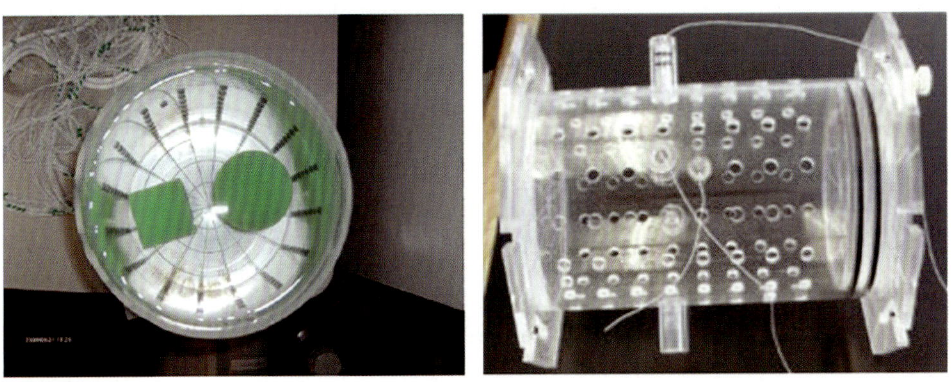

FIGURE 5.8 Phantom development. (Left) Cylinder tank for EIT. (Right) Hermetic cylinder tank for MREIT scaled to fit an MRI head coil and populated by 128 EEG electrodes in addition to 4 recessed MREIT electrodes. Courtesy of Dr. Sergei Turovets, Electrical Geodesic Inc.

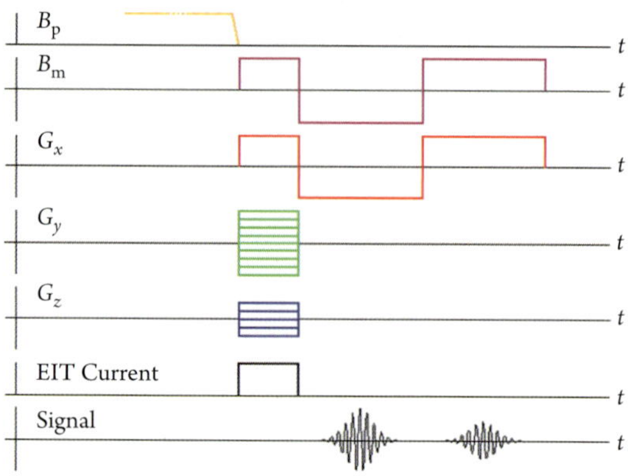

FIGURE 5.9 Gradient echo pulse sequence with DC MREIT current.

present to align the spins with the more uniform B_m field. The precession is then initiated by a $\pi/2$ pulse. This approach might help improve phase stability.

While the phantom was not optimized for the ULF application, resulting in nonideal geometries, we obtained clear signal from the phantom. Figure 5.10 (upper) shows the amplitude image at 94μT with the approximate SQUID sensor pattern superposed (dotted circles) and the injecting electrode locations indicated by arrows. This image is an integrated depth view from the top. In the center and lower panels we see phase images for positive and negative current injection at 10mA. Data are differenced from the zero current case. The effect of the current is clearly evident with the largest phase-shift (0.2 rad) measured beneath SQUID 5, which was closest to the electrodes.

Using a gradient-echo protocol we found a phase noise of 0.05 rad over a single image. The phase images shown in Figure 5.10 represent five averages acquired over ~5 minutes and are differentiated to zero current collections acquired separately. A phase drift also of about 0.05 rad was observed (producing the underlying "stripe" artifacts). Using these data and Eqn. 5.1 we can estimate sensitivity to applied fields (B_z) at ~5nT.

The major impediments found in most recent demonstrations of HF MREIT have been related to low SNR, long imaging time, and the need to inject currents higher than clinically acceptable (>1mA) to obtain a measurable signal. While the spatial resolution we can achieve at ULF currently lags that of HF MRI (resolution in Fig. 5.10 is 3 × 3mm^2), this resolution is adequate for MREIT, and the relevant figures of merit for acceptable current injection levels appear achievable based on our preliminary data.

Sadlier et al. [98] recently presented a theoretical and experimental study of noise considerations for MREIT based on measurement of B_z (phase-shift in the DC/off-resonant current injection). Their work demonstrated ~7nT noise at a voxel size of 1 × 1 × 1mm^3 for four averages using a 3T scanner. They concluded that a carefully designed MREIT study at 3T could attain sensitivity to applied field (B_z) ~ 0.25nT at a voxel size of 3 × 3 × 3mm^3. The authors believe that at these noise levels MREIT using currents below 5mA (which they assess to be acceptable) would be feasible. We can extrapolate their excellent noise analysis framework from the HF regime to interpret the expected performance of our ULF MREIT approach. This analysis indicates we are roughly 20 times less sensitive than required by this analysis to reach a clinically relevant level of noise. However, an improvement of this magnitude seems well within the reach of current technology and techniques considering the very rudimentary nature of this first proof-of-principle experiment.

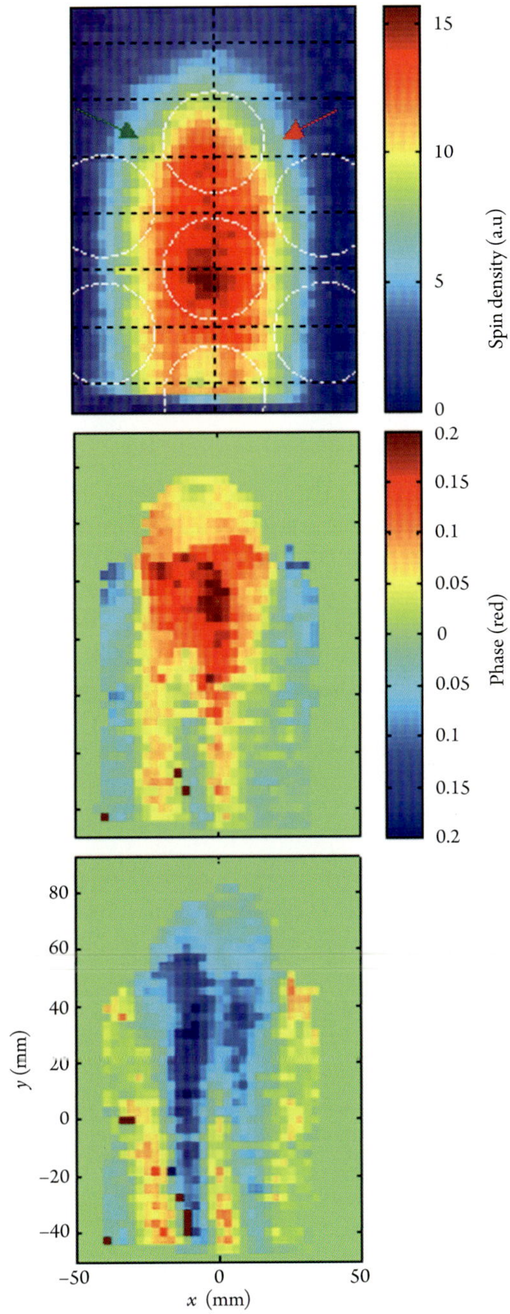

FIGURE 5.10 ULF MRI of the EGI MREIT phantom. (Upper) Amplitude weighted image with the dashed circles indicating the locations of the pickup loops and arrows indicating the MREIT current injection locations. (Middle) Phase image for 10mA. (Lower) Phase image for -10mA.

The issue of sensitivity in the resonant method approach requires a different analysis. Eqn. 5.2 describes the deflection of magnetization, not a phase shift. Based on our preliminary data acquired with the EGI phantom, we calculate that 10mA produced an angular tip of ~0.03 rad. The relevant noise for resonant detection is not phase noise or stability but rather the SNR of our images, which is currently about 100. This leads us to estimate that our present (nonoptimal) system could readily image angular tip down to 0.01 rad, which would be sufficient to detect the expected angular tip.

Improving sensitivity for either phase-shift or resonant MREIT would be realized by increasing signal (via enhanced pre-polarization), reducing system noise (which is currently ~3fT/Hz$^{1/2}$), and optimizing the current injection and pulse sequence. Again, given the rudimentary instrumentation and poorly optimized conditions, such improvements seem eminently possible.

5.3 MAGVIZ AND ULF NMR RELAXOMETERS

One interesting application of ULF MRI has been to relaxometry. As we saw in Chapter 4, the ability to vary the magnetic field strength enables the measurement of T_1 (or T_2) at essentially any field between B_p and B_m. There are commercial implementations of such devices, known as field-cycling (FC) relaxometers. These devices can measure relaxation dispersion over a wide range of frequencies. For example, the Stelar SMARtracer™ [99] can measure dispersion profiles for T_1 from a few kHz to 10MHz.

One implementation of ULF NMR/MRI methods was to develop a SQUID-based relaxometer for the inspection of liquids in a security checkpoint. In this case, a commercial instrument like the Stelar wasn't adequate, primarily because of the return to high frequencies for readout employed by standard FC relaxometers, which makes measuring through unopened streams-of-commerce (SOC) bottles of any shape, size, and material a challenge. The ULF approach, however, has readout at very low magnetic fields, so signals can penetrate most packaging (including aluminum cans) owing to large skindepths, and field uniformity is not an issue.

The issue of inspection of liquids at a security checkpoint was motivated by a 2006 terrorist plot that targeted airplanes by liquid explosives that would be carried aboard disguised as drinks [100]. The plot, thwarted by intelligence before it could be executed, illustrated the challenge of detecting liquids by traditional screening approaches such as x-ray. Most threatening and benign liquids appear the same to conventional x-ray systems, which are best suited for detecting changes in density. At the time of this writing, owing to a lack of a suitable high-throughput screening method, passengers flying into or out of the United States are limited to carrying on aircraft only liquids in 100-mL bottles that fit within a single clear 1-quart bag.

One area of research to address this problem has been NMR, which is very well suited to the study of the chemical properties of liquids. Ideally, chemical shift spectroscopy could be used, but this requires very high and uniform magnetic fields. Relaxometry, however, is also a reliable method for studying chemical properties. By moving to ULF, the magnetic fields are low, safe for the public, and tolerant of screening through most kinds of SOC packaging, including aluminum cans. Also, as we have discussed in Chapters 3 and 4, relaxation information at ULF can often be more informative than at HF.

An imaging relaxometer known as MagViz was developed with the support of the Department of Homeland Security Science and Technology Directorate and was used to demonstrate the inspection of liquids by relaxometry [31,103,101]. By measuring T_1 in the pre-polarization field (~2MHz) using different polarization times, while measuring T_2 at the much lower measurement field (~2kHz), we are able to discriminate between many different liquid types using dispersion (recall that at 2kHz $T_1 \sim T_2$) and comparison to a database.

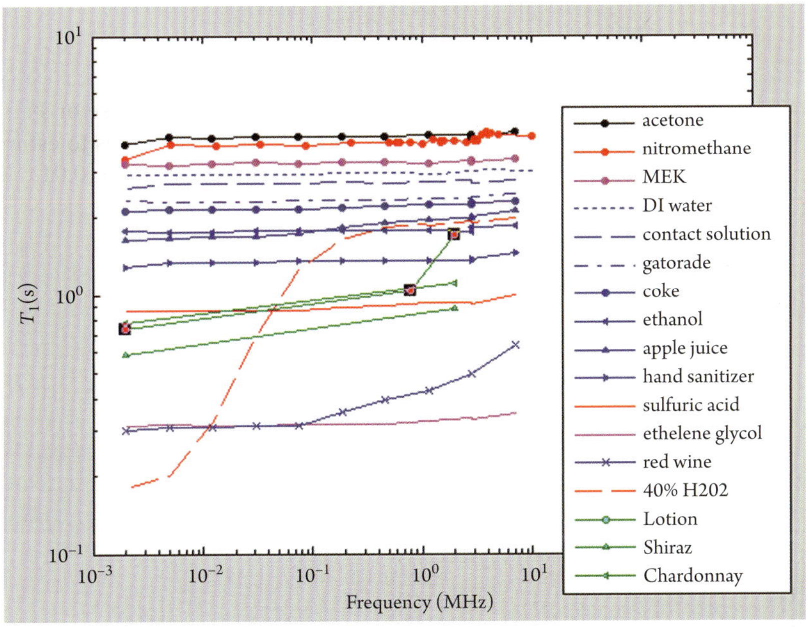

FIGURE 5.11 T_1 dispersion data for a variety of liquids from 2kHz through 10MHz. Data are adapted from [101] with permission from IOP Publishing.

Examples of dispersion data are shown in Figure 5.11. In these data we can see that for many liquids T_1 is relatively flat. However, for some materials, such as lotion, wine, and 40% hydrogen peroxide in hair bleach, there is interesting dispersion associated with changing molecular dynamics as a function of frequency.

Sample images from MagViz are shown in Figure 5.12. The color scheme is normalized such that materials with T_1 close to water or benign substances appear blue, while T_1 close to known threatening material properties would appear yellow or red. This device used

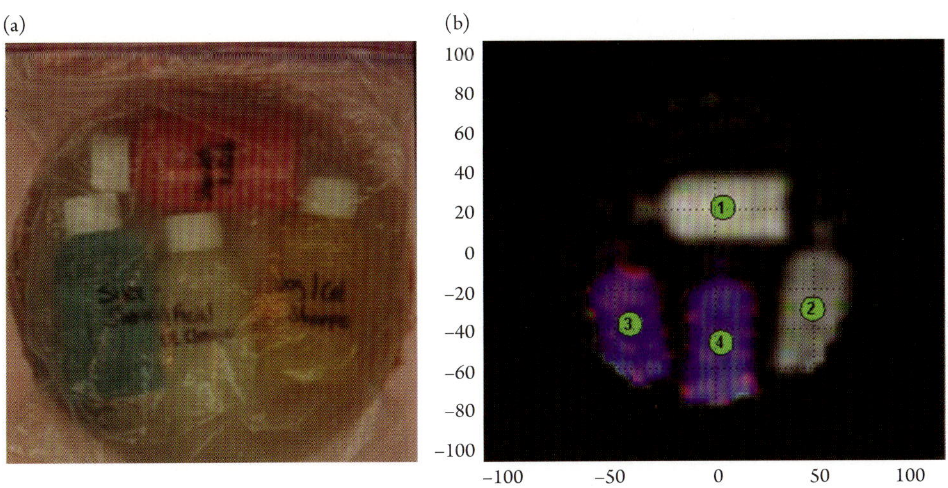

FIGURE 5.12 Data and relaxation-weighted images from a ULF MRI system designed to detect threatening liquids. (a) Photographs of items. (b) Relaxation-weighted 2D ULF MRI image.

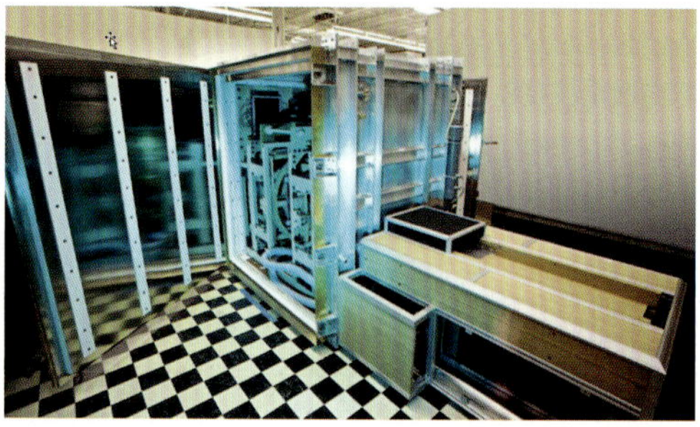

FIGURE 5.13 The MagViz hardware. Shown is the MSR (with door open), conveyor exiting the system, and the imaging coil set inside the MSR.

seven SQUIDs and was not dissimilar from our approach to brain imaging at ULF. One issue with the instrument was the relatively long scan times, ~1 minute per group of bottles. However, it is likely that the use of dense sensor arrays will shorten this time. A photograph of the MagViz hardware are shown in Figure 5.13. Subsequent incarnations of MagViz have been able to move away from the requirement to use SQUIDs [102], and most recently small units devoted to single-bottle screening are being developed [103].

5.4 A FINAL WORD

We have only begun to scratch the surface of ULF MRI. In terms of practice, we have presented the foundational principles that underlie ULF MR and the methods and techniques our group and others have used thus far to apply (or deal with) those principles in exploring various phenomena. Beyond the rigorous physics, we have also attempted to share bits of our practical experience, some of which may be poorly understood in terms of the underlying physics or causes. We also shared a sampling of ideas from our team and those that have been discussed openly in the community about new and as yet untried methods, approaches, and applications. There is a wealth of unexplored territory in ULF NMR and MRI, and we are confident that new discoveries await in this emerging field.

REFERENCES

1. Regan D (1989). *Human brain electrophysiology: Evoked potentials and evoked magnetic fields in science and medicine*. New York: Elsevier Science Publishing.
2. Hämaläinen M, Hari R, Ilmoniemi RJ, et al. (1993). Magnetoencephalography—theory, instrumentation, and applications to noninvasive studies of the working human brain. *Rev Mod Phys 65*(2): 413–497.
3. Logothetis NK, Pauls J, Augath M, et al. (2001). Neurophysiological investigation of the basis of the fMRI signal. *Nature 412*: 150–157.
4. Logothetis NK (2002). The neural basis of the blood-oxygen-level-dependent functional magnetic resonance imaging signal. *Philos Trans R Soc Lond B Biol Sci 357*: 1003–1037.
5. Feichtinger M, Holl A, Korner E, et al. (2002). Future aspects of the presurgical evaluation in epilepsy. *Advances in Epilepsy Surgery and Radiosurgery 84*: 17–26.
6. Lopes da Silva FH, Wieringa HJ, Peters MJ (1991). Source localization of EEG versus MEG: Empirical comparison using visually evoked responses and theoretical considerations. *Brain Topog 4*(2): 133–142.
7. Funke M, Constantino T, Van Orman C, Rodin E (2009). Magneto encephalography and magnetic source imaging in epilepsy. *Clin EEG Neurosci 40*(4): 271–280.

8. Mosher JC, Spencer ME, Leahy RM, Lewis PS (1993). Error bounds for EEG and MEG dipole source localization. *Electroenceph Clin Neurophys 86*: 303–320.
9. Mosher JC, Leahy RM, Lewis PS (1999). EEG and MEG: forward solutions for inverse methods. *IEEE Trans Biomed Eng 46*(3): 245–259.
10. Xia H, Ben-Amar Baranga, Hoffman D, Romalis MV (2006). Magnetoencephalography with an atomic magnetometer. *Appl Phys Lett 89*: 211104.
11. Adjamian P et al. (2004). Co-registration of MEG with MRI using bite-bar fiducials and surfacematching. *Clin Neurophys 115*: 691.
12. Poghosyan V, Ionnides AA (2007). Precise mapping of early visual responses in space and time. *Neuroimage 35*(2): 759–770.
13. Macovski A, Conolly S (1993). Novel approaches to low cost MRI. *Magn Reson Med 30*: 221–230.
14. McDermott R, Trabesinger AH, Mück M, et al. (2002). Liquid state NMR and scalar couplings in microtesla magnetic fields. *Science 295*: 2247–2249.
15. Mößle M, Myers W, Lee S-K, et al. (2005). SQUID detected in vivo MRI at microtesla magnetic fields. *IEEE Trans Appl Supercond 15*(2): 757–760.
16. Matlachov AN, Volegov PL, Espy M, et al. (2005). Instrumentation for simultaneous detection of low field NMR and biomagnetic signals. *IEEE Trans Appl Supercond 15* (2): 676–679.
17. Volegov P, Matlachov AN, Espy M, et al. (2004). Simultaneous magnetoencephalography and SQUID detected nuclear MR in microtesla magnetic fields. *Magn Reson Med 52* (3): 467–470.
18. Zotev VS, Matlachov AN, Volegov PL, et al. (2008). Microtesla MRI of the human brain combined with MEG. *J Magn Reson 194*(1): 115–120.
19. Magnelind PE, Gomez JJ, Matlashov AN, et al. (2011). Co-registration of interleaved MEG and ULF MRI using a 7 channel low-T_c SQUID system. *IEEE Trans Appl Supercond 21*(3): 456–460.
20. Vesanen PT et al. (2012). The spatial and temporal distortion of magnetic fields applied inside a magnetically shielded room. *IEEE Trans Magn 48*(1): 53–61.
21. Nieminen JO et al. (2011). Avoiding eddy-current problems in ultra-low-field MRI with self-shielded polarizing coils. *J Magn Reson 212*:154–160.
22. Pruessmann KP, Weiger M, Scheidegger MB, Boesiger P (1999). SENSE: Sensitivity encoding for fast MRI. *Magn Res Med 42*(5): 952–962.
23. Zotev VS, Volegov PL, Matlashov AN, et al. (2008). Parallel MRI at microtesla fields. *J Magn Reson 192*(2): 197–208.
24. http://www.megmri.net/
25. Matlashov AN, Burmistrov E, Magnelind PE, et al. (2012). SQUID-based systems for co-registration of ultra-low field nuclear magnetic resonance images and magneto encephalography. *Physica C* 482:19–26.
26. Nieminen J (2012). Doctoral dissertation: Ultra low field MRI: techniques and instrumentation for hybrid MEG-MRI. http://lib.tkk.fi/Diss/2012/isbn9789526046457/isbn9789526046457.pdf. Aalto University publication series.
27. Vesanen PT, Nieminen JO, Zevenhoven KCJ, et al. (2013). Hybrid ultra-low-field MRI and MEG system based on a commercial whole head neuromagnetometer. Magn Reson Med 69(6): 1795–1804.
28. Espy M, Magnelind P, Matlashov A, et al. (2013). Toward high resolution images with SQUID-based ultra-low field magnetic resonance imaging. *IEEE Trans Appl Supercond.* 23(3): 1603107 (7 pages).
29. Ahonen AI, Hämäläinen MS, Knuutila JET, et al. (1993). 122-channel SQUID instrument for investigating the magnetic signals from the human brain. *Physica Scripta T49*: 198–205.
30. Nieminen JO, Vesanen PT, Zevenhoven KCJ, et al. (2011). Avoiding eddy-current problems in ultra-low-field MRI with self-shielded polarizing coils. *J Magn Reson 212*(1): 154–160.
31. Espy M, Flynn M, Gomez J, et al. (2010). Ultra-low-field MRI for the detection of liquid explosives. *Supercond Sci Technol* 23(3): 034023.
32. Nieminen JO, Voigt J, Hartwig S, et al. (2013). Improved contrast in ultra-low-field MRI with time-dependent bipolar prepolarizing fields: theory and NMR demonstrations. Metrol Meas Syst XX(3): 327–336.
33. Dale AM, Halgren E (2001). Spatiotemporal mapping of brain activity by integration of multiple imaging modalities. *Cogn Neurosci 11*: 202–208.

34. Baillet S, Mosher JC, Leahy RM. (2001). Electromagnetic brain mapping. *IEEE Sig Proc Mag* 14–30.
35. Kim S-G, Bandettini P (2010). Chapter 1, Principles of Functional MRI. In SH Faro, FB Mohamed (Eds.), BOLD *fMRI: A Guide to Functional Imaging for Neuroscientists*. Springer.
36. Scholvinck ML, et al. (2010). Neural basis of global resting-state fMRI activity. *Proc Natl Acad Sci USA 107*(22):10238.
37. Kayser C, Logothetis NK (2010). Chapter 4, The Electrophysiological Background of the fMRI Signal. In S Ulmer, O Jansen (Eds.), *fMRI: Basics and Clinical Applications*. Springer Berlin Heidelberg: Berlin, Heidelberg.
38. Laufs H (2012). A personalized history of EEG–fMRI integration. *NeuroImage 62*(2): 1056–1067.
39. Kim S-G (1995). Quantification of relative cerebral blood flow change by flow-sensitive alternating inversion recovery (FAIR) technique: application to functional mapping. *Magn Reson Med 34*: 293–301.
40. Kwong KK, Chesler DA, Weisskoff RM, et al. (1995). MR perfusion studies with T_1-weighted echo planar imaging. *Magn Reson Med 34*: 878–887.
41. Schwarzbauer C, Morrissey S, Haase A (1996). Quantitative magnetic resonance imaging of perfusion using magnetic labeling of water proton spins within the detection slice. *Magn Reson Med* 35: 540–546.
42. Magnelind P, George J, Gomez J, et al. (2011). Towards functional magnetic resonance imaging at ultra-low fields. Presented at the Superconductivity Centennial Conference in The Hague, The Netherlands.
43. Adrian ED, Matthews HG (1934). The Berger rhythm: Potential changes from the occipital lobes in man. *Brain* 57: 255–285.
44. Bodurka J, Bandettini PA (2002). Toward direct mapping of neuronal activity: MRI detection of ultra-weak transient magnetic fields changes. *Magn Reson Med 47*: 1052–1058.
45. Bodurka J, Jesmanowicz A, Hyde JS, et al. (1999). Current-induced magnetic resonance imaging. *J Magn Reson 137*: 265–271.
46. Bandettini PA, Petridou N, Bodurka J (2005). Direct detection of neuronal activity with MRI: fantasy, possibility, or reality. *Appl Magn Res 29*(1): 65–88.
47. Kraus R, Volegov P, Matlachov A, Espy M (2008). Toward direct neural current imaging by resonant mechanisms at ultra-low field. *NeuroImage 39*: 310–317.
48. Cassará AM, Maraviglia B (2008). Microscopic investigation of the resonant mechanism for the implementation of nc-MRI at ultra-low field MRI. *NeuroImage 41:* 1228–1241.
49. Cassará AM, Maraviglia B, Hartwig S, Trahms L, Burghoff M (2009). Neuronal current detection with low-field magnetic resonance: simulations and methods. *Magn Reson Imag 27*: 1131–1139.
50. Xiong J, Fox PT, Gao JH (2003). Directly mapping magnetic field effects of neuronal activity by magnetic resonance imaging. *Hum Brain Mapp 20:* 41–49.
51. Parkes LM, de Lange FP, Fries P, et al. (2007). Inability to directly detect magnetic field changes associated with neuronal activity. *Magn Reson Med* 57: 411–416.
52. Espy M, Flynn M, Gomez J, et al. (2009). Applications of ultra-low field magnetic resonance for imaging and materials studies. *IEEE Trans Appl Supercond 19*(3; pt.1): 835–838.
53. Logothetis NK (2002). The neural basis of the blood-oxygen-level-dependent functional magnetic resonance imaging signal. *Philos Trans R Soc Lond B Biol Sci 357*: 1003–1037.
54. Henrie JA, Shapley R (2005). LFP power spectra in V1 cortex: the graded effect of stimulus contrast. *J Neurophysiol 94*: 479–490.
55. Logothetis NK, Pfeuffer J (2004). On the nature of the BOLD fMRI contrast mechanism. *MRI 22*: 1517–1531.
56. Baillet S, Mosher JC, Jerbi K, Leahy RM (2000). Hybrid MEG Source Characterization by Cortical Remapping and Imaging of Parametric Source Models. *Proc 12th Intl Conf Biomagnetism,* Helsinki, Finland.
57. Truccolo WA, Ding M, Knuth KH, et al. (2002). Trial-to-trial variability of cortical evoked responses: implications for the analysis of functional connectivity. *Clin Neurophysiol 113*: 206–226.
58. Gilad O et al. (2009). A method for recording resistance changes non-invasively during neuronal depolarization with a view to imaging brain activity with electrical impedance tomography. *J Neurosci Methods 180*: 87–96.

59. Gilad O, Holder DS (2009). Impedance changes recorded with scalp electrodes during visual evoked responses: Implications for electrical impedance tomography of fast neural activity. *Neuroimage 47*: 514–522.
60. Holder D (Ed.) (2005). *Electrical Impedance Tomography: Methods, History and Applications.* Bristol: Institute of Physics Publishing.
61. Romsauverva A, McEwan A, Horesch L, et al. (2006). Multi-frequency electrical impedance tomography (EIT) of the adult human head: initial findings in brain tumors, arteriovenous malformations and chronic stroke, development of an analysis method for calibration. *Physiol Meas 27*: S147–S161.
62. Barber DC, Brown BH (1984). Applied potential tomography. *J Phys E Sci Instrum 17*: 723–733.
63. Webster JG (Ed.) (1990). *Electrical Impedance Tomography.* Bristol, UK: Adam Hilger.
64. Metherall P, Barber DC, Smallwood RH, Brown BH (1996). Three-dimensional electrical impedance tomography. *Nature 380*: 509–512.
65. Cheney M, Isaacson D, Newell JC (1999). Electrical impedance tomography. *SIAM Rev 41*: 85–101.
66. Zhang N (1992). Electrical impedance tomography based on current density imaging. MSc Thesis, University of Toronto, Toronto, Canada.
67. Woo EJ, Lee SY, Mun CW (1994). Impedance tomography using internal current density distribution measured by nuclear magnetic resonance. *Proc SPIE 2299*: 377–385.
68. Birgul O, Ider YZ (1995). Use of the magnetic field generated by the internal distribution of injected currents for electrical impedance tomography. *Proc 9th Int Conf Elec Bio-Impedance (Heidelberg, Germany).* 418–419.
69. Woo EJ, Seo JK (2008). Magnetic resonance electrical impedance tomography (MREIT) for high-resolution conductivity imaging. *Physiol Meas 29*(10): R1–R26.
70. Joy MLG, Scott GC, Henkelman RM (1989). *In vivo* detection of applied electric currents by magnetic resonance imaging. *Magn Reson Imag 7*: 89–94.
71. Eyuboglu M, Birgul O, Ider YZ (2001). A dual modality system for high resolution-true conductivity imaging. *Proc XI Int Conf Elec Bioimpedance (ICEBI).* 409–413.
72. Kwon O, Lee JY, Yoon JR (2002a). Equipotential line method for magnetic resonance electrical impedance tomography (MREIT). *Inverse Problems 18*: 1089–1100.
73. Kwon O, Woo EJ, Yoon JR, Seo JK (2002). Magnetic resonance electrical impedance tomography (MREIT): simulation study of *J*-substitution algorithm. *IEEE Trans Biomed Eng 48*: 160–167.
74. Birgul O, Ider YZ (1996). Electrical impedance tomography using the magnetic field generated by injected currents. *Proc 18th Ann Int Conf IEEE EMBS (Amsterdam, Netherlands).* 784–785.
75. Ider YZ, Birgul O (1998). Use of the magnetic field generated by the internal distribution of injected currents for electrical impedance tomography. *Elektrik 6*: 215–225.
76. Oh SH, Lee BI, Woo EJ, et al. (2003). Conductivity and current density image reconstruction using harmonic B_z algorithm in magnetic resonance electrical impedance tomography. *Phys Med Biol 48*: 3101–3116.
77. Joy ML (2004). MR current density and conductivity imaging: the state of the art. *Conf Proc IEEE Eng Med Biol Soc 7*: 5315–5319.
78. Dinghui W, DeMonte TP, Weijing M, et al. (2009). Multislice radio-frequency current density imaging. *IEEE Trans Med Imag 28*(7): 1083–1092.
79. Scott GC (2010). Challenges & prospects of rf current density imaging. *Proceedings of the International Workshop on MR-based Impedance Imaging* 8–10, Yonsei and Kyung Hee University, Korea. http://iirc.khu.ac.kr/mrii/
80. Gabriel S, Lau RW, Gabriel C (1996). The dielectric properties of biological tissues: II. Measurements in the frequency range 10 Hz to 20 GHz. *Phys Med Biol 41*: 2251–2269.
81. Jeong WC, Kim YT, Minhas AS, et al. (2010). *In vivo* conductivity imaging of human knee using 3 mA injection current in MREIT. *J Phys Conf Ser 224*: 012148.
82. Nitsche M, Liebetanz D, Lang N, et al. (2003). Safety criteria for transcranial direct current stimulation (tCDS) in humans. *Clin Neurophysiol 114*: 2220–2222.

83. Wagner T, Valero-Cabre A, Pascual-Leone A (2007). Noninvasive human brain stimulation. *Ann Rev Biomed Eng* 9: 527–565.
84. Patriciu A, Yoshida K, Struijk JJ, et al. (2005). Current density imaging and electrically induced skin burns under surface electrodes. *IEEE Trans Biomed Eng* 52: 2024–2031.
85. Agnew WF, McCreery DB (1987). Considerations for safety in the use of extracranial stimulation for motor evoked potentials. *Neurosurgery 20*: 143–147.
86. Lee S, Mossle M, Myers W, et al. (2005). SQUID-detected MRI at 132 μT with T_1- weighted contrast established at 10 μT-300 mT. *Magn Reson Med* 53: 9–14.
87. Zotev VS, Matlashov AN, Savukov IM, et al. (2009). SQUID-based microtesla MRI for in vivo relaxometry of the human brain. *IEEE Trans Appl Supercond 19*(3; pt.1): 823–826.
88. Hartwig S, Voigt J, Scheer H-J, et al. (2011). Nuclear magnetic relaxation in water revisited. *J Chem Phys 135*: 054201.
89. Holmes MD, Miles AN, Dodrill CB, et al. (2003). Identifying potential surgical candidates in patients with evidence of bitemporal epilepsy. *Epilepsy 44*(8):1075–1079.
90. LuuLuu P, Tucker DM, Englander R, et al. (2001). Localizing acute stroke-related EEG changes: assessing the effects of spatial undersampling. *J Clin Neurophys 18*(4): 302–317.
91. Jorden RC (1983). Pathophysiology of brain injury. *Critical Care Quarterly* 5: 1–12.
92. Vespa PM, Gobin YP (1997). Endovascular treatment and neurointesive care of ruptured aneurysms. *Critical Care Clinics 15*(4): 667–684.
93. Abragam A (1961). *Principles of Nuclear Magnetism*. Oxford: Oxford University Press.
94. Joy MLG, Lebedev VP, Gati JS (1999). Imaging of current density and current pathways in rabbit brain during transcranialelectrostimulation. *IEEE Trans Appl Biomed Eng 46*(9): 1139–1149.
95. Zotev VS, Matlashov AN, Volegov PL, et al. (2007). SQUID-based instrumentation for ultra-low-field MRI. *Supercond Sci Technol 20*(11): S367–S373.
96. Zotev VS, Matlachov AN, Volegov PL, et al.(2007). Multi-channel SQUID system for MEG and ultra-low field MRI. *IEEE Trans Supercond 17*(2): 839–842.
97. Esler B, Lyons T, Turovets SI, Tucker D (2010). Instrumentation for low frequency EIT studies of the human head and its validation in the phantom experiments. *J Phys Conf Ser 224*: 012007.
98. Sadleir RJ, Grant SC, Zhang SU, et al. (2005). Noise analysis in magnetic resonance electrical impedance tomography at 3 and 11T field strengths. *Physiol Meas 26*: 875–884.
99. http://www.stelar.it/2010/mainpage.php?folder=products&page=smartracer.php
100. 2006 transatlantic aircraft plot. (n.d.). Retrieved from http://en.wikipedia.org/wiki/2006_ transatlantic_ aircraft_plot
101. Espy M, et al. (2011). Progress on detection of liquid explosives using ultra-low field MRI. *IEEE Trans Appl Supercond 21*(3, pt. 1): 530–533.
102. Matlashov AN, Espy MA, Kraus RH, et al. (2011). SQUIDs vs. Faraday coils for ultra-low nuclear magnetic resonance: Experimental and simulation comparison. *IEEE Trans Appl Supercond 21*(3, pt. 1): 465–468.
103. Austin R, Espy M, Matlashov A, et al. (forthcoming). *MagViz: A Bottled Liquids Scanner Using Ultra-low Field NMR Relaxometry*. Springer: NATO Science for Peace and Security Series.

INDEX

AC current
  AC field skin depth (*See* penetration skin depth)
  magnetic resonance electrical impedance tomography, 218–222
acquisition time, ULF-MRI sequence, 135–137
active shielding, external magnetic fields, 74–76
adiabatic field manipulation
  basic principles, 89–96, 132–134
  ghost artifacts, multiple gradient-echo, 162–165
  polarization field (B_p) removal, 165–167, 211
  precession and spin reorientation, ULF-MRI sequence, 133–135
adiabatic ramp-down
  pre-polarization in magnetically shielded rooms, 211
  ULF MRI, 53–55
adiabatic theorem, 91–96
aluminum shielding, SQUID devices, 28–29
ambient fields, ULF-MRI, ghost artifacts, 160–165
amplitude distortion, concomitant gradients, ULF-MRI, 152–159
anatomical imaging techniques, 124–128
angular frequency
  adiabatic rotation, 92–96
  alternating magnetic fields, 96–99
  nonlinear effects, NMR, 99–110
angular velocity, magnetic field rotation, 92–95
arterial spin labeling (ASL) techniques, 213
atomic magnetometers, 6–10
auditory evoked magnetic field mapping, 204–210

bandwidth parameters, ULF-MRI imaging techniques, 126–128, 145–146
Bloch equation
  concomitant gradients, ULF-MRI, 155–159
  pickup coil size optimization, SQUID systems, 64–66
Bloch-Siegert shift, nonlinear effects, NMR, 100–110
BOLD (blood oxygen level-dependent) fMRI, 212–213
Boltzmann distribution
  NMR, 8–10
  relaxometry theory, 121–122
B_p field and coil optimization, ULF-MRI
  power handling and coil cooling, 53–54
  sensor systems, 55
  signal-to-noise ratio increase, 51–53
brain imaging
  direct neural current imaging, 213–216
  magnetic resonance electrical impedance tomography at ULF, 216–222
  MEG and flow-based fMRI at ULF, 212–213
  signal-to-noise ratio, ULF-MRI, 141–145
  ULF MRI, 47–48, 202–222
bulk magnetization, NMR signal, 8–10

circular polarized field, nonlinear effects, 109–110
classical mechanics, spin evolution, 86–87
coil design
  close voxels, SNR, parallel imaging, 179–180
  concomitant gradients, ULF-MRI, 146–159
  cooling, 53–54
  dense sensor arrays, combined ULF-MRI/MEG, 169
  distant voxels, SNR, parallel imaging, 176–179
  image acceleration, SENSE (sensitivity encoding) system, 170–173
  pickup coil size optimization, SQUID systems, 65–66

coil design (*Cont.*)
pre-polarization in magnetically shielded rooms, 210–211
SQUID system, 60–62
ULF MRI, 58, 68–70, 129–130
commutation relationships
electromagnetic radiation-nuclear spin interaction, 115–120
nonlinear effects, NMR, 101–110
computed tomography (CT), contrast-to-noise ratio, 24–25
concomitant gradients, ULF-MRI, 146–159
algebraic reconstruction, ULF-MRI, 155–159
conductivity image, magnetic resonance electrical impedance tomography, 217–222
conductor materials, susceptibility artifacts, 188–189
contrast phenomena
advantages of ULF-MRI, 180–182
dead time minimization, optimization of ULF MRI, 167–168
dispersion contrast, arbitrary relaxation time measurement, 191–194
magnetic resonance imaging applications, 2–5
ULF-MRI imaging techniques, 125–128, 189–191
contrast-to-noise ratio (CNR)
challenges for ULF-MRI, 194–196
contrast in ULF MRI, 191
NMR, 20, 25
ULF-MRI SQUID sensors, 32–33
correlated noise, distant voxels, SNR, parallel imaging, 178–179
correlation time, contrast in ULF MRI and, 189–191
counter-rotating fields
alternating magnetic field interactions, ULF-MRI, 98–99
nonlinear effects, 99–110
cryostats, 66–67
Curie's law, NMR, 9–10
current switching and control
magnetic resonance electrical impedance tomography, 220–222
superconducting quantum interference devices, 62–64
ULF MRI, 55

damping resistors, current switching and control, 55
data acquisition
bandwidth issues, ULF-MRI imaging techniques, 145–146
ULF-MRI, 70–71

d*B*/d*t*, B_p maximization, ULF-MRI, 51–53
DC current, magnetic resonance electrical impedance tomography, 218–222
DC SQUID
basic properties, 59–62
ULF NMR, 26–29
dead time minimization, optimization of ULF-MRI, 167–168
deflected magnetization, magnetic resonance electrical impedance tomography, 222
dense sensor arrays, combined ULF-MRI/MEG, 169
density operator, electromagnetic radiation-nuclear spin interaction, 114–120
dephasing mechanisms, NMR spin relaxation, 13–15
dipole-dipole coupling, ULF phenomena, 84–86
Dirac notation
concomitant gradients, ULF-MRI, 152–159
electromagnetic radiation-nuclear spin interaction, 111–120
direct linear inversion, concomitant gradients, 157–159
direct neural current imaging (DNI), ULF applications, 213–216
discrete Fourier transform, ULF-MRI imaging techniques, 126–128
dispersion contrast, 32–33
arbitrary relaxation time measurement, 191–194
MAGVIZ and ULF NMR relaxometers, 222–224
distortion artifacts, concomitant gradients, ULF-MRI, 150–159
double resonance, ^{1}H and ^{14}N coupling, 193–194
dynamic magnetic fields, 160–165
Dyson time-ordering operator
concomitant gradients, ULF-MRI, 155–159
electromagnetic radiation-nuclear spin interaction, 113–120

echo pulses, encoding and acquisition, 135–137. *See also* field echo, gradient echo and spin echo
eddy-current effects
magnetic shielding, noise issues, 76–77
superconducting quantum interference devices, 63–64
effective magnetic field, adiabatic/non-adiabatic rotation, 89–96
eigenvalues/eigenvectors
electromagnetic radiation-nuclear spin interaction, 111–120
rotation generator matrices, NMR phenomena, 87–89

electrical impedance tomography (EIT)
magnetic resonance EIT, 217–222
medical imaging applications, 216
electrical permittivitiy, magnetic resonance imaging, 35–36
electrical resistance, signal-to-noise ratio, 20–23
electroencephalography (EEG), brain imaging applications, ULF-MRI *vs.*, 202–210
electromagnetic fields, relaxometry theory, 120–122
electromagnetic radiation
nuclear spin interaction, 111–120
nuclear spins at ULF, 86–110
encoding period. *See also* phase-encoding gradient
concomitant gradients, ULF-MRI, 146–159
dead time minimization, ULF-MRI, 168
ULF-MRI sequence, 135–137
equilibrium magnetization, pre-polarization, ULF-MRI sequence, 131–132
evolution operator
concomitant gradients, ULF-MRI, 155–159
electromagnetic radiation-nuclear spin interaction, 113–120
ghost artifacts, 160–165
external magnetic fields, shielding, 72–76

Faraday coil induction sensors
NMR signal sensing, 16–18
nuclear magnetic resonance signal, 6–10
signal-to-noise ratio, 22–23
"fast" field rotation, alternating magnetic field interactions, 97–99
feedback circuit
pre-polarization in magnetically shielded rooms, 210–211
SQUID system, 60–62
field-cycling MRI
dispersion contrast, arbitrary field measurements, 191–194
ULF-MRI imaging comparisons, 127–128
field-echo sequences
adiabatic/non-adiabatic magnetic field rotation, 96
encoding and acquisition, ULF-MRI sequence, 135–137, 96
field homogeneity requirement, precession and spin reorientation, ULF-MRI process, 134–135
field-of-view (FOV) images
bandwidth issues, ULF-MRI imaging techniques, 145–146
concomitant gradients, ULF-MRI, 157–159
image acceleration, 170–173
sensor arrays and parallel imaging, 168–180
spatial encoding, NMR signal, 20
ULF-MRI image reconstruction, spatial resolution and, 137–140
field orientation flexibility, ultra-low field (ULF) MRI, 183–184
flipping, NMR pulse sequences, 15–16
flow-sensitive alternating inversion recovery (FAIR), brain imaging, 213
flux density, NMR signal sensing, 16–18
flux noise, pickup size optimization, SQUID systems, 64–66
Fourier imaging sequence
concomitant gradients, ULF-MRI, 151–159
encoding and acquisition, ULF-MRI, 135–137
ghost artifacts, multiple gradient-echo, 160–165
precession and spin reorientation, ULF-MRI, 133–135
spatial resolution and field-of-view, ULF-MRI image reconstruction, 137–140
ULF MRI, 126–130
free induction decay (FID)
brain imaging, ULF-MRI, 204–210
image reconstruction and spatial resolution, ULF-MRI, 137–140
NMR relaxation, 12–15
frequency domain
NMR signal, 6–10
ULF-MRI imaging techniques, 126–128
full width at half maximum (FWHM), spatial encoding, NMR signal, 19–20
functional MRI (fMRI)
brain imaging applications, ULF-MRI *vs.*, 202–210
MEG and flow-based fMRI at ULF, 212–213

geometric factor
distant voxels, SNR, parallel imaging, 176–179
NMR signal, 10
geometric phase effect, magnetic field rotation, 93–96
ghost artifacts
adiabatic/non-adiabatic magnetic field rotation, 96
ULF-MRI, 160–165
giant magnetoresistance (GMR) sensors, 69–70
Golay coil
concomitant gradients, 147–159

gradient echo
concomitant gradients, ULF-MRI, 154–159
dead time minimization, optimization of ULF MRI, 167–168
encoding and acquisition, 135–137
ghost artifacts, multiple gradient-echo, 160–165
magnetic resonance electrical impedance tomography, 219–222
gradient fields
bandwidth issues, 146
gradients
concomitant gradients, 146–159
image reconstruction and spatial resolution, 139–140
spatial encoding, NMR signal, 20
ULF-MRI, 56–58
gradient tensor, concomitant gradients, 147–159
gradiometer pickups
SQUID systems, 28–29, 60–62
gray matter (brain)
gray/white matter, contrast data, 195
gray/white matter, NMR signal, 166–168
relaxation data, 192
Gyromagnetic ratio, 6–10

Hamiltonian operator,electromagnetic radiation-nuclear spin interaction, 112–120
hardware requirements
MAGVIZ and ULF NMR relaxometers, 223–224
simplicity of, 180–182
ULF-MRI, 49–50, 127–128
harmonic motion, nonlinear effects, NMR, 106–110
Hermitian operator, electromagnetic radiation-nuclear spin interaction, 111–120
high-field (HF) MRI systems
advantages of ULF-MRI *vs.* HF, 180–182
alternating magnetic field interactions, 96–99
bandwidth issues, 145–146
concomitant gradients, 146–159
dead time minimization, 167–168
historical background, 26
magnetic field direction, 86
MR inverse imaging (InI), 174
polarization measurement, 10–12
safety issues, 196–197
SENSE (sensitivity encoding), 169–173
signal sensing, 16–18
spatial encoding, 19–20
SQUID sensors, 31–33
susceptibility artifacts, 184–189
ULF-MRI imaging comparisons, 40–41, 48, 126–128
Hilbert space, electromagnetic radiation-nuclear spin interaction, 111–120
hyperpolarized gases, 184–189

image acceleration, 169–173
PILS sensor system, image acceleration, 170–173
SENSE (sensitivity encoding) system, 170–173
SMASH sensor system, image acceleration, 170–173
image reconstruction, 137–140
image resolution, 49
imaging techniques, ULF-MRI, 124–197
induced currents and fields, 34–36
induced heating effect, 36–37
infinitesimal generator, NMR phenomena, 87–89
inhomogeneous measurement field
NMR spin relaxation, 13–15
pulse sequence, 16
instantaneous magnetization frequency, nonlinear effects, 108–110
instrumentation, ULF-MRI
magnetic field interaction, 76
simplicity of, 180–182
inverse Fourier transform, concomitant gradients, 157–159
isotope scaling, NMR signal, 6–10

Jacobian matrices, concomitant gradients, 152–159
Johnson noise
B_p coil optimization, 55
signal-to-noise ratio, 20–23
Josephson junctions
DC SQUID systems, 59–64
ULF-MRI signal sensing, 17–18

"ket" vectors, electromagnetic radiation-nuclear spin interaction, 111–120
k-space
concomitant gradients, ULF-MRI, 150–159
image reconstruction and spatial resolution, ULF-MRI, 137–140

LANL systems
brain imaging, ULF-MRI/MEG applications, 207–210
magnetic resonance electrical impedance tomography, 218–222

Larmor frequency
adiabatic magnetic field rotation, 92–95
bandwidth issues, ULF-MRI, 146
concomitant gradients, ULF-MRI, 149–159
contrast in ULF MRI, 189–191
direct neural current imaging, ULF techniques, 213–216
electromagnetic radiation-nuclear spin interaction, 120
flexibility and strength of magnetic fields, 183–184
free induction decay, 12–15
ghost artifacts, multiple gradient-echo, 161–165
magnetic resonance electrical impedance tomography, 217–222
NMR signal, 6–10, 25
nonlinear effects, NMR, 100–110
spatial encoding, NMR signal, 18–20
ULF-MRI imaging techniques, 85–86, 127–130
ULF NMR, SQUID devices, 27–29
Levi-Civita symbols, nonlinear effects, NMR, 102–110
linear polarized field, nonlinear effects, 109–110
line width measurements, spatial encoding, 19–20
liquid helium cryostat, 66–67
liquid nitrogen cryostat, 66–67
liquid screening
MAGVIZ and ULF NMR relaxometers, 222–224
susceptibility artifacts, 189
Lissajous curve, nonlinear effects, NMR, 106–110
Litz wire, B_p coil maximization, ULF-MRI, 54
local magnetic fields, 84–86
longitudinal relaxation
NMR, 13–15
relaxometry theory, 121–122
low-field (LF) MRI systems
concomitant gradients, 146
development of, 3–5
external magnetic fields, shielding, 75–76
superconducting quantum interference devices, 27–30

magnetically shielded room (MSR)
compatibility with ULF-MRI, 49
external magnetic fields, 72–76
noise issues, 76–77
pre-polarization in, 210–211
magnetic dipole moment
dipole-dipole coupling, 84–86
electromagnetic radiation-nuclear spin interaction, 116–120
evolution of, 86–87
NMR signal, 8–10
relaxation mechanisms and theory, 13–15
magnetic fields
adiabatic/non-adiabatic rotation, 89–96
brain imaging, ULF-MRI applications, 202–210, 212–213
directional changes, ULF-MRI, 89–96
flexibility and strength, 183–184
magnetic resonance imaging, 34–36
magnetic relaxation dispersion (MRD) profile, 85–86
magnetic resonance current density imaging (MRCDI), electrical impedance tomography, 217–222
magnetic resonance electrical impedance tomography (MREIT)
brain imaging, ULF techniques, 216–222
ULF-MRI applications, 183–184
magnetic resonance imaging (MRI)
alternating magnetic field interactions, 96–99
contrast-to-noise ratio, 20, 23–25
defined, 1
effects, 33–38
fundamental principles, 1–5
induced heating effect, 36–37
induced neurostimulation, 37–38
material conductivities, 34
signal-to-noise ratio, 20–23
trends in U.S. installations, 4–5
ULF, historical background, 25–26
ULF imaging techniques, 124–197
magnetic shielding
alternative techniques, 77–78
external magnetic fields, 72–76
instrumentation interaction, 75
noise issues, 76–77
ULF-MRI, 71–78, 182–183
magnetocardiography (MCG), 31–33
magnetogyric ratio, electromagnetic radiation-nuclear spin interaction, 116–120
magnetomyography, 31–33
MAGVIZ relaxometer, 222–224
material conductivity
induced heating effect, 36–37
selected material properties, 34
Maxwell coil
concomitant gradients, 147–159
phase-encoding gradients, 56–57

measurement field (B_m)
basic properties, 5–6
direct neural current imaging, 215–216
non-adiabatic magnetic field rotation, 93–96
precession and spin reorientation, 133–135
ULF NMR phenomena, 56
MEG imaging systems
brain imaging applications, 202–210
concomitant gradients, ULF-MRI, 152–159
dense sensor arrays, combined ULF-MRI/MEG, 169
magnetic shielding, 77–78
MEG and flow-based fMRI at ULF, 212–213
ULF-MRI and, 31–33, 49, 51, 211–212
MEGMRI system
functional brain imaging, 207–210
pre-polarization in magnetically shielded rooms, 210–211
metal artifacts, ULF-MRI in presence of, 184–189
mixed sensors, 69–70
molecular processes, ULF-MRI timescales, 84–86
moving reference frame, adiabatic/non-adiabatic rotation, 89–96
MR inverse imaging (InI), 174
multimodal brain imaging, 202–210
multiplicative distortion, concomitant gradients, 151–159

NEMA standard, signal-to-noise ratio, 142–145
neural activity, ULF-based direct imaging, 38–39
neurostimulation, MRI induction, 37–38
noble gas isotopes, 6–10
noise-cancellation methods, magnetic shielding, 78
noise sources
parallel imaging, signal-to-noise ratio, 174–176
signal-to-noise ratio, 20–23, 144–145
SQUID systems, 61–62
ULF-MRI, 49, 126–128
non-adiabatic field manipulation
directional changes, ULF-MRI, 89, 93–96
ghost artifacts, multiple gradient-echo, 161–165
polarization field (B_p) removal, 165–167
precession and spin reorientation, ULF-MRI sequence, 133–135
pre-polarization, ULF-MRI process, 132
nonresonant spin-tipping, precession and spin reorientation, ULF-MRI sequence, 133–135
nuclear magnetic resonance (NMR)
alternating magnetic field interactions, 96–99
history, at ULF, 2
in MRI, 3–5
nonlinear effects, 99–110
polarization measurement, 10–12
pulse sequences, 15–16
relaxation, 12–15
signal characteristics, 6–20
spatial encoding, 18–20
SQUID-based ULF NMR, 26–29
ULF phenomena, 83–110
nuclear magnetization evolution, ghost artifacts, 160–165
nuclear quadrupole resonance (NQR), dispersion contrast, 193–194
nuclear spin properties
electromagnetic radiation at ULF and, 86–120
null detectors, SQUID systems, 59–62
Nyquist theorem, image reconstruction and spatial resolution, 138–140

Ohmic heating, magnetic resonance imaging, 36–37
one-dimensional NMR
image acceleration, SENSE (sensitivity encoding) system, 170–173
ULF-MRI imaging techniques, 126–128
optimization of ULF-MRI, 165–180
close voxels, SNR, parallel imaging, 179–180
dead time minimization, 167–168
dense sensor arrays, 169
distant voxels, SNR, parallel imaging, 176–179
image acceleration, 169–173
MR inverse imaging (InI), 174
sensor arrays and parallel imaging, 168–180
orthogonal matrices, nonlinear effects, NMR, 105–110

"pancake" echo
encoding and acquisition, ULF-MRI process, 135–137
ghost artifacts, multiple gradient-echo, 163–165
parallel imaging
distant voxels, SNR, 176–179
near voxels, signal-to-noise ratio, 179–180
sensor arrays, optimization of ULF MRI, 168–180
signal-to-noise ratio, 174–176
paramagnetic susceptibility, ULF-MRI optimization, 185–189
penetration skin depth, 35–36
perturbative expansion, nonlinear effects, 103–110

phantom data
concomitant gradients, ULF-MRI, 153–159
magnetic resonance electrical impedance tomography, 219–222
phase correction algorithm, concomitant gradients, 157–159
phase-encoding
concomitant gradients, 148, 154–159
ghost artifacts, multiple gradient-echo, 162–165
image reconstruction and spatial resolution, 137–140
ULF-MRI, 56–57
ULF-MRI, encoding and acquisition, 125–126, 135–137
phase shifts
direct neural current imaging, ULF techniques, 214–216
magnetic resonance electrical impedance tomography, 218–222
pickup coils
close voxels, SNR, parallel imaging, 179–180
concomitant gradients, 156–159
distant voxels, SNR, parallel imaging, 176–179
size optimization, 64–66
SQUID system, 60–62
PILS sensor system, image acceleration, 170–173
polarization field (B_p). *See also* pre-polarization field generation
adiabatic/non-adiabatic rotation, 91–95
basic properties, 5–6
non-adiabatic magnetic field rotation, 93–96
optimization of ULF-MRI and removal of, *Bp*, 165–167
polarization measurement, NMR signal, 10–12
positron emission tomography (PET), brain imaging applications, 202–210
power handling, 53–54
precession
adiabatic/non-adiabatic rotation, 90–96
NMR relaxation, 13–15
pre-polarization, ULF-MRI sequence, 132
spin reorientation, ULF-MRI sequence, 133–135
pre-polarization field
dispersion contrast, arbitrary field measurements, 194
magnetically shielded rooms, 210–211
optimization of ULF-MRI, 166–167
signal-to-noise ratio, ULF-MRI, 143–145
superconducting quantum interference devices, 62–64
ULF-MRI imaging technique, 51–55, 130–132
projection imaging, magnetic field flexibility and strength, 183–184
projection operator
dead time minimization, 167–168
electromagnetic radiation-nuclear spin interaction, 113–120
proportional-integral-differential (PID) controllers, external magnetic fields, shielding, 75–76
proton spin
contrast in ULF MRI and, 189–191
direct neural current imaging, ULF techniques, 214–216
dispersion contrast, arbitrary field measurements, 193–194
magnetic resonance imaging applications, 1–5
ULF-MRI SQUID sensors, 33
ULF-NMR, 25
pulse sequences
adiabatic/non-adiabatic rotation, 89–96
encoding and acquisition, ULF-MRI process, 135–137
ghost artifacts, multiple gradient-echo, 162–165
image reconstruction and spatial resolution, 137–140
NMR, 15–16
precession and spin reorientation, ULF-MRI process, 133–135
pre-polarization, ULF-MRI, 130–132
ULF-MRI and imaging techniques, 50, 128–165

Q spoilers, SQUID devices, 28–29
quenching, polarization measurement, 11–12

Rabi frequency
alternating magnetic field interactions, 98–99
electromagnetic radiation-nuclear spin interaction, 119–120
nonlinear effects, NMR, 99–110
radiofrequency interference (RFI)
shielding devices, SQUID sensors, 66–67
signal-to-noise ratio, ULF-MRI, 144–145
ULF-MRI RF screening, 184–189
rare-earth-barium-copper-oxide (REBCO) coil, signal-to-noise ratio increase, 53
readout gradient
concomitant gradients, 152–159
dead time minimization, optimization of ULF MRI, 167–168
ghost artifacts, multiple gradient-echo, 162–165

readout gradient (*Cont.*)
image reconstruction and spatial resolution, 139–140
ULF-MRI, 56
receptivity, nuclear magnetic resonance signal, 10
reciprocal space vector, ULF NMR imaging procedures, 129–130
reflective shielding, external magnetic fields, 73–76
relative permeability, magnetic resonance imaging, 35–36
relaxation times
adiabatic magnetic field rotation, 92–95
contrast in ULF MRI and, 189–191
dead time minimization, optimization of ULF-MRI, 167–168
dispersion contrast, arbitrary field measurements, 191–194
limitations, ULF-MRI, 146
MAGVIZ and ULF NMR relaxometers, 223–224
NMR, 12–15
relaxometry theory, 121–122
ULF NMR, SQUID devices, 29
relaxometry
magnetic field dependence, 120–122
MAGVIZ and ULF NMR relaxometers, 222–224
resistive heating, magnetic resonance imaging, 36–37
resonance conditions, nonlinear effects, NMR, 100–110
resonant effect, direct neural current imaging, ULF techniques, 215–216
resonant spin-tipping, precession and spin reorientation, ULF-MRI process, 133–135
reversible geometric distortion, concomitant gradients, ULF-MRI, 151–159
Rodrigues' identity, rotation generator matrices, NMR phenomena, 89
root-mean-square (RMS) Johnson voltage noise, signal-to-noise ratio, 22–23
rotating magnetic field ($\mathbf{B}_{RF}$)
adiabatic/non-adiabatic rotation, 89–96
direct neural current imaging, ULF techniques, 214–216
nonlinear effects, NMR, 100–110
polarization measurement, 11–12
ULF-MRI applications, 183–184
rotating-wave approximation
alternating magnetic field interactions, 99
nonlinear effects, NMR, 101–110
rotational frequency, NMR, 6–10
rotation generator matrix
alternating magnetic field interactions, 96–99
spin evolution, 87–89
R-space, image reconstruction and spatial resolution, ULF-MRI, 138–140

safety issues, ULF-MRI, 196–197
sample noise, signal-to-noise ratio, 20–23
scalar operators, electromagnetic radiation-nuclear spin interaction, 116–120
Schrödinger equation, electromagnetic radiation-nuclear spin interaction, 112–120
second-feedback, SQUIDs, 62–64
security applications, MAGVIZ and ULF NMR relaxometers, 222–224
self-adjoint operator, electromagnetic radiation-nuclear spin interaction, 111–120
SENSE (sensitivity encoding) method
image acceleration using, 169–173
MR inverse imaging (InI), 174
parallel imaging and, 169–180
signal-to-noise ratio, 174–176
spatial encoding, NMR signal, 20
sensitivity values
isotope scales, 6–8
magnetic resonance electrical impedance tomography, 222
sensor design
B_p coil maximization, 55
brain imaging, ULF-MRI/MEG applications, 207–210
dense arrays, combined ULF-MRI/MEG, 169
MR inverse imaging (InI), 174
NMR signal sensing, 17–18
optimization of ULF-MRI, 168–180
pickup size optimization, SQUID systems, 66
pre-polarization in magnetically shielded rooms, 210–211
signal-to-noise ratio, 20–23
ULF-MRI, 67–70
Shielding
magnetic (*See* magnetic shielding)
radiofrequency (RF) (*See* radiofrequency interference (RFI))
signal parameters
signal-to-noise ratio, acquisition challenges, 141–145
ULF-MRI imaging techniques, 124–128
signal sensing
NMR, 16–18
ULF-MRI, 49, 58–71

signal-to-noise ratio (SNR)
B_p maximization, ULF-MRI, 51–53
close voxels, parallel imaging, 179–180
contrast in ULF MRI and, 189–191
contrast-to-noise ratio (CNR) challenges and SNR, 194–196
distant voxels, parallel imaging, 176–179
image acceleration, SENSE (sensitivity encoding) system, 172–173
magnetic resonance electrical impedance tomography, 220–222
NMR, 6–10, 20–23
parallel imaging, ULF-MRI optimization, 174–176
pickup size optimization, SQUID systems, 64–66
sensor arrays and parallel imaging, 168–180
single voxel, 141
ULF-MRI and imaging techniques, 49, 126–128, 141–145
ULF-MRI SQUID sensors, 32–33
simultaneous signals, ULF NMR, SQUID sensors, 29
single-collection EEG/fMRI, brain imaging, 213
single image technique, signal-to-noise ratio, 142–145
singular value decomposition (SVD), concomitant gradients, ULF-MRI, 157–159
skew-symmetric matrices, spin evolution, 86–89
skin depth, 35–36
"slice select" gradient, ULF NMR imaging procedures, 129–130
"slow" field rotation, alternating magnetic field interactions, 97–99
SMASH sensor system, image acceleration, 170–173
spatial encoding
NMR signals, 18–20
ULF-MRI procedures, 128
spatial resolution
MRI, 2–5
precession and spin reorientation, ULF-MRI techniques, 134–135
signal-to-noise ratio, 141–145
ULF-MRI image reconstruction, 137–140
specific absorption rate (SAR), 57–58
spectral decomposition, electromagnetic radiation-nuclear spin interaction, 114–120
spectral density, contrast in ULF MRI, 189–191
spin-echo sequence
encoding and acquisition, ULF-MRI techniques, 135–137
NMR relaxation, 12–16
susceptibility artifacts, 186–189
spin-flip pulses
precession and spin reorientation, ULF-MRI techniques, 133–135
ULF-MRI, 57
spin-lattice interactions, relaxometry theory, 122
spin-lattice relaxation
NMR, 13–15
pulse sequence, 16
relaxometry theory, 121–122
spin-lock mode, nonlinear effects, NMR, 106–110
spin populations
direct neural current imaging, ULF techniques, 214–216
electromagnetic radiation at ULF, 86–110
NMR, 8–10
polarization field (B_p) removal, 166–167
recruitment, ULF-MRI sequence, 131–132
relaxation times, 146
relaxometry theory, 120–122
spin properties
magnetic resonance imaging applications, 1–5
NMR signal, 10
ULF phenomena, 83–86
spin reorientation, precession, ULF-MRI sequences, 133–135
spin-spin interactions, relaxometry theory, 122
spin-spin relaxation
NMR, 13–15
pulse sequence, 16
SQUID. *See* superconducting quantum interference devices
static magnetic fields
alternating magnetic field interactions, ULF-MRI, 96–99
ghost artifacts, 160–165
static nuclear susceptibility, relaxometry theory, 121–122
Stern-Gerlach experiment, 114–120
stray field problems, 146–165
streams-of-commerce (SOC) bottles, MAGVIZ and ULF NMR relaxometers, 222–224
superconducting quantum interference devices (SQUIDs)
basic properties, 59–62
cryostats and radiofrequency interference shielding, 66–67

superconducting quantum interference devices (*Cont.*)
dense sensor arrays, combined ULF-MRI/MEG, 169
direct neural current imaging, 216
external magnetic field shielding, 72–76
magnetic resonance electrical impedance tomography, 220–222
magnetic shielding, noise issues, 76–77
MAGVIZ and ULF NMR relaxometers, 222–224
MEG instrumentation, 203–210
NMR, 6–10
non-adiabatic magnetic field rotation, 93–96
parallel imaging, 168–180
pickup coil size optimization, 64–66
pre-polarization field exposure, 62–64
signal-to-noise ratio, 22–23, 144–145
spatial encoding, NMR signal, 19–20
ULF-MRI signal sensing, 17–18, 59–67
ULF NMR, 26–29
superposition principle, electromagnetic radiation-nuclear spin interaction, 111–120
susceptibility artifacts
direct neural current imaging, 213–216
ULF-MRI, 184–189

Tesla regime, high-field MRI, 3–5
thermal shields, SQUID sensors, 67
three-dimensional imaging
Fourier imaging pulse sequences, ULF NMR imaging procedures, 129–130
ghost artifacts, Fourier multiple field echo imaging, 160–165
spatial encoding, 20
three-dimensional Lissajous curve, nonlinear effects, NMR, 106–110
time-dependent state vector, electromagnetic radiation-nuclear spin interaction, 117–120
time evolution operator
electromagnetic radiation-nuclear spin interaction, 112–120
functional MRI, 2–5
timescales
contrast in ULF MRI, 189–191
dead time minimization, optimization of ULF MRI, 167–168
dispersion contrast, 191–194
magnetic resonance electrical impedance tomography, 220–222
signal-to-noise ratio, 144–145
ULF-MRI, 84–86
time-varying magnetic fields, MRI-induced neurostimulation, 37–38
total flux density, NMR signal, 10
transient pulses, pre-polarization in magnetically shielded rooms, 210–211
transverse relaxation
NMR, 13–15
relaxometry theory, 122
time constant, 14–15
two-dimensional imaging, image reconstruction and spatial resolution, ULF-MRI, 138–140

ULF-MRI
advantages of, 180–197
alternating magnetic field interactions, 96–99
alternative imaging techniques, compatibility, 49
brain imaging applications, 202–222
challenges in application, 141–165
comparisons with HF-MRI, 40–41, 48
concomitant gradients, 147–159
contrast-to-noise ratio (CNR), 23–25, 194–196
current switching and control, 55
data acquisition, 70–71
direct neural current imaging, 213–216
dispersion contrast, arbitrary field relaxation time measurements, 191–194
electromagnetic radiation-nuclear spin interaction, 86–110
external magnetic fields, shielding, 72–76
field and gradient properties, 55–58
flexible field orientation and strength, 183–184
fundamental principles, 1–5
ghost artifacts, 160–165
historical background, 25–26
image reconstruction, spatial resolution and field of view, 137–140
imaging procedure guidelines, 128–165
instrumentation, magnetic field interaction, 76
magnetic resonance electrical impedance tomography, 216–222
magnetic resonance phenomena, 83–86
magnetic shielding, 71–78
MAGVIZ and ULF NMR relaxometers, 222–224
measurement field generation, 56
MEG and flow-based fMRI at ULF, 211–213
multimodal brain imaging, 202–210
neural activity imaging, 38–39
NMR at, 25

optimization techniques, 165–180
phase-encoding gradient, 56–57
physics principles in, 38–39
polarization measurement, 10–12
power handling and coil cooling, 53–54
pre-polarization field generation, 51–55
pulse sequences, 16
readout gradient, 56
research trends in, 47–48
safety issues, 196–197
sensor properties, 67–70
signal, noise, and SNR, 20–23, 49, 125–128, 141–146, 168–180
signal sensing, 17–18, 58–71
spatial encoding, NMR signal, 19–20
spin-flip pulses, 12–16, 57
SQUID sensors, 30–33, 59–67
stray field problems, 146–165
summary of properties, 39–40
susceptibility artifacts and RF screening, 184–189
system overview, 49–50
ULF NMR, SQUID sensors, 26–29
uncorrelated noise, parallel imaging, 176–179

vacuum permeability, dipole-dipole coupling, 84–86
vector rotation, nonlinear effects, NMR, 108–110
voltages, MRI-induced neurostimulation, 37–38
voxels
close voxels, SNR, parallel imaging, 179–180
distant voxels, SNR, parallel imaging, 176–179
encoding and acquisition, ULF-MRI process, 136–137
NMR signal, 10
pickup size optimization, SQUID systems, 64–66
signal-to-noise ratio, 141
ULF-MRI, 49
ULF-MRI imaging techniques, 125–128

water phantom imaging
first reports, 26–27, 29–30
ghost artifacts, multiple gradient-echo, 163–165
white matter
contrast with gray matter, 24, 189–196
relaxation and signal loss, 166–168
white noise spectrum for SQUIDs, 61

x-ray-based imaging, contrast-to-noise ratio, 24–25

Zeeman interaction, NMR, 8–10